# COPING WITH CHRONIC ILLNESS
## OVERCOMING POWERLESSNESS

**Judith Fitzgerald Miller, M.S.N., R.N.**
Associate Professor, Nursing
Marquette University College of Nursing
Milwaukee, Wisconsin

 **F. A. Davis Company, Philadelphia**

Copyright © 1983 by F. A. Davis Company

Second printing 1983
Third printing 1984
Fourth printing 1985
Fifth printing 1986
Sixth printing 1987

**Library of Congress Cataloging in Publication Data**

Miller, Judith Fitzgerald.
    Coping with chronic illness.

    Includes bibliographies and index.
    1. Nursing—Psychological aspects. 2. Chronic diseases—Psychological aspects. 3. Sick—Psychology. 4. Adjustment (Psychology) I. Title. [DNLM: 1. Sick role. 2. Chronic disease—Rehabilitation. 3. Nurse—Patient relations. 4. Models, Psychological. 5. Chronic disease—Nursing. WY 152 M648c]
RT86.M5                          610.73'61                          82-4982
ISBN 0-8036-6191-6                                                  AACR2

TO PATRICK AND OUR CHILDREN,
KIM, ELIZABETH, AND PATRICIA

# PREFACE

The uncertainty that accompanies illness, particularly chronic illness, precipitates within patients a feeling of being unable to control what is happening to them. If the perception of powerlessness continues and is not contained, a cycle of low self-esteem, depression, and hopelessness is begun. This mental state significantly affects a lack of physical improvement. If the perception of powerlessness (helplessness) is not halted, physical deterioration can occur as though it were invited by the ill person.

This book is offered as a resource for nurses to enable them to alleviate patients' perceived lack of control. Nursing strategies identified, although specified for patients with particular health problems, are applicable to any patient who has the nursing diagnosis powerlessness.

The purposes of this book are threefold: (1) to help nurses develop an understanding of powerlessness in chronic illness; (2) to contribute to nursing's body of knowledge as it relates to the concept of powerlessness by sharing the process of concept development; and (3) to analyze coping and provide means by which the nurse facilitates patient coping with powerlessness in illness.

This book is divided into four parts. Part 1 provides a foundation for understanding the concepts of coping and powerlessness. Part 2 includes a discussion of powerlessness during vulnerable periods of human development. Specific chronic health problems and patient-perceived control are analyzed in Part 3. Part 4 contains suggested strategies for nurses to use to alleviate powerlessness in patients.

Clinical data, based on systematic observation, are included. These data enliven the theoretical propositions and facilitate real-world applications. It is hoped that nurses who read this book will be able to overcome their own sense of powerlessness when caring for the chronically ill.

J.F.M.

# ACKNOWLEDGMENTS

Thank you to my graduate students whose evolving insights spearheaded this project. I am grateful to Dr. Lorraine Machan, Professor of Biology, University of Lesotho, Africa, who, while at Marquette University, helped me realize that a book of this nature needed to be written. I appreciate the efforts of Beverly Thomas, Richard Thomas, Polly Ryan, and the late Helen Harrington, not only for their reviews of parts of this manuscript but also for their continuing expressions of confidence and encouragement.

J.F.M.

# LIST OF CONTRIBUTORS

**Diann Recker Baumann, M.S.N., R.N.**
Maternal Child Clinical Nurse Specialist
Joint Practice—OB/GYN, S.C.
Milwaukee, Wisconsin

**Pamela Miller Gotch, M.S.N., R.N.**
Assistant Director, Continuing Education in Nursing
Assistant Professor, Nursing
Marquette University College of Nursing
Milwaukee, Wisconsin

**Diane A. Hellenbrand, M.S.N., R.N.**
Clinical Nurse Specialist
Formerly, Visiting Nurse Association
Milwaukee, Wisconsin

**Bonnie Hildebrandt Howe, M.S.N., R.N.**
Staff Development and Clinical Supervisor, Critical Care
Consultant, Critical Care Staff Development
Holy Family Hospital
New Richmond, Wisconsin

**Judith Fitzgerald Miller, M.S.N., R.N.**
Associate Professor, Nursing
Marquette University College of Nursing
Milwaukee, Wisconsin

**Christine Bohm Oertel, M.S.N., R.N.**
Instructor
St. Luke's Hospital School of Nursing
Racine, Wisconsin

**Kathy Pfister-Minogue, M.S.N., R.N.**
Private Practitioner and Instructor
University of Oregon Health Sciences Center, School of Nursing
LaGrande, Oregon

**Patricia S. Schroeder, M.S.N., R.N.**
Clinical Nurse Specialist
St. Michael Hospital
Milwaukee, Wisconsin

**Susan R. Stapleton, M.S.N., R.N.**
Nurse Specialist
Polyclinic Medical Center
Instructor
Harrisburg Area Community College
Harrisburg, Pennsylvania

# CONTENTS

# 1

# CURRENT STATUS

A model for understanding nursing care of the chronically ill patient that promotes patient control through development and support of the individual's power resources is presented in Chapter 1. Although it is not possible to enumerate all of the human being's unique strengths that are to be supported by nurses, a common core of patient resources is presented in the power resource model. The model provides a frame of reference for the book.

All persons have capacity for coping. Coping is stimulated in individuals with chronic health problems. Unlike acute crises, during which denial of the impact of the threat is the prevailing means of coping, chronic illness brings about a reorganized confrontation with reality, adaptation, and participation in therapy.[1] The individual must respond to the requirements of the external situation (e.g., adhere to medication regimen, participate in exercises, maintain weight-reduction program, and complete treatments such as self-dialysis), as well as respond to one's own feelings about the situation (powerlessness, depression, or low self-esteem). Coping with perceived powerlessness is a major demand throughout the chronic illness. Other specific coping tasks that have been identified in chronically ill patients are discussed in Chapter 2.

The research base with resulting theoretical propositions and nursing practice speculations are presented in Chapter 3. Although the research base about concepts of powerlessness, locus of control, helplessness, and reactance theory has been derived from behavioral science literature, relevance for nursing is noted. Development of a nursing diagnostic category on powerlessness appears essential and valid for nursing.

# REFERENCE

1. Moos, R. H. and Tsu, V. D.: *Human competence and coping.* In Moos, R. H. (ed.): *Human Adaptation: Coping with Life Stresses.* Lexington Books, Division of D. C. Heath, Lexington, Mass., 1976.

# 1 PATIENT POWER RESOURCES

## JUDITH FITZGERALD MILLER

There *is* a way for individuals with chronic illness to be and feel in control of what is happening to them. Power is a resource for living that is present in all individuals. In the most rudimentary sense, power is the ability to influence what happens to oneself. May[1] described five types of power: exploitative, manipulative, competitive, nutrient, and integrative. The type of power that is relevant for this book is nutrient power. May defines nutrient power in terms of providing for, caring for, or having concern for the welfare of others. For purposes of this book, power will be thought of as nurturative, that is, providing for and caring for self, directing others regarding self-care, and being the ultimate decision maker regarding care. With power is the ability to effect change or prevent it.[1] Power and control will be considered synonymous terms. No differentiation is made between powerlessness and helplessness.

Powerlessness is a perception that one's own actions will not affect an outcome. The greater the individual's expectation to have control and the greater the importance of the desired outcomes to the individual, the greater the perceived powerlessness experienced when the individual does not, in fact, have control.[2] Powerlessness occurs in chronically ill patients for a variety of reasons. The patient may experience uncertain health with remissions and exacerbations or, in some instances, progressive physical deterioration. There are physical and psychologic losses. Overwhelmingly strange, invasive, and threatening experiences may occur as part of ongoing diagnostic and treatment measures. What is routine to the health worker may be devastating to the patient. The esoteric language system of health workers creates an aura of their being sophisticated masters of the situation while patients feel isolated from knowing what is happening to them. Some or all of these factors may influence the chronically ill person's perceived lack of control.

Chronic illness refers to an altered health state that will not be cured by a simple surgical procedure or a short course of medical therapy. Although each chronic illness presents unique demands on the patient and family, two generalizations can be made about chronic illnesses: (1) the person with a chronic illness experiences impaired functioning in more than one—often multiple—body-mind[3] and spirit systems; and (2) the illness-related demands on the individual are never completely eliminated.

The patient is subjected to close medical scrutiny regarding symptoms, response to therapy, and compliance. Demands on the patient and/or family include developing and refining skills for daily monitoring and management of the health problem. Self-monitoring depends on knowledge of self and therapy. Efforts are directed at keeping the health problem controlled and in remission while controlling anxiety over the threat of full-blown incapacitation during exacerbations.

Reif[4] identified three general features of chronic illness: (1) the disease symptoms interfere with many normal activities and routines; (2) the medical regimen is limited in its effectiveness; and (3) treatment, although intended to mitigate the symptoms and long-range effects of disease, contributes substantially to the disruption of usual patterns of living.

Unpredictable dilemmas characterize chronic illness and promote powerlessness. These dilemmas include symptom exacerbation, failure of therapy, physical deterioration despite adherence to the prescribed regimen, side effects of drugs, iatrogenic alterations, breakdown in patient's family or significant-other support network, and breakdown in the patient's psychologic stamina.

Although the psychodynamics of chronically ill patients have not been well described, Strain[5] identified the following eight categories of psychologic reactions to chronic medical illness:

—perceived threat to self-esteem and body intactness that challenges individuals' beliefs that they are masters of their own bodies;
—fear of loss of love and approval that evolves from patients' fears that illness and dependence on others will cause significant others to withdraw;
—fear of loss of control of achieved body functions and/or parts with resulting loss of independence;
—anxiety resulting from separation from loved ones and familiar environment that provided support, gratification, and a sense of intactness;
—fear of loss of, or injury to, body parts;
—guilt and fear of retaliation for having incurred the health problem in the first place, or for having lost control;
—fear of pain; and
—fear of strangers providing intimate care.

A prevalent theme throughout all these reactions is a lack of control. The lack of control seems to pervade all aspects of chronic illness—from etiology of the disease itself, to events and experiences within the health-care system while the patient seeks treatment for the disease. In some instances, the patient's expectation for control is inadvertently thwarted, for example, by not being included in scheduling of appointments or timing of procedures, or by not receiving acknowledgment of the patient's quest for deeper insights about problems and alternative therapies.

Strain[5] explains that regressive behavior which occurs in children during stress is likely to occur in chronically ill adults. Lack of involvement in care promotes regression in chronically ill patients. The regression to unwarranted dependency and passivity that could occur can be prevented by nursing care. Nursing measures to prevent negative dependency are discussed throughout this book, and specific measures to empower the chronically ill person are described in Part 4.

Feldman[6] used the term readaptation in referring to rehabilitation of chronically ill patients. He stated that readaptation "is coming to terms existentially with the reality of chronic illness as a state of being, discarding both false hope and destructive hopelessness, restructuring the environment in which one must now function." Readaptation for chronically ill patients requires reorganization and acceptance of self on a level that transcends the illness. This is a sizable challenge, in light of the multiple stresses and unpredictable dilemmas that accompany chronic illnesses.

Despite the unpredictable dilemmas of living with illness, chronically ill persons have goals similar to those of any well person, that is, to live life fully and to function optimally in all aspects of life. Specific abilities for which chronically ill individuals may strive to attain *quality of life* include being able to engage in roles that are important to the individual; perceiving themselves as worthwhile; achieving a sense of independence; feeling satisfaction with self, accomplishments, and relationships; and having a sense of well-being despite limitations imposed by illness. Accomplishing the goals depends, to a large extent, on controlling powerlessness.

Maximizing the patient's power resources facilitates coping with the chronic illness. An individual's power resources (Fig. 1-1) include physical strength (physical reserve), psychologic stamina and support network, positive self-concept, energy, knowledge, motivation, and belief system-hope. Individuals with chronic illnesses may have deficits in several power resources, that is, physical strength and energy; therefore, remaining power components may need to be developed to prevent or overcome powerlessness. The patient's unique and varied coping strategies compensate for deficient resources and build up remaining resources such as hope and positive self-concept (specifically self-esteem). Because the power resources are discussed in more detail in chapters throughout this book, each resource will be described only briefly here.

# PHYSICAL STRENGTH

Physical strength refers both to the individual's ability for optimal physical functioning and to physical reserve. When any body system is compromised by illness, the individual's power to act is decreased. The present status of an individual's physical strength—whether the patient is on a downward course with more physical symptoms arising (a deteriorating health state) or whether the patient is improving physically—will influence the patient's power. Physical reserve is the ability of the body to maintain physical

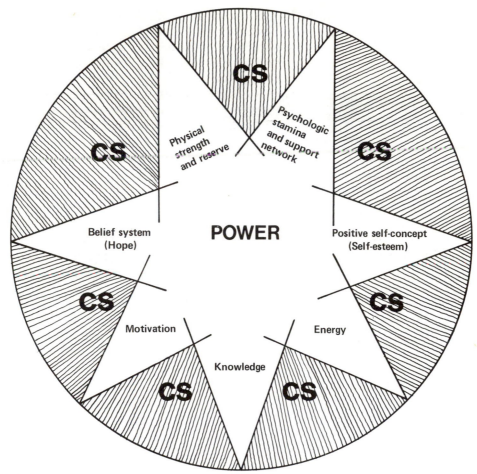

**FIGURE 1-1.   Patient power resources. CS refers to the individual's unique coping strategies utilized when resources are compromised.**

balance when confronted with threats or extra demands. For example, individuals on long-term therapy with immunosuppressive drugs have less reserve in fighting infection than do persons not taking these drugs. Persons with arthritis may need several days' rest after engaging in some unusual event or exercise because their energy reserves are depleted.

## PSYCHOLOGIC STAMINA

Psychologic stamina refers to a unique resiliency present in human beings. Despite the crisis of illness and day-to-day uncertainty, some patients are able to maintain psychologic equilibrium. Somehow, events that could be viewed as threats are interpreted as being meaningful. At the other extreme, chronic illness may cause psychologic imbalance. Depression and anxiety are two prevalent symptoms in chronically ill individuals that may require psychotherapy.[7] The patient with a chronic health problem may need help to maintain a positive outlook and to prevent or alleviate paralyzing anxiety, depression, and hopelessness.

The support network provided by family helps maintain psychologic stamina as a power resource. Dimond[8] studied adaptation to chronic illness, specifically in patients on hemodialysis. She found positive correlations between presence of social support (in terms of family environment, spouse, and confidant) and morale of the 36 chronically ill patients studied. Pattison[9] found that the life spans of patients with chronic obstructive lung disease were not predicted by the amount of remaining respiratory function (extent of pathology), but rather depended on their having someone in their social network who cared about them.

Family members themselves need support in coping with the burden of caring for and worrying about their chronically ill family member.

## POSITIVE SELF-CONCEPT

Self-concept is the individual's total thoughts and feelings about oneself.[10] Components of the self-concept include physical self (body image), functional self (role performance), personal self (moral self, self-ideal, and self-expectancy),[11] and self-esteem (self-worth). Epstein states, "There is a basic need for self-esteem which relates to all aspects of the self systems, and in comparison to which, almost all other needs are subordinate."[12] Self-esteem is therefore a very crucial component of self-concept and a determinant of functioning. Feeling worthwhile is basic to taking action to achieve improved health.

Chronic illness has an impact on how the person perceives self. The illness may promote a feeling of being "permanently different"[7] or of having less worth, akin to a defective mechanical device being worthless when one part is nonfunctional. Cooper[13] refers to the world of chronic illness as the "fourth world." The fourth world is made up of millions of persons alienated from desired everyday life and denied desired interaction with life because of the effects of the disease and its treatment.

Self-concept reconstruction, then, is one facet of adjusting to the illness. The goal in self-concept reconstruction is to integrate an accurate perception of the altered body part into a positive concept of self, while understanding that the ability or potential ability for managing care of the health problem resides within the self. Having the illness completely engulf the individual (taxing every thought and activity) must be avoided. Allowing the illness to be the dominant component in defining self needs to be avoided. In other words, individuals with multiple sclerosis may need nurses' help to define themselves in terms of continuing roles, strengths, abilities, and goals, rather than simply in terms of the neurologic impairment. Chapter 15 discusses enhancement of self-esteem (one component of self-concept) as a method of alleviating powerlessness.

The nature of an individual's personality influences self-concept. One personality characteristic that is directly related to the subject of this book is locus of control. Unlike powerlessness, which is a situationally determined perception that outcomes are beyond the individual's control, locus of control is a stable tendency to perceive events and outcomes to be within or outside the person's own control regardless of the situation. Persons with internal loci of control tend to perceive positive and negative life events as being a result of their own actions—under personal control.[14,15] Persons with external loci of control tend to perceive life events as being unrelated to their own behavior but rather as being contingent on chance, fate, or powerful others.[14,15] This particular trait is important in determining the individual's usual perceptions of life events, and how much or how little control and/or involvement in self-care management the ill individual needs. In caring for chronically ill patients, nurses need to be concerned with whether or not the individual with an internal locus of control experiences more intense feelings of powerlessness when dealing with the illness than does an individual with an external locus of control. Locus of control is discussed in more detail in Chapters 6, 8, and 9.

# ENERGY

Energy is a force capable of doing work or being stored. There must be a balance between energy uptake and energy expenditure. Energy sources include nutrients, water, rest, and motivation. Energy is expended to restore or heal physical states, to actively cope with daily living demands, and to cope with unusual stress. Energy is also spent for growth through learning, work, and play.[16] Absence of energy for the most basic levels of energy utilization, referred to as the compensatory level needed for physical balance,[16] contributes to powerlessness of the individual and prevents energy utilization for higher-level expenditure needs, for example, growth and learning. Action is possible if strength and energy are present. Actions of the ill person include measures initiated by the person to protect and/or improve health. Coping with uncertainty of energy availability is discussed in Chapter 11.

# KNOWLEDGE AND INSIGHT

Having knowledge and insight about what is happening to an individual is an enabling factor for patient control. The anxiety of uncertainty is controlled by knowledge about the nature and timing of anticipated events. It has been documented many times that patients who were informed of the sensory experiences and had accurate expectations about the anticipated experience would exhibit less anxiety during the stress event.[17-21]

The care regimens chronically ill persons are required to implement are difficult in that they require learned skills, are time consuming to execute, usually require changes in habits and routines, and entail physical and psychologic stress.[22] The regimen's difficulty is not only due to the individual's having to learn psychomotor skills as an injection technique or having to learn technical content as action of drugs, but also due to the individual's having to cope with psychologic reactions to the health problem. Engaging in the learned therapy is a constant reminder of being different and of having the chronic illness.

Patient knowledge allows for involvement in decision making. Knowledge of a situation means that patients are aware of the alternatives and the anticipated consequences of each alternative course of action. Lack of understanding contributes to lassitude and inaction, both of which are characteristic of powerlessness. See Chapters 12 and 13 for more information.

Internal awareness[23] is a concept appropriate for discussion in relation to the power resource knowledge-insight. Internal awareness is the ability to detect and interpret physical and psychologic cues so as to take appropriate action to control symptoms and maintain psychologic balance.[24] This refers to developing a sensitivity to an individual's own body and means having an accurate perception of alterations in health such as changes in fatigue, pain, appetite, skin color, elimination, mood states, tension, anger, depression, guilt, and other physical and psychologic states. For example, a young patient with insulin-dependent diabetes may discover that circumoral numbness is the earliest symptom of impending insulin shock. Taking the appropriate action—ingesting glucose, then a protein food—could avoid an emergency-room visit. Internal awareness also means knowing the desired effect of the therapy and monitoring self in light of this effect. The patient with congestive heart failure on diuretics who noted daily weight was increasing by 2 pounds would be aware of the seriousness of this sign and would contact the physician. The patient would *not* wait a week until the respiratory distress could be severe. Having this sensitivity to know one's own signs and symptoms and reactions to therapy empowers the person to take action to control symptoms and avert crises.

# MOTIVATION

The theory of motivation based on competence and self-determination was reviewed by Deci.[25] This theory of motivation is congruent with approaches proposed in this book, namely, to develop the patient's sense of control over self and environment. Competence theory refers to the individual's ability to deal effectively with the environment by manipulating the environment not only to meet personal needs (as for food and comfort) but also to have a feeling of efficacy.[25]

Kagan[26] describes the human being as having a motive for mastery. He proposed that the origins of mastery were human beings' desire to achieve standards, predict the future, and define themselves. Reduction of uncertainty is a component of Kagan's concept.

In the same sense, deCharms[27] states that individuals strive to be their own causal agents (for producing change in the environment, as well as in self and self-behavior). The desire to control one's destiny influences all other human motives. Deci also describes competence behaviors as being geared to "dissonance" reduction. That is, the individual strives to reduce the amount of incongruity among beliefs, expectations, and actual actions and outcomes of events.

Deci[25] concludes his review of motivational theories by stating that intrinsically motivated behaviors enable persons to feel competent and self-determining. He summarizes intrinsically motivated behaviors as two kinds: (1) those seeking stimulation, and (2) those reducing incongruity (dissonance).

In chronic illness, motivation is important in maximizing potential, promoting social and work roles, and developing self-confidence through risk taking (e.g., being able to risk rejection when applying for a new job despite the chronic illness). Motivation is also needed to learn new skills and engage in therapies.

The reader should note that a complete overview of theories of motivation is beyond the scope of this book. Humanistic theories especially relevant for nurses are discussed in Chapter 13. The power resource of motivation is addressed as one aspect of enabling behaviors in Chapter 13.

## BELIEF SYSTEM

The belief system of the individual encompasses belief in God to provide strength and ability to cope with stress and overcome it; belief in therapeutic regimens, with the accompanying autosuggestion that the therapy will be effective; belief in care givers; and belief in self, that is, confidence in one's own capabilities. Kraines[28] stated if the patient believes strongly in a care giver, by that very belief the patient obtains moral support and can face problems with a new degree of equanimity. Frank[29] describes how patients' expectations for therapy influence outcomes. Patients' self-suggestions about success of therapy may have self-fulfilling prophecy effects. The psychiatric patients' expressed optimism about treatment was a determinant in their symptomatic improvement in a 6-week course of therapy.[30]

Spiritual malaise does not appear to be conducive to healing.[29] The chronically ill person needs relief from the isolation of suffering. Having a relationship with God alleviates the aloneness. The definition of chronic illness affecting mind, body, and spirit systems directs nurses' attention to developing spiritual well-being. "Spiritual well-being is the affirmation of life in a relationship with God, self, community, and environment that nurtures and celebrates wholeness."[31] Some individuals may find meaning in the misfortune of chronic illness through religion-faith. A new hope is derived from renewed spiritual well-being.

The presence of faith and hope empowers an individual to have a perceived sense of control and may enhance therapeutic results. Inspiring hope is discussed in detail in Chapter 16.

The more power resources that are compromised in an individual patient, the more nursing strategies will be needed to help the patient overcome a lack of control. These nursing strategies must consider the individual's unique coping strategies and must focus on specific deficient power resources.

## SUMMARY

The continuous ups and downs of chronic illness present a threatening sense of uncertainty. The uncertainty may range from being unable to predict whether the individual will have enough physical energy for an upcoming event, pain or comfort, nausea resulting from chemotherapy, or the internal motivation needed to follow through with an expectation. Not being able to know about these and several other factors often prevents the individual from planning and engaging in social activities. Because social activities play a role in the development of a positive self-concept, these types of interactions are especially important for chronically ill persons. However, the uncertainty that accompanies the illness may cause ill individuals to isolate themselves. Eventually, the cure-oriented medical profession may demonstrate its own discouragement to the patient.

The lack of improvement in the chronically ill patient's condition may threaten the physician's narcissistic integrity.[5] Any tendency to give up by medical staff due to physician helplessness is counteracted by deliberate nursing that focuses on quality-of-life interventions. Many uncertainties interfere with quality of life.

An ultimate uncertainty of "When will this end in death?" is with the patient. How much more loss the family and patient will suffer before the final departure of death is a query seldom voiced by the patient and family, yet it is quietly with them. Psychologic stability and a support network help patients balance these fears with recognition of abilities and potential in their lives.

Patients who are chronically ill need to have power to be managers of their care. They should not forfeit this role to health-care personnel. Nurses can maximize patients' resources for power. Nurses help patients with deficits in one or more of the power resources by developing remaining intact power resources, as well as by supporting the patients' select coping strategies.

The power resources model provides the general framework for this book. Chapters are devoted to examining causes, indicators, and measurement of power resource deficits in specific health problems and/or age-groups. Strategies to alleviate powerlessness are described for specific chronic health problems. Empowerment strategies specific to components of the power resources model are developed in this book; individual chapters are devoted to enhancing self-esteem, inspiring hope, overcoming energy deficits, and developing enabling strategies (motivation and knowledge), all of which are directed at alleviating powerlessness of chronic illness. The many explicit challenges confronting chronically ill patients are discussed in Chapter 2. A typology of coping tasks for chronically ill patients is presented in Chapter 2.

# REFERENCES

1. May, R.: *Power and Innocence: A Search for the Sources of Violence.* W. W. Norton & Co., New York, 1972.
2. Wortmann, C. and Brehm, J.: *Responses to uncontrollable outcomes: An integration of reactance theory and the learned helplessness model.* In Berkowitz, L. (ed.): *Advances in Experimental Social Psychology, Vol. 8.* Academic Press, New York, 1975, pp. 277-336.
3. Turk, D., et al.: *A sequential criterion analysis for assessing coping with chronic illness.* J. Human Stress 6(2):35, 1980.
4. Reif, L.: *Beyond medical intervention strategies for managing life in face of chronic illness.* In Davis, M., Kramer, M., and Strauss, A. (eds.): *Nurses in Practice: A Perspective on Work Environments,* C. V. Mosby, St. Louis, 1975, p. 263.
5. Strain, J.: *Psychological reactions to chronic medical illness.* Psychiatric Quarterly 51:173, 1979.
6. Feldman, D.: *Chronic disabling illness: A holistic view.* J. Chronic Dis. 27:287, 1974.
7. Adams, J. and Lindemann, E.: *Coping with long-term disability.* In Coelho, G., Hamburg, D., and Adams, J. (eds.): *Coping and Adaptation.* Basic Books, New York, 1974, pp. 127-138.
8. Dimond, M.: *Social support and adaptation to chronic illness: The case of maintenance hemodialysis.* Research in Nursing and Health 2:101, 1979.
9. Pattison, E. M.: *Psychosocial predictors of death prognosis.* Omega 5:145, 1974.
10. Rosenberg, M.: *Conceiving the Self.* Basic Books, New York, 1979.

11. Driever, M.: *Theory of self-concept.* In Roy, Sister Callista (ed.): *Introduction to Nursing: An Adaptation Model.* Prentice-Hall, Englewood Cliffs, N.J., 1976, pp. 169-191.
12. Epstein, S.: *The self-concept revisited: Or a theory of a theory.* Am. Psychol. 28:404, 1973.
13. Cooper, I. S.: *Living with Chronic Neurologic Disease.* W. W. Norton & Co., New York, 1976.
14. Rotter, J. B.: *Generalized expectancies for internal versus external control of reinforcement.* Psychol. Monogr. 80:1, 1966.
15. Lefcourt, H. M.: *Belief in personal control: Research and implications.* J. Individ. Psychol. 22:185, 1966.
16. Ryden, M. B.: *Energy: A crucial consideration in the nursing process.* Nurs. Forum 16:71, 1977.
17. Johnson, J.: *The effect of structuring patients' expectations on their reactions to threatening events.* Nurs. Res. 21:499, 1972.
18. Johnson, J.: *Effects of accurate expectations about sensation on the sensory and distress components of pain.* J. Pers. Soc. Psychol. 27:261, 1973.
19. Johnson, J., Morrissey, J., and Leventhal, H.: *Psychological preparation for an endoscopic examination.* Gastrointest. Endosc. 19:180, 1973.
20. Johnson, J. and Rice, V.: *Sensory and distress components of pain: Implications for the study of clinical pain.* Nurs. Res. 23:203, 1974.
21. Johnson, J., Kirchhoff, K., and Endress, M. P.: *Altering children's distress behavior during orthopedic cast removal.* Nurs. Res. 24:404, 1975.
22. Reif: *op. cit.,* p. 264.
23. Kinsman, R., et al.: *Patient variables supporting chronic illness.* J. Nerv. Ment. Dis. 163:159, 1976.
24. Miller, J. F.: *Categories of self-care needs of ambulatory patients with diabetes.* Journal of Advanced Nursing (in press).
25. Deci, E.: *Intrinsic Motivation.* Plenum Press, New York, 1976.
26. Kagan, J.: *Motives and development.* J. Pers. Soc. Psychol. 22:51, 1972.
27. DeCharms, R.: *Personal Causation: The Internal Affective Determinants of Behavior.* Academic Press, New York, 1968.
28. Kraines, S. H.: *The Therapy of Neuroses and Psychoses.* Lea & Febiger, Philadelphia, 1943.
29. Frank, J.: *Persuasion and Healing.* Schocken Books, New York, 1975.
30. Uhlenhuth, E. H. and Duncan, D. B.: *Subjective change with medical student therapists: II. Some determinants for change in psychoneurotic outpatients.* Arch. Gen. Psychiatry 18:532, 1968.
31. Moberg, D.: *Spiritual Well-Being: Sociological Perspectives.* University Press of America, Washington, D.C., 1979, p. 5.

# SELECTED READINGS

Anderson, S. V. and Bauwens, E.: *Chronic Health Problems: Concepts and Application.* C. V. Mosby, St. Louis, 1981.
Carlson, C. and Blackwell, B. *Behavioral Concepts and Nursing Intervention,* ed. 2. J. B. Lippincott Co., Philadelphia, 1978.
Fordyce, W. *Behavioral Methods for Chronic Pain and Illness.* C. V. Mosby, St. Louis, 1976.
Gaylin, W.: *Caring.* Alfred A. Knopf, New York, 1976.
Lambert, V. and Lambert, C.: *The Impact of Physical Illness and Related Mental Health Concepts.* Prentice-Hall, Englewood Cliffs, N.J., 1979.
Moos, R.: *Coping With Physical Illness.* Plenum Medical Book, New York, 1977.
Roberts, S.: *Behavioral Concepts and Nursing Throughout the Life Span.* Prentice-Hall, Englewood Cliffs, N.J., 1978.
Shontz, F.: *The Psychological Aspects of Physical Illness and Disability.* Macmillan, New York, 1975.
Strauss, A.: *Chronic Illness and the Quality of Life.* C. V. Mosby, St. Louis, 1975.
Watson, J.: *Nursing: The Philosophy and Science of Caring.* Little, Brown & Co., Boston, 1979.
Weisman, A.: *Coping With Cancer.* McGraw-Hill, New York, 1979.
Werner-Beland, J.: *Grief Responses to Long-Term Illness and Disability.* Reston Publishing, Reston, Va., 1980.

Wilkerson, S.: *Factors influencing the relationship between the nurse and the client/patient.* In Leonard, B. and Redland, A. (eds.): *Process in Clinical Nursing.* Prentice-Hall, Englewood Cliffs, N.J., 1981, pp. 43-73.

Wu, R.: *Behavior and Illness.* Prentice-Hall, Englewood Cliffs, N.J., 1973.

# 2
# COPING WITH CHRONIC ILLNESS

## JUDITH FITZGERALD MILLER

The human potential for resilience in situations of extreme threat is indeed remarkable. Psychologic equilibrium can be maintained in the midst of severe trauma. The individual's ability to withstand trauma and strengthen intact power resources depends on coping ability. Coping is a term used frequently in everyday language; however, the concept deserves careful analysis by health-care professionals. Members of helping professions need to develop insight into patients' coping styles. Nurses are required to sustain patients during stress and to help mobilize power resources, such as by promoting significant other's support. Patients have vast capacities for coping; however, nurses who do not recognize helpful coping behaviors may be less than adequate in helping patients confront the tasks that accompany illness. Nurses must develop understanding of coping behavior in order to have greater insights into their patients' overall behavior and reactions throughout chronic illness.

Chronically ill persons look to nurses to help them face the challenge of long-term health problems. Chronic illness taxes the resources of individuals to continue with all of life's demands. Nurses play a major role in helping patients meet the demands. Consider the following comments of a middle-aged woman with multiple sclerosis: "How can I face this deterioration, this physical destruction, this waning ability to get around? Look at me, a mother, wife, and businesswoman, now unable to care for myself. I am totally dependent on others, a characteristic I find intolerable!" These words challenge our very beings as helping professionals. How do nurses help patients cope with states of powerlessness? Nurses need to identify coping styles of individuals and determine the effectiveness of the unique coping behavior a patient has chosen. Nurses also need to help patients discover their own individual repertoires of coping strategies.

This chapter analyzes the definition of coping, coping tasks of the chronically ill, coping strategies and styles, and specific coping strategies identified in chronically ill patients. The more coping tasks confronting the individual, the greater likelihood that powerlessness will occur.

# COPING DEFINED

Coping is defined by Lipowski[1] as all cognitive and motor activities a sick person uses to preserve bodily and psychic integrity, to recover reversible impaired function, and to compensate to the limit for any irreversible loss. In terms of psychologic stress theory, Lazarus[2] defined coping simply as strategies used to deal with threat. Psychologically, threats need to be diminished to prevent psychologic immobilization. Lazarus describes coping as a process, not a single act. Coping is cognitive activity in the form of cognitive appraisal of events and reactions, then determination of a course of action based on reappraisal. Coping activity is stimulated by the cognition, "My life, health, wealth, or cherished social relationships are in danger."[3] However, coping may be defined broadly in terms of achieving life goals and meeting life demands.[4-6] Coping is viewed as problem solving, that is, confronting the realities of a problem while still maintaining integrity of functioning.[7] Coping is what one does about a problem to bring about relief, reward, quiescence, and equilibrium.[8] Coping is a dynamic process of actions (cognitive and psychomotor) that is different from defending. Defense mechanisms (defending) may be rather rigid psychologic mechanisms despite the problem presented,[8] whereas coping is an open system that permits new information to be taken in and utilized and behavior to be modified in light of continuous reappraisals of reality.[9] Although there is a difference between defending and coping, defense mechanisms may be a part of an individual's coping behavior.

Throughout this chapter, *coping* refers to dealing with situations that present a threat to the individual so as to resolve uncomfortable feelings such as anxiety, fear, grief, and guilt. Problems precipitating these uncomfortable affects may be thought of as *coping tasks*. Coping tasks are external stimuli such as dealing with pain, threat of surgery, and impending death, as well as internal psychic phenomena such as threatened body image, perceived alterations in role function, and unresolved anger. *Coping strategies* are the specific techniques a sick person selects to deal with the illness and its consequences. An individual's coping style is one's enduring disposition to deal with challenges and stress by employing a specific group of techniques.[1] Weisman[10] states, "Coping combines perception, performance, appraisal, correction, followed by further activity and directed motivated behavior." The aim of coping is mastery, control, or resolution.[11]

## Effective Coping

Coping behavior is effective when the behavior utilized resolves the uncomfortable feeling associated with threat and/or loss, preserves the integrity of the individual, and preserves the ability of the individual to function effectively in relationships, life roles, and maintenance of a positive self-concept. Visotsky and coworkers[12] described coping as being effective when it (1) kept distress within manageable limits, (2) generated encouragement and hope, (3) maintained or restored a sense of personal worth, (4) maintained or restored relationships with significant others, (5) enhanced prospects for physical recovery, and (6) enhanced prospects for favorable situations (interpersonal, social, and economic). Caplan[13] identified effective coping strategies such as actively exploring reality issues and searching for information; freely expressing both positive and negative feelings, and having tolerance for frustration; actively invoking help from others; breaking problems into manageable bits and working them through one at a time; being aware of fatigue and tendencies toward disorganization, pacing activities, and engaging in problem-solving efforts; mastering feelings when possible and accepting the inevitable when not; trusting in oneself and others, and maintaining optimism about the outcome.

## Variables Affecting Coping

The same variables that shape the ego have an impact on coping. Categories of variables that affect coping include intrapersonal, environmental, and illness-related factors.[1] *Intrapersonal factors* may include age, personality, intelligence, specific self-care skills, values, beliefs, emotional state, and cognitive capacity. *Environmental factors* may include presence of support network of significant others and friends, access to health services, physical resources for living, and financial resources. *Illness-related factors* include the type of illness, its location, degree of impairment, meaning of the illness to the individual, rate of onset, and stage of progression.[1]

In analyzing the stages of progression of an illness, differences in coping energy utilization can be easily understood. Charmaz[14] presented a three-stage progression of chronic disease. *Stage 1* is labeled interrupted time, when daily activities are temporarily adjusted to obtain a diagnosis. *Stage 2* is the time intrusion phase, when daily activities need to be adjusted to control the effect of the disease. The illness consumes time and energy. *Stage 3* is time encapsulation, during which the individual is consumed by the illness; the individual is engulfed with care management throughout the day.

The meaning of the illness to the individual affects coping behavior. Differences in coping can be expected if one individual perceives the illness to be a threat to sexual role functioning and another views the illness as insignificant. Illness may be viewed as a loss or gain, or of no significance.

Perceiving illness as a loss refers to loss of pleasures, role fulfilment, functional abilities, self-esteem, self-satisfaction, love, recognition, and normalcy. Illness may be viewed as a threat to life. Grief and anxiety accompany the perception of illness as a loss.

Illness may be perceived by some as a gain. Illness may provide relief from stress of other life roles. The suffering of illness may be viewed as having spiritual value for the individual. Illness may be viewed as an opportunity for the individual to relieve guilt, repent for felt past offenses, and accept this plight as a punishment. Illness may provide respite from intrapersonal conflict or an opportunity to withdraw and resolve conflict.

Illness may also afford some individuals the opportunity to receive kindness, attention, and signs of affection that are otherwise absent.

If the individual views the illness as insignificant, little importance is assigned to the symptoms[15] or possible consequences of the illness and treatment.

The meaning of the illness to the individual influences the amount of coping energy needed to deal successfully with problems. The nurse's understanding of the patient's perception of the illness will enhance the nurse's ability to identify and support the coping strategy the patient selects. Clear differences in coping would exist between individuals perceiving illness as a threat or loss and those perceiving illness as a gain or being insignificant.

# COPING TASKS OF CHRONICALLY ILL INDIVIDUALS*

Coping tasks are those particular challenges that must be faced and overcome so that the individual preserves integrity, restores or maintains a positive concept of self, and functions effectively in relationships and life roles. Individuals with chronic health problems may be challenged to cope with multiple complex tasks.

Kiely[16] categorized three types of stresses that initiate coping responses: (1) loss or threat of loss of psychic "objects," that is, personal relationships, body functions and image, and social roles; (2) injury or threat of injury to body involving notions of pain or mutilation; and (3) frustration of biologic drive satisfaction—especially nurturant or libidinal drives—as well as frustration over lack of avenues for aggressive discharge.

To identify the coping tasks of chronically ill persons, nursing diagnoses of 118 chronically ill patients were reviewed. These nursing diagnoses were made by 44 graduate nursing students enrolled in a graduate nursing practicum course entitled "Nursing Strategies for Adults: Long-Term Health Problems." Each student studied and cared for a small caseload of patients (no more than three) for the duration of the academic semester. Coping tasks were also identified in literature review and through Stapleton's[17] and my clinical practice. Table 2-1 lists the coping tasks identified.

Each coping task will be discussed briefly.

## Striving to Feel Normal

Maintaining a sense of normalcy includes keeping signs and symptoms of illness under control or out of view from persons surrounding the individual. It includes a mental review of existing abilities and functions. When the chronically ill individual engages in a personal reaffirmation of being as capable as coworkers or individuals in the person's social network, the ideal of being and feeling normal (having abilities similar to others in the social network) is fostered.

Wiener[18] described how individuals with rheumatoid arthritis used the normalizing strategies of covering up, keeping up, and pacing. Covering up means keeping signs of

*Recognition and gratitude are expressed to Susan Stapleton, M.S.N., R.N., who as a Research Assistant at Marquette University College of Nursing, under HEW Grant No. 1 D23 NU00038-03, participated in identifying an original typology of coping tasks.

**TABLE 2-1. Typology of Coping Tasks of Chronically Ill Adults***

| Broad Task Category | Subconcepts in the Category |
| --- | --- |
| 1. Maintaining a sense of normalcy. | Hiding, minimizing illness, and/or responding to curious inquiries of others. Living as normally as possible despite daily therapy and obvious symptoms. |
| 2. Modifying daily routine, adjusting life-style. | Including therapy and symptom control in daily routine. Providing for safety. |
| 3. Obtaining knowledge and skill for continuing self-care. | Having internal awareness. Monitoring effects of therapy. |
| 4. Maintaining a positive concept of self. | Integrating illness into self-concept. Maintaining or enhancing self-esteem. |
| 5. Adjusting to altered social relationships. | Experiencing loneliness and social isolation. Undergoing patient- or other-initiated disengagement. Preserving relationships with friends and family who satisfy dependency needs. Maintaining family solidarity. |
| 6. Grieving over losses concomitant with chronic illness. | Losing physical abilities, function. Losing status. Losing income and social relationships. Losing roles and dignity. Dealing with financial losses. |
| 7. Dealing with role change. | Losing roles—social, work, family. Gaining roles—dependent help seeker, self-care agent, chronically ill patient. |
| 8. Handling physical discomfort. | Handling illness-induced discomfort. Handling pain caused by therapy. |
| 9. Complying with prescribed regimen. | |
| 10. Confronting the inevitability of one's own death. | |
| 11. Dealing with social stigma of illness or disability. | |
| 12. Maintaining a feeling of being in control. | Exerting cognitive control. Exerting behavioral control. Exerting decisional control. |
| 13. Maintaining hope despite uncertain or downward course of health. | Experiencing effects of hope. Finding meaning in physical changes. |

*Supported by HEW Grant No. 1 D23 NU00038-62.

disability and pain hidden. It may include not using an assistive device—cane or other external sign of handicap (wheelchair). Controlling evidence of discomfort and fatigue is an imperative behavior for successful covering up. Chronically ill individuals expend much energy covering up, not only to maintain a sense of normalcy but also to avoid questions from curious onlookers and to avoid making those around them feel uncomfortable. Persons interacting with the chronically ill individual may feel uncomfortable about not knowing how much assistance with mobility to provide, how to respond to obvious evidence of pain, and how to minimize their own vigor and vitality so as to lessen the discrepancy between their health and the chronically ill person's impairment. Covering up is not a form of denial; it is a rejection of the disability as interfering with social interactions.

Keeping up refers to the ill individual's successful carrying through with a planned event,[18] while covering up, expending increased energy, and causing overwhelming fatigue and perhaps exacerbation of symptoms. Events such as hosting the family get-together or preparing a holiday meal call for frantic keeping-up activity.

Pacing refers to balancing the activities of covering up and keeping up with rest so as to avoid unnecessary periods of immobilization that would be needed to restore energy wasted in covering up and keeping up. Pacing results from the individual's understanding limitations and abilities and appropriately engaging in activities over a time span that satisfy ego needs without causing undue exhaustion.

## Modifying Routines and Life-Styles

To control symptoms and live as normally as possible, the individual may need to alter habits and routines. Habits of overeating, getting no exercise, having no form of relaxation, or smoking may need to be modified. Daily routines may need to be interrupted to obtain needed therapy for the chronic disease, for example, postural drainage and intermittent positive-pressure breathing for individuals with emphysema. Activities that exacerbate symptoms must be learned and avoided. (The elementary teacher with rheumatoid arthritis may need to avoid playground duty on cool, damp days.)

## Obtaining Knowledge and Skill for Continuing Self-Care

Self-care is a key concept for the chronically ill individual's maintenance of optimal health. Achieving desired outcomes depends on the patient's self-care practices and not on the health-care team's power. Being competent in ministering to self means acquiring the necessary skills, knowledge, and motivation. It also means having an awareness of body cues, interpreting physical changes accurately, and taking appropriate action either to alter therapy or to seek help from the health-care system to prevent a crisis.

## Maintaining a Positive Concept of Self

When previous abilities are gone, energy and ability to successfully engage in desired activities that satisfy ego needs have disappeared, and changes in physical self have occurred, maintaining a positive concept of self is a major coping task. The individual must avoid allowing the disability or illness to become one's entire identity. Instead, the illness, related changes, and therapies must be integrated into a positive concept of self that helps the individual maintain a sense of competence and normalcy. Activities that enhance self-esteem need to be identified; the remaining personal strengths need to be emphasized. Helping the patient review accomplishments and remaining intact roles enhances self-esteem. Balancing the self-ideal with the altered body image is necessary to maintain a positive self-concept and self-esteem (see Chapter 15).

## Adjusting to Altered Social Relationships

Chronic illness may cause social isolation and loneliness. The sick person may withdraw because of depleted energy reserve or poor self-concept, feeling unworthy of previous social contacts or simply physically unable to participate in former social events. As the illness encapsulates more of the person's time, thought processes may be dominated by the illness, controlling symptoms, and obtaining relief. Only the most loyal friends may persist in being supportive during this repetitive pattern of interaction. In other words, isolation may be initiated by significant others' withdrawal to obtain relief from the difficult scene of physical deterioration. Davis[19] quotes a chronically ill woman as saying, "Anyone who is sick for longer than 6 months won't be remembered except for birthdays and holidays."

The ill individual may need to adjust to having fewer interactions with fewer people and to receiving decreased confirmation of being a capable individual. The ill person must also strive to preserve relationships with those friends and family members who satisfy physical and emotional dependency needs.

## Grieving over the Losses of Chronic Illness

Chronically ill individuals grieve over multiple losses. Loss of physical abilities includes losses of mobility, organ functioning, energy availability, physical stamina, sexual attractiveness, and sexual function. Other losses may include losses of self-esteem, role performance, and social relationships. Grief work takes place to deal with these losses and to preserve a sense of personal integrity and dignity. The cumulative effect of significant losses may create doubts in ill persons' minds about their own ability to maintain quality of life. Reformulating goals and examining aspirations requires coping skills.

## Dealing with Role Change

Role changes of chronically ill persons may be analyzed as losses and gains. The role losses may include loss of social roles (church participant, member of bowling team, officer in a community group) and employment role, and diminishment of role as family decision maker, and disciplinarian. The individual has to take on roles of being chronically ill, dependent help seeker, self-care agent, and client of a complex health-care system.

Role change encompasses giving up roles accompanied by grief work, as well as taking on new roles accompanied by role insufficiency. "Role insufficiency is any difficulty in the cognizance and/or performance of a role or of the sentiments and goals associated with the role behavior as perceived by self or by significant others."[20] In adoption of the role of self-care agent, rehearsal of role enactment may be an important prelude to actual role taking. Kassebaum and Baumann[21] point out that Parsons' sick-role theory[22] is inadequate when referring to the chronically ill person because of Parsons' emphasis on the *temporary* surrendering of roles and the person's desire to get *well*. Kassebaum and Baumann[21] identified four dimensions of the sick role in chronically ill persons. The dimensions include dependence, reciprocity (mutual expectations for exemption from some role obligations), role-performance alteration, and denial of sick role. The incapacity for role performance is not a total, temporary incapacity as described by Parsons, but rather may be a partial permanent alteration in roles and performance of roles.[21]

Learning the role of dependent help seeker, maintaining a positive dependence, is another component of this coping task. Positive dependency "requires honest acceptance of one's differentness and the special needs and conditions it imposes."[23] Seeking help for physical and emotional needs without feeling weak and inadequate is necessary. The patient is challenged to resolve feelings of conflict over wanting to be totally independent yet needing to be dependent at a time in adult life when independence is expected. Manipulating a complex health-care system to have needs met is also a challenge to the individual. Accepting the role of being chronically ill and having a less-than-ideal state of health is included in coping with role change.

## Handling Physical Discomfort

Virtually all chronic illnesses are accompanied by some discomfort, either from the disorder itself (e.g., joint pain of arthritis) or from the prescribed therapy (e.g., insulin injections or hemodialysis treatment). The individual needs to discover personally satisfying and adequate means of dealing with pain. Modalities adjunctive to medications that have been effective include relaxation, autosuggestion, distraction (as with music), and biofeedback.

As pain becomes chronic, the sufferer devotes time and energy describing the discomfort so as to reinforce with others that the pain is legitimate. The pain of a specific chronic illness such as arthritis is not as overt as pain of a fracture or surgical incision. When the pain experience is prolonged and the chronically ill patient's pain experience is not congruent with health-care workers' perception of the usual course of pain, the patient may need constantly to reaffirm that the pain is real.

## Complying with the Prescribed Regimen

It is one thing to make temporary adjustments in habits and daily patterns and quite another to alter life-style and change habits for the rest of a lifetime. Acquiring new behaviors, taking medications, and so forth are less difficult compliance problems than altering personal habits and routine behaviors of smoking, drinking, and eating.[24]

Helping sick individuals realize their actions will result in desired outcomes is a challenge to health professionals, especially when the actions demand discipline and result in uncomfortable side effects (see Chapter 12).

# Confronting the Inevitability of One's Own Death

Having a chronic illness causes reflection on life's accomplishments and a direct realization of the temporary nature of earthly existence. There may be thoughts of having "little time left," especially in comparison with the life expectancies of healthy friends. The goal is to confront this task, interpreting it as a challenge to make the most of life instead of giving in to paralyzing depression and anticipating one's own annihilation.

# Dealing with Social Stigma

How does the chronically ill individual handle the second looks, the stares from children, and the embarrassment of being unable to enter buildings or use toilet facilities unassisted? Wright[25] describes three types of responses of individuals to stigmatizing behavior: (1) bury head in the sand—ignore it; (2) overreact with rage, retaliation, and overt hostility; and (3) use humor, causing further self-depreciation. It is hoped that nurses can help chronically ill persons develop mature acceptance of self and undaunted confidence in self despite the disability.

# Maintaining a Feeling of Being in Control

Seligman states, "What produces self-esteem and a sense of competence, and protects against depression, is not only the absolute quality of the experience, but the perception that one's own actions controlled the experience."[26]

Chronically ill persons may find it difficult to maintain control because of intrusions into privacy by health-care teams and the sharing of intimate information on medical records for all interested onlookers to review. As one patient with brittle diabetes put it, "It's as though you're a butterfly with a pin stuck through you. The MDs come around to view you as a specimen on exhibit." The ability to control environmental intrusion while maintaining a sense of privacy preserves personal dignity.

Controlling a deteriorating physiologic state may not always be possible, even in the best of compliance situations. Enhancing the patient's knowledge of what is happening—physiologic changes and improvements, and effects of therapy—increases a sense of control. Having the patient make decisions about routine timing of therapy and altering habits gives the patient psychologic control.

Nurses can plan for increasing patient control according to Averill's[26] categories: (1) behavior control—the individual's direct action on the environment; (2) cognitive control—the way in which an event is interpreted or appraised by the individual; and (3) decisional control—the opportunity to choose among various courses of action.

# Maintaining Hope Despite Uncertain or Downward Course of Illness

As the chronic health problem progresses, and as physiologic deterioration and loss of function continue, hope is a sustaining force that helps the individual avoid despair and actually "prolongs life against all odds."[27] The course of events is unpredictable in chronic illness, in which remissions and exacerbations occur. There may be uncertainty in day-to-day functioning; for example, patients with rheumatoid arthritis may find planning ahead impossible owing to unexpected pain and stiffness. To augment and confirm an individual's values and purposes in life and to help the individual establish realistic goals are challenges to the nurse and the individual's significant others. Pattison studied three types of predictors of death prognoses in 12 men with pulmonary emphysema over an 18-month period. He found that neither the physiologic measures (blood gases and pulmonary studies) nor the psychologic measure (Inpatient Multidimensional Psychiatric Scale) was correlated with death or clinical improvement. The only measure that correlated with death was the sociologic tool that determined the nature of family and friend relationships. Clinical improvement correlated with an intact and positive family relationship; death correlated with disruption and negative family relationships.[28] "Hope for life and the will to live is related to having something and someone to live for."[29]

Although chronic illness has been discussed in general, predominant themes or coping tasks may be apparent with particular chronic illnesses. For example, Hinton[30] identified six major stressors experienced by 100 patients with cancer. These major stressors included pain, disfigurement, concern over future (fear of dying), loss of work role, dependency, and alienation.

When the coping tasks are examined collectively, the challenges for the ill person are overwhelming and produce powerlessness. Yet human beings are resourceful and adaptable. Individuals have a unique repertoire of behaviors to use in confronting the tasks.

## COPING STYLES

The repeated manner in which the chronically ill individual responds to the presenting coping task is the individual's coping style. Coping style can be identified by noting the individual's range of behaviors over time. An important role for the nurse is to identify the individual's coping style.

Coping styles described by various authors[1,2,15,31,32] can be divided into three categories of styles: approach, avoidance, and nonspecific defenders. The term approach[2] is synonymous with the style Goldstein and coworkers[31] labeled as sensitizer and the style Lipowski labeled as vigilant focuser. The term avoidance is synonymous with minimization[1] and repression.[32] Figure 2-1 illustrates the coping continuum.

Individuals who practice avoidance use repression, denial, projection, and any strategy that minimizes the threat. Avoidance includes intellectual strategies that diminish the seriousness of the threat for the individual. Selective inattention and ignoring or rationalizing the facts or consequences of the illness are avoidance strategies.[16]

Approach behaviors on the other end of the coping continuum include tackling, vigilant focusing, and sensitizing. Tackling is an energetic fighting of the illness and an active engaging in therapy. Vigilant focusing refers to an obsessional alertness and compulsive attention to details of therapy. Vigilant focusers need detailed explanations of procedures and treatment.[16] Vigilant focusers have more evident anxiety than do minimizers. Sensitizers are those who readily acknowledge threatening emotions of

**Approach**                    **Nonspecific defenders**                    **Avoidance**
(Vigilant focuser)                                                          (Minimizer)
(Sensitizer)                                                               (Repressor)

FIGURE 2-1.   Continuum of coping styles with synonymous terms identified.

hate, fear, disgust, and love.[33] They are on the approach end of the coping continuum because of their direct confrontation with emotional states.

Neutrals, or nonspecific defenders, use combinations of approach and avoidance strategies. On the Mainord Coper-Avoider Sentence Completion Test (an instrument to measure coping), the individuals classified as neutrals score in the middle; they are neither avoiders nor sensitizers.[33] Other tools to determine coping style need to be developed so that nurses' clinical impressions can be validated and care suited to the patient's coping style can be designed. Patients can also develop insights about their own coping styles based on test results. This would be of value to patients in preparation for confronting future stress.

# COPING WITH CHRONIC ILLNESS: A STUDY

A study of 56 chronically ill adults was undertaken to determine the specific coping strategies used to deal with the tasks of being ill. The study sample consisted of the caseloads of 19 graduate students enrolled in a seminar-practicum course entitled "Nursing Strategies for Adults: Long-Term Health Problems" during two academic semesters. The graduate students, with the author's guidance, cared for and studied the patients for a 3-month period. The students used field notes to record the impact of chronic illness on the patient's life; daily activities of leisure and work, family interaction, role disturbances, self-esteem, patterns of self-care, and grief work were noted. Coping behaviors were documented and summarized from a review of field notes that were recorded throughout the semester. The coping strategies were recorded on a data collection tool "Impact of Chronic Illness." The aim of this tool was to enhance the students' understanding of the world of chronically ill persons as well as to collect data about coping.

Adults with chronic health problems hospitalized during exacerbations in a 700-bed metropolitan hospital were included in the sample. Patients in the sample ranged from ages 20 to 79, with the largest number being in the 40 to 69 age group. Twenty-five subjects were men and 31 were women (Table 2-2).

The medical diagnoses reported in Table 2-3 are the patients' major presenting diagnoses, which caused problems and/or incapacitation at the time of the study. Many patients had multiple diagnoses, that is, patients with coronary artery disease also had underlying diabetes. Only one diagnosis was tabulated for each patient. The most frequent diagnoses were cancer, 12 patients; diabetes, 9 patients; coronary artery disease, 9 patients; and ostomies, 5 patients. See Table 2-3 for complete tabulation.

Data on coping from the Impact of Chronic Illness tool were analyzed to determine the various coping strategies 56 patients utilized. The intent was not to categorize the patients as minimizers, focusers, or neutrals, but rather to discover as many effective

**TABLE 2-2. Sample Age and Sex Characteristics**

| Age | Number of Men | Number of Women |
|-----|---------------|-----------------|
| 20–29 | 2 | 5 |
| 30–39 | 2 | 3 |
| 40–49 | 5 | 7 |
| 50–59 | 7 | 6 |
| 60–69 | 6 | 8 |
| 70–79 | 3 | 2 |
| Total | 25 | 31 |

coping strategies as possible. Coping strategies were considered effective if they met any one of the criteria listed in Figure 2-2 as modified from Visotsky and coworkers.[12] More than one strategy has been identified for each patient. The coping behaviors were categorized as approach or avoidance strategies. Approach strategies are behaviors that indicated a willingness to confront the realities of the threat, an awareness of personal reactions and feelings, and an attempt to deal with these feelings. Avoidance strategies are behaviors that protect the individual from conscious confrontation with the threat. Table 2-4 summarizes the approach and avoidance behaviors.

## Approach Strategies

The approach strategy most frequently used to deal with the tasks of chronic illness had to do with *seeking information*. Being attentive to the details of care and symptom control, participating in managing requirements of the illness, and raising questions without hesitation are examples of this approach strategy.

**TABLE 2-3. Number of Prevalent Chronic Diseases**

| Chronic Disease* | Number |
|------------------|--------|
| Cancer | 12 |
| Coronary artery disease | 9 |
| Diabetes | 9 |
| Ostomies | 5 |
| Congestive heart failure | 4 |
| Arthritis | 3 |
| Chronic renal failure | 3 |
| Multiple sclerosis | 3 |
| Amputation | 2 |
| Paraplegia | 2 |
| Cerebral vascular accident | 1 |
| Hypertension | 1 |
| Peripheral vascular disease | 1 |
| Systemic lupus erythematosus | 1 |
| Total | 56 |

*Many patients in the sample had multiple diagnoses. Only the major presenting diagnosis of each patient that is causing problems at this time is listed.

Uncomfortable feelings
(anxiety, fear, grief, or guilt) contained

Hope generated

Self-esteem enhanced

Relationships with others maintained

State of wellness (self-actualized well-being)
maintained or improved

FIGURE 2-2. Criteria for effective coping.

*Enhancing one's spiritual life* was the second most frequently used approach strategy. Specifically, individuals renewed their faith in God, prayed for strength to endure the threats, and received a sense of peace and hope as a result of "asking God for help." Patients related that they felt God's love and had strong convictions about His goodness to all earthly creatures. They felt God would challenge them with tasks He knew they could handle. When individuals interpreted handling the challenge as an expectation of God, they established a self-expectation to be successful.

Methods of self-distraction—diverting attention from illness to other facets of living—included submerging oneself in work and performing mental exercises such as solving problems and meditating. More passive self-distraction activities were watching television and doing needlework. Self-distraction was classified as an approach strategy when the patient consciously selected these activities as a means of dealing with otherwise continuous thoughts about the illness.

Another approach strategy is being keenly aware of emotions and reactions to personal dilemmas and sharing these feelings with a helper.

Some patients coped with stress by using a specific routine of physical relaxation exercises. Other specific approach strategies are listed in Table 2-4.

## Avoidance Strategies

The mental mechanisms of *denial,* repression, and suppression are included in the most frequently used avoidance strategies. These influence all the avoidance strategies; that is, if the individual denies the fact that diabetes is serious, participation in treatment may be haphazard, or no help will be sought when assistance is needed. Both of the latter are other avoidance strategies. One patient who was blind because of retinopathy of diabetes believed her eyesight would return.

Patients avoid the serious nature of their illness by *minimizing* symptoms and therapy, playing down consequences of their illness. This is noted in the way the patients describe the illness and refer to their being little affected by it.

TABLE 2-4. Approach and Avoidance Coping Strategies of 56 Chronically Ill Adults

| Approach Coping Strategies | Number Using Strategy | Avoidance Coping Strategies | Number Using Strategy |
|---|---|---|---|
| 1. Seeks information. | 14 | 1. Uses denial, suppression, repression. | 11 |
| —Focuses vigilantly on details of care. | | 2. Minimizes problems, signs, and symptoms of illness. | 9 |
| —Eagerly learns illness-related modifications in habits, diet. | | 3. Social isolation. | 6 |
| —Questions rationale for therapy. | | —Disengages from previous activities and social relationships. | |
| —Compares staff responses to same questions. | | —Becomes preoccupied with self. | |
| 2. Gains strength from spirituality. | 13 | —Withdraws. | |
| —Prayer. | | 4. Avoids talking about self, feelings or thinking about health problem. | 6 |
| —Faith. | | 5. Passive acceptance. | 5 |
| 3. Diverts attention. | 10 | —Belief in spiritual predestination. | |
| —Recognizes when becoming anxious; engages in extreme physical exertion or compulsive activity. | | —It's God's will; nothing can be done. | |
| —Meditation. | | —Shows little or no emotional concern over existing problems. | |
| —Pain distraction. | | 6. Sleeping. | 3 |
| Television. | | 7. Delays decision making on personal health matters. | 2 |
| Needlework. | | 8. Considers alternative modes of therapy. | 2 |
| 4. Expresses feelings and emotions. | 8 | —Unconventional diets. | |
| —Cries. | | 9. Blames others. | 2 |
| —Expresses hostility, anger. | | —Physician. | |
| —Describes powerlessness. | | 10. Refuses to participate in treatment. | 1 |
| 5. Uses relaxation exercises. | 6 | 11. Excessive dependence on significant other. | 1 |
| 6. Maintains control. | 5 | | |
| —Of environment. | | | |
| —Of daily activity schedules in hospital. | | | |
| —Of ostomy care. | | | |
| —Of advice-giving to spouse and nurse. | | | |
| 7. Verbalizes concerns. | 4 | | |

8. Maintains a positive healthy dependence on others. — 4
   —For physical needs (shopping, housework).
   —For emotional needs (love, support).
9. Uses positive thinking techniques. — 4
   —Tries to see good in every situation.
   —Autosuggestion for pain relief.
10. Seeks help. — 4
    —From diabetes nurse-specialist when patient determines it is needed.
11. Maintains realistic independence. — 4
    —Completes self-care activities within the limitations of illness.
    —Relates past health experiences to future actions in caring for self (responding to insulin reactions).
    —Manipulates prescribed therapy, tranquilizers.
    —Has realistic expectations for outcome of therapy.
12. Maintains social activities. — 3
    —Retirement activities.
    —Church activities.
13. Sets goals, strives to achieve them. — 3
    —Attacks problems, "digs in" to get things done.
14. Reminisces over past accomplishments. — 3
    —Life review.
15. Conserves energy. — 3
    —Analyzes daily activity; saves energy for most desirable activity.
    —Daily rest periods.

12. Manipulates others. — 1
    —Significant other performs care tasks the patient could do.
13. Sets unrealistic goals. — 1
14. Unrealistic hope for future. — 1
    —Functional abilities to return.
    —Remission.
15. Does not actively seek help. — 1
16. Uses cigarettes, drugs, alcohol. — 1

**TABLE 2-4.** *Continued*

| *Approach Coping Strategies* | *Number Using Strategy* | *Avoidance Coping Strategies* | *Number Using Strategy* |
|---|---|---|---|
| 16. Uses humor. | 3 | | |
| 17. Intellectualization. | 3 | | |
| —Mental mechanisms used to devise rational, personally meaningful explanations for occurrences (physical deterioration). | | | |
| 18. Engages in activities covering up disability, discomfort. | 2 | | |
| 19. Role rehearsal. | 2 | | |
| —Visualizes what it will be like as illness progresses. | | | |
| —Rehearses a variety of personal outcomes as a result of therapy. | | | |
| 20. Utilizes problem-solving approach. | 2 | | |
| 21. Finds comfort in realizing there are other persons who are in the same boat. | 1 | | |

The third most frequent avoidance strategy was *withdrawing* from others, either to avoid disclosure about the impact of the illness or to continue preoccupation with self. Patients use avoidance in not talking about themselves and their health problems with health-care workers. Other specific avoidance strategies are listed in Table 2-4.

Although the isolated strategies have been categorized as either approach or avoidance, it should be noted that many patients are in the center of the approach–avoidance continuum, using combinations of approach and avoidance strategies. Figure 2-3 illustrates a model of coping with chronic illness that identifies the tasks and depicts patients' use of coping strategies that characterize themselves as approachers, avoiders, or nonspecific defenders (combined approach and avoidance). Criteria for effective coping are included in the model.

Weisman and Worden[11] studied coping of 120 patients with newly diagnosed cancer. A tool based on the coping scale of Sidle and coworkers[34] was developed to categorize coping strategies of the patients with cancer. This tool included 15 coping behaviors, such as seeking more information (rational inquiry), sharing concerns (mutuality), making light of the situation (affecting reversal), doing something else (distraction), taking action regarding the problem (confronting), seeking direction (cooperative compliance), and blaming self (masochism). The coping behaviors used by each patient were compared with their scores on three other indices: (1) the patients' total mood disturbance was measured by the Profile of Mood States; (2) patients completed a self-rating revealing how adequately their problem was resolved; and (3) the patients' vulnerability index was determined by a psychologic interview. Weisman and Worden concluded that good copers used confrontation, redefinition of the problem (accepting the problem and looking for positive aspects), and compliance with authority. Good copers had high resolution, low vulnerability, and low total mood disturbance. Poor copers used suppression, passivity, submission, and tension-reducing measures (drinking, drugs), and had low resolution, high vulnerability, and high total mood disturbance.

Weisman[8] described good copers in more detail. Good copers are resourceful and are not rigid. They are characterized by the fact that they avoid denial and take action based on confronting reality; redefine problems into solvable forms, considering alternatives; maintain open communications; seek help and accept support; maintain high morale; and maintain hope.

## Impact on Care

Does being able to recognize individual's coping mechanisms serve any real therapeutic purpose? Identifying individual patients' coping styles and specific coping strategies is imperative for a holistic nursing approach. Nurses need to be sensitized to how the patient is confronting the ups and downs of chronic illness. Nurses may unwittingly stifle helpful patient strategies, making judgments about what the nurse would do in similar circumstances instead of objectively evaluating the effectiveness of the patient's selected strategies and supporting the patient's use of strategies that are effective.

Judgments cannot be made about the value of approach versus avoidance strategies unless criteria for effective coping are used (see Fig. 2-1). Coping is effective if uncom-

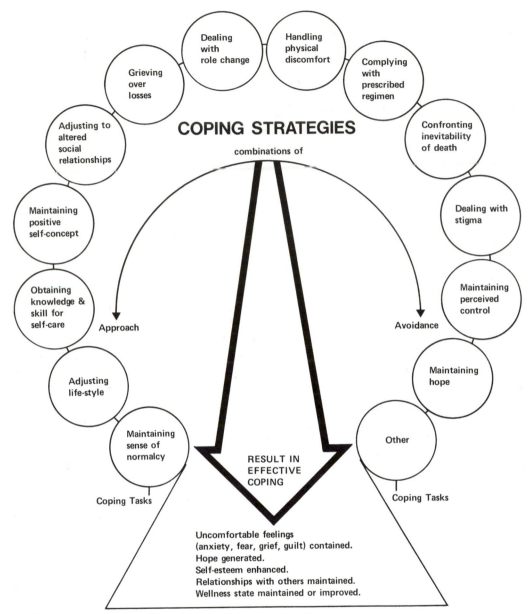

**FIGURE 2-3.  A model of coping with chronic illness.**

fortable feelings of anxiety, fear, grief, or guilt are contained; hope is generated; self-esteem is enhanced; relationships with others are maintained; and state of wellness is maintained or improved. Cohen and Lazarus[35] studied 61 surgical patients to determine the relationship between the mode of coping and recovery from surgery. Patients were classified as using avoidance, vigilance, or both types of behavior as a result of the Andrew version of the Goldstein Coper-Avoider Sentence Completion Test.[36] The variables studied were number of days in the hospital, number of analgesics used, minor medical complications, and negative psychologic reactions. The results indicated that the 10 vigilant patients had slower recoveries that required more days of hospitalization and had more minor complications than did the 14 patients who used avoidance or the 37 patients who manifested both vigilance and avoidance. There were no significant differences in the other variables.[35]

Nurses are to be aware that patients who are vigilant focusers are active seekers of information who master situations in active roles. Persons using this coping style must be kept informed of minute details of care and alternative methods available. The vigilant focuser needs to participate fully in providing care, setting goals, and evaluating progress. Vigilant focusers may test staff by asking several persons the same questions to compare responses and verify information given. These patients need the same approaches used by nurses for various personal-care activities. Variation in approaches will heighten already-present anxiety. Being forced into powerlessness situations of pain and disability may be more devastating to the vigilant patient's self-esteem than to the self-esteem of an avoider.

Andrew[37] completed a study similar to that of Cohen and Lazarus[35] in which she tested a preoperative information-giving technique on 40 patients undergoing hernia surgery. The patients were categorized as sensitizers, avoiders, or neutrals in their coping styles based on a sentence-completion test.[31] Twenty-two patients were given a preoperative instruction audio tape that described origins of hernias, dangers of delaying surgery, the surgery process, and preparation for and consequences of surgery. Eighteen patients were in an unprepared group. The two groups were compared in relation to the number of days hospitalized and number of medications needed. The patients classified as neutrals in the prepared group needed fewer medications and stayed fewer days than those classified as neutrals in the unprepared group. The patients classified as avoiders in the prepared and unprepared groups stayed equal days, and the prepared avoiders used more medications. The prepared and unprepared sensitizers stayed equal days and used equal medications.[37]

Andrew had expected that the sensitizers, who welcome information to reduce stress, would improve because of the instruction tape. Sensitizers in both prepared and unprepared groups may have obtained information about impending surgery on their own; therefore, no significant difference could be noted because of the instruction tape between the prepared and unprepared groups. The unprepared sensitizers had the fewest hospital days (5.50), followed by the prepared neutrals (5.54 days). The prepared sensitizers stayed 6.20 days.

It is particularly relevant for nurses to note that instruction programs need to be tailored to the individual's coping style. To belabor an individual who is an avoider with the meticulous details of an anticipated stress may cause more harm than good. On the other hand, the vigilant focuser needs to feel in control, and the sense of control is rooted in knowledge and competent participation in care. To bombard the avoider with information may diminish ability to cope. To avoid any detail of what will happen to a vigilant focuser would heighten anxiety and diminish coping ability.

Shanan, DeNour, and Garty[38] studied 59 terminally ill renal failure patients who were on hemodialysis and a matched sample of 59 subjects to determine if prolonged stress reduced active coping and to determine the effect of the patient's background on coping. The results of the Shanan Sentence Completion Test indicated that patients on dialysis obtained lower coping scores and had passivity, negative self-perception, and a tendency to withdraw by using denial. The only background variables related to illness and coping were the individual's sex and education. Women were more negative than men. Education helped prepare the patient to cope with specific problems.

Dimond[39] studied the effect of two coping strategies used by 36 patients on hemodialysis to adapt to chronic hemodialysis. The two coping strategies were patient-perceived progress in managing dialysis (cognitive control) and patient use of short-term planning (behavioral control). Adaptation was determined by subjects' morale scores (Behavior-Morale Scale), changes in social function (Sickness Impact Profile), number of medical problems, and stability of physical status. Those subjects who used the two coping strategies had significant higher scores at the 0.05 level on the four measures of adaptation. Dimond[39] emphasized that short-term planning was one way that patients on dialysis could control their daily lives. She suggests that in addition to teaching patients with renal failure about the disease and its treatment, teaching specific skills in short-term planning is important to enhance the patient's perception of personal competence and control.

Does the coping capacity of chronically ill individuals decrease as the illness continues over long periods? Although there is no conclusive answer to this based on research, it seems logical that nurses should generate specific strategies patients can try out as the illness progresses. Determining the combinations of strategies that are appropriate to the patient's coping style and control orientation is the challenge. Much nursing research on the topic of coping is needed.

Langer, Janis, and Wolfer[40] studied the effectiveness of a coping strategy on reducing stress in surgical patients. The coping device was based on use of distraction and perception control. Patients were taught to direct attention toward favorable aspects of the anticipated stressful situation. The patient was made to feel in control by using the strategy of cognitive reappraisal of the anxiety-provoking events and calming self-talk. Patients were taught that it is rarely the events themselves that cause stress, but rather the views people take of events and attention given to these views. Patients were taught to rehearse the positive aspects of hospitalization (improving health, receiving care and attention, having a rare opportunity to relax, and enjoying temporary relief from the pressures of the world).

Sixty patients were divided into four groups of preparation. Group 1 received the coping device described. Group 2 received preparatory information only, that is, preoperative skin preparation instructions and information about medications, anesthesia, and how the patient would feel after surgery, with incisional pain, nausea, and constipation described as possible discomforts. Group 3 received a combination of preparatory information and the coping device. Group 4 served as a control and received only information about hospital routines. Nurses blindly rated the subjects' anxiety and ability to cope with discomfort before and after the researcher intervention. There was a rapid decrease in anxiety and increase in ability to cope in the group given the coping strategy. Postoperatively, the group given the coping device required fewer pain medications and fewer sedatives than the groups not given the device. There was no significant difference among the groups in the number of days of hospital stay.[40]

The strategy described by Langer is appropriate for nurses to use to help patients cope not only with stresses that are short term in nature, such as facing surgery, but also with stresses lasting a lifetime, as in the case of chronic disease.

Specific tasks confronting chronically ill persons can be labeled coping tasks. Individuals have unique means of responding to the tasks (using coping strategies) in order to master, control, or resolve the tasks. Collectively, the coping tasks of chronic illness precipitate powerlessness. Coping facilitates powerfulness.

# REFERENCES

1. Lipowski, Z. J.: *Physical illness, the individual and the coping process.* Psychiatry in Medicine 1:91, 1970.
2. Lazarus, R.: *Psychological Stress and the Coping Process.* McGraw-Hill, New York, 1966, pp. 151-152.
3. *Ibid.*, p. 153.
4. Mechanic, D.: *Medical Sociology.* Free Press, New York, 1968.
5. Coelho, G., Hamburg, D., and Adams, J.: *Coping and Adaptation.* Basic Books, New York, 1974, pp. 127-138.
6. Murphy, L. B. and Moriarity, A.: *Vulnerability, Coping and Growth: From Infancy to Adolescence.* Yale University Press, New Haven, Conn., 1976.
7. Bruner, J.: *Toward a Therapy of Instruction.* Harvard University Press, Cambridge, Mass., 1966.
8. Weisman, A.: *Coping with Cancer.* McGraw-Hill, New York, 1979.
9. Haan, N.: *Coping and Defending: Processes of Self-Environment Organization.* Academic Press, New York, 1977.
10. Weisman: *op. cit.*, p. 27.
11. Weisman, A. and Worden, W.: *The existential plight in cancer: Significance of the first 100 days.* Int. J. Psychiatry Med. 7:1, 1976-77.
12. Visotsky, H., et al.: *Coping behavior under extreme stress.* Arch. Gen. Psychiatry 5:27, 1961.
13. Caplan, G.: *Emotional crises.* In Deutsch, A. (ed.): *The Encyclopedia of Mental Health, Vol. 2.* Franklin Watts, New York, 1963.
14. Charmaz, K.: *Time and Identity: The Shaping of Selves of the Chronically Ill.* Doctoral dissertation, University of California, San Francisco, 1973.
15. Lipowski, Z. J.: *Psychosocial aspects of disease.* Ann. Intern. Med. 71:1197, 1969.
16. Kiely, W. F.: *Coping with severe illness.* Adv. Psychosom. Med. 8:105, 1972.
17. Stapleton, S.: *Coping with chronic illness.* Unpublished paper, Marquette University College of Nursing, Milwaukee, 1978.
18. Wiener, C.: *The burden of rheumatoid arthritis: Tolerating uncertainty.* Soc. Sci. Med. 9:97, 1975.
19. Davis, M.: *Social isolation as a process in chronic illness.* In Davis, M., Kramer, M., and Strauss, A. (eds.): *Nurses in Practice: A Perspective on Work Environments.* C. V. Mosby, St. Louis, 1975, pp. 253-259.
20. Meleis, A. I.: *Role insufficiency and role supplementation: A conceptual framework.* Nurs. Res. 24:264, July-August 1975.
21. Kassebaum, G. and Baumann, B.: *Dimensions of the sick role in chronic illness.* J. Health Hum. Behav. 6:16, 1965.
22. Parsons, T.: *The Social System.* Free Press, New York, 1951.
23. Feldman, D.: *Chronic disabling illness: A holistic view.* J. Chronic Dis. 27:290, 1974.
24. Haynes, R. B.: *A critical review of the determinants of patient compliance with therapeutic regimens.* In Sackett, D. and Haynes, R. B. (eds.): *Compliance with Therapeutic Regimens.* Johns Hopkins University Press, Baltimore, 1976, p. 31.
25. Wright, B.: *Physical Disability: A Psychological Approach.* Harper & Row, New York, 1970.
26. Averill, J.: *Personal control over aversion stimuli and its relationship to stress.* Psychol. Bull. 88:2ᶜ 1973.

27. Korner, I.: *Hope as a method of coping.* J. Consult. Clin. Psychol. 34:134, 1970.
28. Pattison, E. M.: *Psychosocial predictors of death prognosis.* Omega 5:145, 1974.
29. *Ibid.*, p. 157.
30. Hinton, J.: *Bearing cancer.* Br. J. Med. Psychol. 46:105, 1973.
31. Goldstein, M. F., et al.: *Coping style as a factor in psychophysiological response to a tension-arousing film.* J. Pers. Soc. Psychol. 1:290, 1965.
32. Lomont, J.: *The repression-sensitization dimension in relation to anxiety responses.* J. Consult. Psychol. 29:84, 1965.
33. Andrew, J.: *Coping style and declining verbal abilities.* J. Gerontol. 28:179, 1973.
34. Sidle, A., et al.: *Development of a coping scale.* Arch. Gen. Psychiatry 20:226, February 1969.
35. Cohen, F. and Lazarus, R.: *Active coping processes, coping dispositions, and recovery from surgery.* Psychosom. Med. 35:375, 1973.
36. Andrew, J.: *Coping Styles, Stress Relevant Learning and Recovery from Surgery.* Doctoral dissertation, University of California, Los Angeles, 1967.
37. Andrew, J.: *Recovery from surgery with and without preparatory instruction for three coping styles.* J. Pers. Soc. Psychol. 5:223, 1970.
38. Shanan, J., DeNour, A. K., and Garty, S.: *Effects of prolonged stress on coping style in terminal renal failure patients.* J. Human Stress 2:19, December 1976.
39. Dimond, J.: *Patient strategies for managing maintenance hemodialysis.* Western Journal of Nursing Research 2:555, Summer 1980.
40. Langer, E., Janis, I., and Wolfer, J.: *Reduction of psychological stress in surgical patients.* Journal of Experimental Social Psychology 11:155, 1975.

# 3

# CONCEPT DEVELOPMENT OF POWERLESSNESS: A NURSING DIAGNOSIS

## JUDITH FITZGERALD MILLER

Development of the concept of powerlessness is the focus of this chapter. The process of concept development involves distinct phases such as developing a commitment to study the concept as a result of experienced challenges and/or piqued curiosity, defining the concept in a working-definition format, reviewing the literature to substantiate current concept development, making observations in the field, drawing conclusions from own and others' descriptive research, and designing predictive and prescriptive studies. The phases of concept development* emphasized in this chapter include reviewing the literature (deriving theoretical propositions and proposing nursing practice speculations) and reporting field observations.

Developing and validating new nursing diagnostic categories require systematic investigation. A descriptive research approach in developing this concept is used throughout this book. Dubin[1] distinguishes between descriptive and hypothesis-testing research. He states that descriptive research is the questioning, or theory-building, side of research. For purposes of this book, concept development of powerlessness takes place on this side of the model. Hypothesis testing is the answer-seeking, theory-testing side. See Figure 3-1.

Before hypotheses can be formulated and tested, systematic observations of phenomena must take place. Observations of patients in states of powerlessness have been made and are reported in this book. Interest and curiosity have been piqued by these

---

*For another approach to concept development, see Wilson, J.: *Thinking With Concepts,* Cambridge University Press, London, 1970.

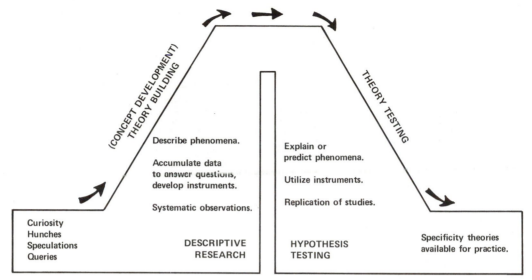

**FIGURE 3-1. Theory building and testing.**

observations of individuals whose physical conditions plunged downward despite strict adherence to prescribed regimens.

Nurses are challenged to help patients achieve a sense of control and avoid or alleviate powerlessness. Nurses need to be able to recognize the nursing diagnosis, determine which patients are vulnerable to diagnoses related to powerlessness, design nursing strategies to alleviate the diagnosis, and evaluate outcomes.

## POWERLESSNESS DEFINED

Powerlessness is the perception of the individual that one's own actions will not significantly affect an outcome. Powerlessness is a perceived lack of control over a current situation or immediate happening. When one or more of the power resources of physical strength, psychologic stamina, self-concept, energy, knowledge, motivation, and belief system are compromised, powerlessness is a potential problem. See Figure 1-1, Chapter 1.

In contrast to locus of control, powerlessness is situationally determined. Locus of control is directly related to powerlessness and is a rather stable personality trait. Locus of control seems to be a long-term tendency or a stable view of why events take place. If events are perceived to be contingent on an individual's own behavior, the individual tends to have an internal locus of control. If events are perceived to be contingent on chance, fate, luck, powerful others, or a complex of forces, the individual tends to have an external locus of control.[2]

The locus of control construct was developed from social learning theory. Rotter[3] was trying to combine stimulus-response theories with cognitive or field theories. Four classes of variables to keep in mind in social learning theory are behaviors, expectancies, reinforcements, and psychologic situations. Rotter states, ''The potential for a behavior to occur in any specific psychological situation is a function of the expectancy that the behavior will lead to a particular reinforcement in that situation.''[4] The value of the reinforcement to the individual must also be noted.

By 1975, Rotter[3] estimated that more than 600 studies on locus of control had been done. These did not include doctoral dissertations, master's studies, or unpublished reports. In nursing's concept development, this fund of research cannot be ignored.

The studies on locus of control and powerlessness were analyzed in the following categories: powerlessness and learning; individual's beliefs or illusions and control; effects of no control on animals; effects of no control on human beings' physiologic response and problem solving; control in select health-illness situations; and powerlessness as a precipitant of death.

For each section of literature reviewed, theoretical propositions[5] will be deduced. Theoretical propositions are translations and conclusions drawn from research findings. Some interpretation for nursing practice will be included in each section. These interpretations are labeled practice speculations. They are derived from theoretical propositions, and although they have logical practice relevance, they need to be tested.

# LITERATURE REVIEW

## Powerlessness and Learning

Seeman[6] concluded that powerlessness leads to poor learning of control-relevant information. Patients hospitalized with tuberculosis who were high in powerlessness knew fewer facts about the disease and maintaining health than did a matched sample low in powerlessness. The low powerless patients were less satisfied with information given by staff and were rated by the staff as being more knowledgeable about their illness. In Seeman's study of prisoners,[7] there was no difference between high powerless and low powerless prisoners' knowledge of life in the correctional institution; however, prisoners who were low in powerlessness had more knowledge about parole matters, that is, how to get out on parole, conditions while on parole, and so forth. The premise for Seeman's studies is that ''an individual's generalized expectancy for control of his outcomes governs attention to and acquisition of information available in the environment.''[8] Seeman also correlated high powerlessness with low political awareness[9] and low nuclear survival knowledge.[10]

Phares[11] studied acquisition and utilization of information in subjects with internal or external locus of control. Both groups were taught information until they had perfect recall. Then the subjects had to use the information in a computer simulation task. He found that the internals and externals did not differ in the acquisition of material; internals provided significantly more reasons for decisions made during the simulation task than did the externals; differential retention of the information did not explain the internals' superior utilization of the information.

Nineteen externals and 21 internals were given personality tests and informed of reports containing negative and positive information about their personalities. The externals had greater recall of the negative information given to them about themselves than did internals. The internals were more willing to try remedial behaviors to improve than were the externals.[12]

Giving learners a choice, such as determining the series in which to take a test,[13] resulted in lower anxiety as indicated by palmar sweating than did not giving individuals a choice. Perlmuter and Monty[14] demonstrated that the group given the choice of lists for word memorization did better than the group given no choice. The theoretical propositions (translation and conclusion statements) and practice speculations are presented in Figure 3-2.

## DISCUSSION OF PRACTICE SPECULATIONS

The phrase "start patient teaching where the patient is" has new meaning when we look beyond motivation, psychologic readiness, and ability to grasp concepts to determine the patient's feelings of powerlessness. Patients with low powerlessness may need multiple avenues of content presentation. They should be encouraged to compare methods of self-care and be given freedom to question and pursue alternate modes of meeting needs for care. Those patients who tend to have an internal locus of control may need added emphasis on information that would give them a sense of control. This may even involve explicit verbalization by the nurse, such as, "Knowing this will give you added ability to be in control of the situation." High powerless patients, however, may need structured approaches. This could mean teaching self-care in small increments so that patients feel a sense of accomplishment when they are successful with these scaled-down, yet realistic, goals.

A feeling of being controlled by fate, destiny, or others is not conducive to learning new skills such as self-care.[15] Patients with this orientation may believe that learning a self-care skill—such as learning a low-salt and calorie-restricted diet, as well as monitoring the effects of the rest of the antihypertensive regimen—will do no good because what was meant to happen will happen despite patient involvement. Despite their locus-of-control tendency, perhaps all patients must perceive some sense of situational control before they can learn health-control information.

# Illusions of Control

In situations where personal competence can affect outcomes, individuals tend to perform more actively and competently than in situations that appear beyond their control. What effect does the individual's *belief* in having control have on arousal, anxiety, and so forth? The reviewed studies on perceived control all report that subjects who believed they had control of an aversive stimulus such as an electric shock or noise manifest less anxiety and tolerate noxious stimuli better than subjects who believed they had no control.

Geer, Davison, and Gatchel[16] studied autonomic responses of 20 men who perceived they had control over electric shock and 20 men who perceived no control. The subjects in the perceived-control group were led to believe that they could decrease the duration of the shock from 6 to 3 seconds if they pushed a reaction switch with each electric shock. The no-perceived-control group was not given this information. Both groups were told the researcher was interested in reaction time between receiving the shock and pushing a switch. Even though the perceived-control group did not affect the duration of the shock, their perception of being in control influenced the results. The

| Theoretical Propositions | Practice Speculations |
|---|---|
| 1. Perceived powerlessness leads to poor learning of control relevant information. | Before beginning patient teaching, determine the patient's feelings of powerlessness. |
| 2. Involving learners in decision making regarding content to be learned enhances learning. | Patients with an internal locus of control need emphasis on information that gives them a sense of control. |
| 3. The personality trait locus of control influences ability to utilize control-relevant information. | High-powerless patients may need structured approaches, teaching of self-care in small increments so patients can feel a sense of control without being overwhelmed with care demands. |
| | Involve patients by having them determine what aspects of care they are ready to learn and when they want to learn them. |

FIGURE 3-2. Powerlessness and learning.

perceived-control subjects rated the shocks as less painful than did the no-perceived-control subjects; the perceived-control subjects had less galvanic skin response, suggesting they were less aroused by the shocks than were the no-perceived-control subjects. This study was replicated by Glass and coworkers[17] on 48 college students. The perceived-control group rated their pain as less and performed better on the Stroop Color Word Test than did the no-perceived-control group. Contrary to the findings of Geer, Davison, and Gatchel,[16] there was no significant difference in autonomic response as measured by the galvanic skin response between the two groups.

Glass and Singer[18] studied the response to belief of control over aversive stimuli. The subjects received 18 electric shocks while trying to solve graphic puzzles. Half of the group was given soluble puzzles, whereas the other half was given unsoluble puzzles. All subjects received the same number of shocks but were told that solving the puzzles would prevent the next scheduled shock. The subjects who perceived control performed better on postshock tasks, making fewer errors on a proofreading test and having shorter reading times than the subjects who perceived no control.

Procedures that give subjects the choice of avoiding or not avoiding aversive stimuli are equivalent to giving them perceived control over the potential stress of threat.[19] Forty subjects were divided into two groups: an escape group, which had the choice instructions, and a no-escape group, which had no choice instructions. The escape group was instructed to press a button to escape white noise if the noise became uncomfortable. The choice was up to them. The no-escape subjects were told not to push the button unless the noise "became so uncomfortable you must." The galvanic skin response was used as an indicator of physiologic arousal. The escape group had less arousal than did the no-escape group. The escape group also rated the discomfort as less than did the no-escape group.[19] A sense of control influences how threats are appraised. This study suggests that choice is a variable that can reduce the aversive quality of the stimulus.

Houston[20] studied the effects of an illusion of control on anxiety and physiologic arousal as measured by the Zuckerman Affect Adjective Check List and heart rate, respectively. He also used no-control situations to compare the physiologic arousal of individuals with internal locus of control with the arousal in individuals with external locus of control. The 20 subjects in the avoidable-shock group were led to believe that they could avoid an electric shock by not making mistakes on a memory task. The 20 subjects in the unavoidable-shock group were told there was no way to avoid the shock. Despite the fact that both groups received the same number and intensity of shocks, subjects in the latter group reported more anxiety but demonstrated less physiologic arousal. Contrary to Houston's expectations, the group with external locus of control manifested less physiologic arousal than did the group with internal locus of control. This could be attributed to the effects of placing individuals with an internal-locus personality trait in no-control situations. More anxiety, as measured by physiologic arousal, may be caused in subjects with an internal locus of control because they are *not* resigned to events being contingent on external forces. See Figure 3-3.

## DISCUSSION OF PRACTICE SPECULATIONS

The illusion of patient control has benefits for patients in terms of creating less anxiety and physiologic arousal and greater ability to learn than does the perception of no control. Helping patients know when specific events will take place provides an illusion of control. The events may be diagnostic tests or treatments such as a dressing change. Patients can achieve some sense of control by knowing about alternatives for self-care and feeling free to make decisions about the alternatives. Nurses need to help patients become aware of alternatives and enable them to make decisions. An example is having the new patient with diabetes realize that a 1200-calorie diet restriction involves freedom and variety in meal planning. Good selections will now enhance the patient's nutritional state because food of no nutritional value is not included in the selection of six food exchange lists.

Helping the patients and families be as informed as health-care personnel about their health states seems so fundamental. Yet this obvious principle and patient right is oftentimes overlooked.

# Effects of No Control on Animals

"The mere knowledge that one can exert control, then serves to mitigate the debilitating effects of aversive stimuli."[21] The reported aversive quality of a stimulus decreases when subjects exercise control over that stimulus.

| Theoretical Propositions | Practice Speculations |
|---|---|
| 1. An illusion of control causes less physiologic arousal during stress events than perceived no control. | Providing patient with alternatives so as to make choices provides an illusion of control. |
| 2. An illusion of control causes threats to be evaluated as less harmful than perception of no control. | Containing anxiety and aversive physiologic arousal is desirable in all phases of health-illness. Helping patients feel a sense of control achieves this end. |
| 3. When individuals are provided with freedom to make choices, an illusion of control is created. | Help the patient feel control over aspects of the immediate environment, personal effects, plants, and so forth. |

FIGURE 3-3. Illusions of control.

The original study of control by Mowrer and Viek[22] demonstrated that rats exhibited less fear of an aversive stimulus (electric shock) if they could exercise control (leap into the air when shocked to terminate the shock). A significant difference in eating inhibition was noted in the group that had no control over the shock. (The animals were presented with food; if they did not eat within 10 seconds, the behaviors were labeled an inhibition). Mowrer and Viek observed the 20 animals for 15 consecutive days. They described the no-control animals as being helpless, having lost their will, and not actively providing for their self-interest, for example, satisfying hunger.

The effects of subjecting animals to no-control situations have also been documented in a series of studies by Seligman, Maier, and Solomon[23]; Overmier and Seligman[24]; Overmier[25]; and Seligman and Maier.[26] In these studies, dogs were restrained in a cloth hammock and given electric shocks by electrodes attached to their feet. The intensity and duration of the shocks varied in the experiments. Another series of shocks was given to the same dogs while they were in an escapable shuttle box. The animals were shocked by a wire grid on the bottom of the box. If the animal crossed the shoulder-high barrier in the center of the box, the shocks would be stopped. Overmier and Seligman[24] compared responses of dogs that received inescapable shocks and those that received no aversive pretreatment but were placed in the escapable shuttle box. Those animals that had been restrained and shocked when placed in the escape box displayed helpless behavior; at first, they ran around frantically for approximately 30 seconds, then they lay down and quietly whined. After a few seconds, the dogs seemed to give up and passively accept the shock.

The helplessness induced by the inescapable shock was eliminated if the animal had some experience controlling the shock.[26,27] Seligman[28] tried to overcome the helplessness in dogs previously shocked in no-escape conditions by calling the animal over a lowered barrier in the box to the no-shock side. One in four dogs crossed the barrier. The other three were then leashed and forced to the escape side. The animals were pulled across the barrier 20 times. It then took 20, 35, and 50 trials for the dogs to escape the shock on their own. The animals' behavior was explained as resulting from learned helplessness. Their having learned a lack of control over reinforcement was difficult to reverse.

Not all animal studies reported that the control subjects have the advantage. Brady and coworkers[29] reported that the four monkeys who pressed levers to escape electric shocks developed ulcers. The paired monkeys who had no control did not develop gastrointestinal lesions. The control monkeys were labeled by Brady and coworkers as "executive" monkeys. The findings were refuted by Weiss' study[30] of 180 rats, in which ulcers were more common and more extensive among the animals with no control.

Seligman and Meyer[31] studied the effects of unpredictable shock on rats' bar-pressing behavior for food. A variable number of unpredictable shocks were given to 20 rats. Suppression of bar pressing occurred. After being given a fixed number of otherwise unpredictable shocks in each session, rats resumed bar pressing after the last shock, using its occurrence as a safety signal. Bar pressing resumed more quickly in rats that received milder predictable shocks than in rats that received the mild unpredictable shocks. Fear, measured by the suppression of bar pressing, correlated with the amount of gastric ulceration found in the unpredictable-shock animals. See Figure 3-4.

The implications of this research and these propositions will be discussed at the end of the next section.

## Effect of No Control on Humans

When subjects administered shocks to themselves and selected the level of intensity of shock, they reported less discomfort at higher levels of shock and endured stronger shock intensity than did matched subjects who were administered shocks by the investigator.[32] The predictability of self-administered shocks diminished the threat of aversive stimuli.[33-35] On a second series of shocks, both control and no-control groups now had shocks administered to them; the group that previously had control declined in tolerance for shocks and rated shocks as more painful than when they had control. The ability to predict events may reduce the subjective experience of helplessness, even when control is not possible, and may thereby reduce tension or anxiety. When ability to terminate aversive stimuli is lacking, predictability may reduce the impact of the stimuli; and when the ability to predict is lacking, perceived ability to terminate aversive stimuli may have a similar effect.[32]

To determine the effect of control over environmental stressors on frustration tolerance and task performance, two groups of subjects were exposed to random noise played on a tape recorder at 110 decibels.[36] One group had control over the noise through use of a button; the other group had no control. The response to the noise stressor was measured by use of the galvanic skin response readings, number of errors made on cognitive tasks, tolerance for frustration by the number of trials made at insoluble puzzles, and a postexperimental questionnaire requesting ratings from the subjects on how distracting, irritating, and unpleasant they felt the noise to be. The group that had control demonstrated much greater tolerance for frustration based on a larger number of trials at solving insoluble puzzles. The percentage of proofreading errors was less for the group with control. The group with control also rated the noise as less aversive than did the group with no control.

| Theoretical Propositions | Practice Speculations |
|---|---|
| 1. Repeated exposure to threat and/or harm induces a state of helplessness in animals. | See "Effect of No Control on Humans," Figure 3-5. |
| 2. Reversal of learned helplessness is difficult but can take place with forceful success experiences provided by someone controlling the situation. | |
| 3. Predictability of aversive stimuli decreases the threat of the stimuli. | |

FIGURE 3-4. Effects of no control on animals.

Kanfer and Seidner[37] studied the effectiveness of self-controlling response in 45 women undergraduate students. The subjects were divided into three groups, all of whom had one hand immersed in ice water. Subjects in group 1 viewed travel slides that they advanced at their own desired rate. Group 2 had the slides advanced by the experimenter. No slides were used for group 3. Duration of ice-water tolerance was greater for subjects who advanced the slides at their own rate (significant at the 0.01 level). The researchers did not attribute the tolerance for ice water to self-distraction techniques that may have been used by the group controlling the slides. The conclusion was that the self-controlling responses increased tolerance for the aversive stimuli.

Thornton and Jacobs[38] were able to replicate learned helplessness in humans as had been done in previous animal studies. After pretreatment in which the subjects had no control, humans transferred helplessness to a second task in which they had control, just as the animals had done. Eighty subjects were divided into four groups. One group could avoid the electric shock by pushing a button in a 30-second reaction time; the second and third groups could not avoid the shock. The second group received a fixed shock; the third, a variable shock. The fourth group was given no shock pretreatment. The variable-shock group that had less predictability experienced more stress. Groups 1, 2, and 3 transferred their helplessness to a task in which they had control. In this second phase, pushing a button could eliminate the shock. Fewest attempts to control the shock were made by the variable-shock pretreatment group.

The learned helplessness is due to learning that reinforcement and responding are independent of one another. Miller and Seligman,[39,40] in comparing depression and laboratory-induced learned helplessness, determined that learning that reinforcement and responding are independent is central to the symptoms and etiology of both learned helplessness and depression. Seligman[41] draws a parallel between the behaviors of depression and those of learned helplessness, stating that in both there is:

1. A lowered initiation of voluntary responses—animals and men who have experienced uncontrollability show reduced initiation of voluntary responses.
2. A negative cognitive set—helpless animals and men have difficulty learning that responses produce outcomes.
3. A time course—helplessness dissipates in time when induced by a single session of uncontrollable shock; after multiple sessions, helplessness persists.
4. Lowered aggression—helpless animals and men initiate fewer aggressive and competitive responses, and their dominance status may diminish.
5. Loss of appetite—helpless animals eat less, lose weight, and are sexually and socially deficient.
6. Physiologic changes—helpless rats show norepinephrine depletion, and helpless cats may be cholinergically overactive.

Hiroto and Seligman,[42] and Gatchel, McKinney, and Koebernick[43] found that depressed subjects and nondepressed subjects exposed to inescapable noise exhibit similar deficits in attempting to solve anagram puzzles.

Johnson and Kilmann[44] studied the relationship between locus of control and perceived problem-solving ability in 20 internal men, 20 internal women, 20 external men, and 20 external women. Men who were internal rated themselves as more confident in problem-solving ability than did men who were external. No significant difference was found between internal and external women.

Anderson[45] studied 90 owner-managers of small businesses that were damaged by a hurricane to determine the relationship among locus of control, perceived stress, coping behaviors, and performance. Externals perceived higher stress than did internals. The externals responded with more defensiveness and less task-oriented coping behavior than did internals. The task-oriented coping behaviors of the internals were more successful in solving the problems created by the stressful event, since the performance of the internals' organizations were better. (Coping was determined by evaluating the economic position of the company. If the company returned to preflood status, coping was considered effective.) Kahn and coworkers'[46] categorization of coping behaviors was employed to categorize coping. Class I coping responses are aimed at dealing with the objective task situation. In Class I, coping behavior included problem-solving efforts such as obtaining resources to counter the initial loss. Class II coping behaviors deal with emotional or anxiety reactions to the stimulus. Examples include withdrawal, group affiliation, hostility, and aggression. See Figure 3-5.

## DISCUSSION OF PRACTICE SPECULATIONS

Helplessness is a syndrome of behaviors that mimic depression.[47] A challenge to the nurse is to be aware of how helplessness can be induced in patients in order to take measures to prevent it. This involves the nurse being sensitive to the patient's response to a strange language system, strange environment, uncertainty of health-illness and treatment situations, and unpredictability of therapy outcomes. Planning for patient control by enabling patient decision making and participation is crucial. Determining patients' preferred coping strategies and not suggesting strategies that could be in conflict with their related locus-of-control tendency must also be kept in mind.

| Theoretical Propositions | Practice Speculations |
|---|---|
| 1. Repeated no-control experiences precipitate a state of helplessness. | Be sensitive to how helplessness is induced in patients: strange language system, strange environment, uncertainty of health-illness and treatment situations, unpredictabilty of therapy outcomes. |
| 2. Observed behaviors of helpless animals parallel behaviors of depressed human beings. | |
| 3. Coping behaviors may vary depending on the personality trait locus of control. | Eliminate unpredictability of events by informing patients of scheduled tests and procedures. |
| 4. When aversive stimuli are predictable the stimuli are interpreted by the subject as less threatening than when the stimuli are unpredictable. | Helping patients be aware of the sensory events that may accompany a threatening procedure will decrease the perception of threat. Recognize that individuals' coping styles will vary. |
| | Recognize that no control or helplessness in one aspect of the patient's life may be transferred to all aspects, creating generalized helplessness. Help the patient be aware of those aspects that are patient controlled. Prevent generalized helplessness, which is difficult to reverse. |

FIGURE 3-5. Effects of no control on humans.

Eliminating unpredictability of events is possible for most patients. This may involve keeping patients informed of scheduled tests, anticipated sensations during an examination or test, and the expected outcomes. It may involve, for example, helping the patient and family plan for discharge from a health setting to home. The certainty of knowing the date of discharge gives the patient a sense of control. Knowledge about anticipated events allows the patient to direct activities within the family to prepare for the events.

## Control in Health-Illness Situations

MacDonald and Hall[48] studied the relationship of locus of control and perception of disability. The Rotter Locus of Control Scale and a Disability Scale were completed by 479 subjects. Externally controlled subjects rated physical disabilities as more debilitating than did the internally controlled subjects. Internals rated emotional disorders as being more debilitating than physical disabilities. The emotional disabilities included having irrational fears, being extremely depressed, and being withdrawn. Physical disabilities included internal disorders such as heart problems and diabetes, sensory disorders such as speech loss and deafness, and cosmetic disorders such as obesity and amputations.

Several studies have been done on the relationship of locus of control to anxiety.[49-51] Findings of all these studies are the same; that is, external subjects have higher anxiety than internal subjects. In these studies, anxiety was measured by the Taylor Manifest Anxiety Scale and the Zuckerman Affect Adjective Check List. The Lowery, Jacobsen, and Keane study[51] measured state anxiety in preoperative patients. Both trait and state anxiety are higher in external subjects when self-report is used. Donovan and coworkers[50] also used an unobtrusive measure of anxiety, the Activity Preference Questionnaire. The results of this anxiety measure revealed no difference in anxiety between internals and externals. These authors raise the issue that the Taylor Manifest Anxiety Scale may measure a dimension of neuroticism and/or negative self-concept rather than anxiety. Yet another consideration is that the subjects with internal locus of control may be unwilling to disclose anxiety on tools that overtly measure it.

Kirscht[52] studied perceptions of control and health beliefs in 166 subjects. Those higher on control regard themselves less vulnerable to ill health.

Andrew[53] studied 65 veterans who delayed hernia surgery to determine the relationships among delay of surgery, coping style, control type, and race. Contrary to her expectation, the control type did not relate to delay. When only whites were analyzed, the relationship between externals and delay of surgery did exist. The blacks were significantly more external than the whites. The hypothesis that externals would more often be avoiders was supported only for whites. Those subjects who were neutrals in the coping style, as measured by the Mainord Coper-Avoider sentence completion, delayed surgery longer than did sensitizers and avoiders. Whites delayed surgery longer than blacks.

Internals showed a different response to forearm blood flow during tasks requiring sensory intake and sensory rejection.[54] Internals had less of an increase in forearm blood flow than did externals in the 29 subjects studied. An individual's cardiovascular response may be influenced by a variety of personality factors.

A scale measuring health locus of control was designed by Wallston and coworkers[55] and by Wallston, Wallston, and DeVellis.[56] These instruments are area-specific for health and have been used to study health behavior and predict the most helpful approaches for patients desiring weight reduction. Wallston and coworkers[55] studied 88 subjects and found that internals who valued health sought more information on hypertension as a health risk, by choosing a significantly larger number of pamphlets made available, than did the high- and low-health-value external subjects and the low-health-value internal subjects. The Rokeach[57] value survey served as a model for developing the health-value scale.

In the study of subjects participating in a weight-reduction program, 34 women completed the Health Locus of Control Scale and were randomly assigned to two different types of weight-reduction treatments. The basic difference in the type of treatment program was that one was self-directed and the other was group-oriented. The 8-week program was completed by 22 women. The externals in the group program lost more weight than did the externals in the self-directed program. The internals in the self-directed program lost more weight than did the internals in the group program.[55] The results of this study provide some support for the need to tailor diet and behavior modification programs to match the individual's locus-of-control tendency.

In comparing locus of control to pain tolerance, Craig and Best[58] found that internals had greater pain tolerance to increasing intensities of researcher-administered electric shocks than did the externals. See Figure 3-6.

## DISCUSSION OF PRACTICE SPECULATIONS

Consideration of the unique patient situation and personal meaning of control is necessary for accurate nursing prescriptions. Nurses must recognize that fear of not being in control during pain experiences or of being unable to terminate the pain is a major threat. These fears can be ameliorated somewhat by the nurses sharing information, demonstrating pain relief strategies, and teaching the patients relaxation, use of auto-suggestion, and many self-control techniques.

One of several variables that influence self-disclosure of anxiety is the locus of control tendency. Interpretation of mood states must be validated with the patient and not conclusively interpreted and recorded on care plans. Individuals with internal locus of control do not readily self-report anxiety, yet these patients may have more anxiety than patients with external locus of control.

The Health Locus of Control Scale[55] should be considered for nursing research involving locus of control tendencies in patients. This tool is area specific for health and does not have the global political items that are contained in the Rotter Internal-External Locus of Control Scale.[2] Behavioral indicators of locus of control need to be studied in more detail. An initial study is described in Chapter 8.

As programs of nursing care are prescribed, tailoring the program to patient's control tendency is essential.

# Precipitants of Death

Richter[59] concluded that death in rats resulted from a combination of responses to various stresses occurring in rapid succession, which generates a sense of hopelessness in the animals. In wild (non–laboratory-bred) rats, handling, whisker snipping, and confinement to glass jars to swim without knowing the investigator would save them caused the animals to die. The death was not attributed to an adrenal response. When hopelessness was eliminated by removing the rats from the water and then immersing them again, the rats did not die. Removal of the rats caused them to become aggressive in trying to free themselves, showing no signs of giving up. Such rats swam for 40 to 60 hours, instead of dying within minutes. Animals could not have learned what to do to cause recurrence of the good fortune to be removed from the water and replaced in the water; rather, they perceived the situation not to be hopeless, so they kept swimming and did not die.

Accounts of deaths in humans due to hopelessness are reported by Seligman,[47] Engel,[60,61] Kastenbaum and Kastenbaum,[62] and Lefcourt.[63] A dramatic example of a healthy individual succumbing to hopelessness is reported by Lefcourt:[64]

| Theoretical Propositions | Practice Speculations |
|---|---|
| 1. Control is stress reducing. | Ways of ameliorating fear during pain and strategies to enhance control should be used. |
| 2. Individuals with an external locus of control more readily report anxiety than do those with internal locus of control. | Validation of mood states is necessary in that anxiety may not be disclosed by patients with internal locus of control and therefore may not be treated by the nurse. |
| 3. Effectiveness of treatment programs may depend on tailoring the program to an individual's locus-of-control tendency. | Provide support and behavior therapy to patients considering their locus of control. Externals benefit from a group approach, and internals benefit from a one-to-one approach. |

FIGURE 3-6. Control in health-illness situations.

A female patient who had remained in a mute state for nearly 10 years was shifted to a different floor of her building along with her floor mates, while her unit was being redecorated. The third floor of this psychiatric unit where the patient in question had been living was known among the patients as the chronic, hopeless floor. In contrast, the first floor was most commonly occupied by patients who held privileges, including the freedom to come and go on the hospital grounds and to the surrounding streets. In short, the first floor was an exit ward from which patients could anticipate discharge fairly rapidly. All patients who were temporarily moved from the third floor were given medical examinations prior to the move, and the patient in question was judged to be in excellent medical health though still mute and withdrawn. Shortly after moving to the first floor, this chronic psychiatric patient surprised the ward staff by becoming socially responsive such that within a 2-week period she ceased being mute and was actually becoming gregarious. As fate would have it, the redecoration of the third floor unit was soon completed and all previous residents were returned to it. Within a week after she had been returned to the "hopeless" unit, this patient, who like the legendary Snow White had been aroused from a living torpor, collapsed and died. The subsequent autopsy revealed no pathology of note, and it was whimsically suggested at the time that the patient had died of despair.

Ferrari[65] studied freedom of choice in 75 elderly patients admitted to a nursing home. Of the 17 who said they had no alternative except to move into the nursing home, 8 died after 4 weeks in the home and 16 were dead by the end of 10 weeks. Of the 38 who saw alternatives to being admitted to the nursing home but chose to reside there, only 1 subject died in the 10 weeks. All the deaths were termed unexpected by the nursing home staff. It could be argued that the sicker patients had fewer alternatives and more family pressure to move into a nursing home; yet all the deaths were termed unexpected.

Although skepticism may be expressed by researchers who do not recognize a qualitative approach, it is impossible to validate the happenings with the subjects themselves. To permit these findings to fall on deaf ears would cause needless physiologic deterioration and death in situations in which nurses could intervene by instilling a sense of hope. Is it possible to document the passive surrender of some chronically ill individuals? A case is presented in Chapter 6.

Hopelessness is a feeling of giving up. The individual is filled with despair, a sense of "there is nothing left." A feeling that one is completely responsible for the situation contributes to the feeling that nothing can be done to overcome or change the situation. The individual does not feel worthy of help.[66] Hopelessness is loss of autonomy, with a feeling of despair coming from the individual's awareness of an inability to provide gratification to self.[67] If powerlessness is not contained, a cycle of lowered self-esteem and depression occurs, followed by hopelessness. The patient is immobilized in terms of solving problems, setting goals, and taking action. If this state is permitted to continue, isolation, loneliness, and death may ensue.

Engel[68] has identified five characteristics of a hopelessness complex he labels "giving-in–given-up." This complex includes:

—a feeling of giving up, experienced as helplessness or hopelessness.
—a depreciated image of the self.
—a sense of loss of gratification from relationships or roles in life.

| Theoretical Propositions | Practice Speculations |
|---|---|
| 1. Hopelessness is a temporary failure of mental coping mechanisms. | Helping patients achieve a sense of control, averting a hopeless state, may be vital to their recovery. |
| 2. When helplessness builds over time and results from various situations, a generalized feeling of hopelessness results. | Inspiring hope affects survival. |
| 3. When a cycle of powerlessness, depression, immobility, and hopelessness is not broken, a deteriorated physical health state may result. | Helping patients realize there is someone and/or something to live for prolongs life. |

FIGURE 3-7. Precipitants of death.

—a feeling of disruption of the sense of continuity between past, present, and future.
—reactivation of memories of earlier periods of giving up.

Theoretical propositions on powerlessness and death are listed in Figure 3-7.

## DISCUSSION OF PRACTICE SPECULATIONS

Having someone or something to live for inspires continued life.[69] Building patient endurance and inspiring survival by instilling hope are familiar to nurses. Strategies for inspiring hope are discussed in Chapter 16.

Averill[70] specifies three types of control: behavioral, cognitive, and decisional. Behavioral control is the availability of a response that may directly influence or modify the objective characteristics of a threatening event. Providing the patient control over aspects of the environment is an example of behavioral control. Allowing the patient to carry out a procedure such as a colostomy irrigation, in a self-determined, therapeutically effective way, is another example. Cognitive control is the way in which an event is interpreted, evaluated, or used in a cognitive plan. Patients can be helped to interpret events as being controlled by them. Decisional control is the opportunity to choose

**TABLE 3-1. Factors Decreasing Behavioral, Cognitive, and Decisional Control in Hospitalized Chronically Ill Patients**

| Behavioral Control | Cognitive Control | Decisional Control |
|---|---|---|
| Blind patient was left in a wheelchair in the center of the waiting room and was not told where she was or how long she must wait. | Patient was reprimanded for leaving waiting room to go to restroom after waiting 2 hours. "If you aren't here when we call you, you will miss your turn." | Appointment scheduled in ambulatory care department without asking patient if date and time is convenient. |
| Patient was left alone in x-ray room on hard table, in cold room, only partially covered. | Patient was not informed of his daily lab values, although he had requested that this be done. | Patient in x-ray department told to "try to hold it" when he asked location of bathroom. |
| | Health-care personnel more knowledgeable about patient's illness and treatment than he is. | Diagnostic and treatment procedures scheduled without asking patient or explaining why they were being done. |
| | Health-care personnel walked into patient's room without knocking. | Patient has little or no choice about who will share room. |
| | Health-care personnel talk "over" patient about their personal activities. | Little choice over scheduling activities—eating, sleeping, bathing, and treatments. |
| | Health-care personnel are not wearing name tags. | |

**TABLE 3-2. Factors Increasing Behavioral, Cognitive, and Decisional Control in Hospitalized Chronically Ill Patients**

| Behavioral Control | Cognitive Control | Decisional Control |
|---|---|---|
| Nursing-care Plan: "Allow patient to sleep until breakfast trays arrive; do not awaken for TPR." | Patient informed of weight, blood pressure, lab values. | Patient given access to refrigerator to get own soft drinks. |
| Patient moved to another room at her request because roommate smoked. | Patient taught about medications. | Patient given list of all U. S. dialysis centers and given full responsibility for making own vacation arrangements. |
| Patient in x-ray was told, "We can see you through the window. Hold up your hand if you need something." | Nursing-care Plan: Detailed description of how to do patient's dressing change had been worked out with the patient. | Medications left at bedside for patient to take when ready. |
| After patients were taught specific procedures, expectation given for them to take full responsibility for catheter care, urine testing, dressing change, shunt care. | Patients given feedback about lab values, taught how to record results on a flow sheet. | |

among various alternatives. Patients need to be aware of alternatives and consequences of alternatives. This categorization of control types may be helpful in guiding nurses to provide for patient control so as to avert hopelessness. Helping patients perceive a sense of control may be vital to their recovery.

The review of literature reveals that powerlessness has devasting effects on the person's physical and emotional states. This is a diagnosis that not only is amenable to nursing but also is unique to nursing, dependent upon *nursing* as the professional group to take action to alleviate powerlessness. The speculations derived from a research base provide ideas for testing in practice. Whether the interventions proposed alter the powerlessness state needs to be studied.

# FIELD OBSERVATIONS AS ANOTHER PHASE OF CONCEPT DEVELOPMENT

Making observations in the field verifies or refutes the need for developing the concept of powerlessness. Questions about whether the concept has real-world relevance are answered by initial field observations. These observations were made to identify factors in the health-care environment and actions of health-care providers that could increase or decrease control. Averill's[70] categories defined in this chapter were used to categorize observations of chronically ill patients in one urban hospital. Observations were made for a period of 6 weeks, 2 to 3 hours a week. Examples of factors decreasing and increasing control according to Averill's[70] categories are presented in Tables 3-1 and 3-2.

**TABLE 3-3. Defining Characteristics of Powerlessness**

| Severe | Moderate | Low |
|---|---|---|
| Verbal expressions of having no control or influence over situations. | Nonparticipation in care or decision making when opportunities are provided. | Expressions of uncertainty about fluctuating energy levels. |
| Verbal expressions of having no control or influence over outcomes. | Expressions of dissatisfaction and frustration over inability to perform previous tasks and/or activities. | |
| Verbal expressions of having no control or influence over self-care. | Expressions of uncertainty about treatment outcomes. | |
| Depression over physical deterioration that occurs despite patient compliance with regimens. | Dependence on others that may result in irritability, resentment, anger, and guilt. | |
| Passivity. | Inability to seek information regarding self-care. | |
| | Inability to monitor progress. | |
| | Does not defend self-care practices when challenged. | |
| | Hesitant to plan for future, set goals. | |
| | Expressions of doubt regarding role performance. | |
| | Reluctance to express true feelings, fearing alienation of self from care givers. | |
| | Apathy. | |

These field observations help us conclude that further development and validation of the nursing diagnostic label powerlessness is warranted.

# Indicators of Powerlessness

The indicators or defining characteristics of powerlessness are those signs and symptoms that lead nurses to conclude that powerlessness exists. Indicators of the nursing diagnosis of powerlessness were determined by 27 graduate students enrolled in a clinical nursing course on chronic illness. The students had studied powerlessness as part of the course content and made powerlessness diagnoses on 81 chronically ill patients in their caseloads. The graduate students recorded the indicators that led them to believe their chronically ill patients were experiencing powerlessness. Similar specific signs and symptoms were clustered into 17 categories (broad statements or indicators). The indicators were then rated by a panel of 24 experts (graduate nursing faculty and advanced-standing graduate students), to determine which indicators may be characteristic of severe, moderate, low, or no powerlessness. See Table 3-3.

The indicators rated as "severe" could be termed "critical indicators" of the nursing diagnosis of powerlessness. That is, when any of these indicators are present, nurses could conclude that the patient has a nursing diagnosis of powerlessness. Although the signs and symptoms categorized as "moderate" and "low" are important cues, they may not lead the nurse to conclusively make the diagnosis of powerlessness. Validity and reliability of this tool have not been established.

# SUMMARY

The purpose of this chapter was to review literature on powerlessness and to report work on initial phases of concept development. Harmful effects of powerlessness were identified in each category of literature reviewed: powerlessness and learning, the illusion of control, effects of no control on animals and humans, control in health-illness situations, and powerlessness as a precipitant of death. The practice speculations derived from the theoretical propositions provide direction for nursing and the assurance that alleviation of powerlessness is within the realm of nursing practice.

In developing the concept of powerlessness as a relevant nursing diagnostic category, initial phases of concept development have been completed. Drawing conclusions from other descriptive research is the focus of other chapters in this book.

# REFERENCES

1. Dubin, R.: *Theory Building*. Free Press, New York, 1969.
2. Rotter, J. B.: *Generalized expectancies for internal versus external control of reinforcement*. Psychol. Monogr. 80:1, 1966.
3. Rotter, J. B.: *Some problems and misconceptions related to the construct of internal versus external control of reinforcement*. J. Consult. Clin. Psychol. 43:56, 1975.
4. Ibid. p. 57.
5. Newman, M.: *Theory Development in Nursing*. F. A. Davis, Philadelphia, 1979.
6. Seeman, M.: *Alienation and learning in a hospital setting*. American Sociological Review 27:772, 1962.
7. Seeman, M.: *Alienation and social learning in a reformatory*. American Journal of Sociology 69:270, 1963.
8. Seeman, M.: *Powerless and knowledge: A comparative study of alienation and learning*. Sociometry 30:105, June 1967.
9. Seeman, M.: *Alienation and knowledge-seeking: A note on attitude and action*. Social Problems 20:3, Summer 1972.
10. Seeman 1967, op. cit., entire work.

11. Phares, E. J.: *Differential utilization of information as a function of internal-external control*. J. Pers. 36:649, 1968.
12. Phares, E. J., Ritchie, D. E., and Davis, W.: *Internal-external control and reaction to threat*. J. Pers. Soc. Psychol. 10:402, 1968.
13. Stotland, E. and Blumenthal, A.: *The reduction of anxiety as a result of the expectation of making a choice*. Canad. J. Psychol. 18:139, 1964.
14. Perlmuter, L. C. and Monty, R. A.: *Effect of choice of stimulus on paired associate learning*. J. Exp. Psychol. 99:120, 1973.
15. Zahn, J.: *Some adult attitudes affecting learning: Powerlessness, conflicting needs and role transition*. Adult Education Journal 19:91, 1969.
16. Geer, J., Davison, G., and Gatchel, R.: *Reduction of stress in humans through nonveridical perceived control of aversive stimulation*. J. Pers. Soc. Psychol. 16:731, 1970.
17. Glass, D., et al.: *Perceived control of aversive stimulation and the reduction of stress responses*. J. Pers. 41:577, 1973.
18. Glass, D. and Singer, J.: *Urban Stress: Experiments in Noise and Social Stressors*. Academic Press, New York, 1972.
19. Corah, N. and Boffa, J.: *Perceived control, self-observation, and response to aversive stimulation*. J. Pers. Soc. Psychol. 16:1, 1970.
20. Houston, B. K.: *Control over stress, locus of control and response to stress*. J. Pers. Soc. Psychol. 21:249, 1972.
21. Lefcourt, H.: *The function of the illusions of control and freedom*. Am. Psychol. 28:419, 1973.
22. Mowrer, O. H. and Viek, P.: *An experimental analogue of fear from a sense of helplessness*. J. Abnorm. Soc. Psychol. 43:193, 1948.
23. Seligman, M., Maier, S., and Solomon, R.: *Unpredictable and uncontrollable aversive events*. In Brush, F. R. (ed.): *Aversive Conditioning and Learning*. Academic Press, New York, 1969.
24. Overmier, J. and Seligman, M.: *Effects of inescapable shock upon subsequent escape and avoidance responding*. J. Comp. Physiol. Psychol. 63:23, 1967.
25. Overmier, J. B.: *Interference with avoidance behavior: Failure to avoid traumatic shock*. J. Exp. Psychol. 78:340, 1968.
26. Seligman, M. and Maier, S. F.: *Failure to escape traumatic shock*. J. Exp. Psychol. 74:1, 1967.
27. Seligman, M., Maier, S., and Geer, J.: *The alleviation of learned helplessness in the dog*. J. Abnorm. Soc. Psychol. 73:256, 1968.
28. Seligman, M.: *Chronic fear produced by unpredictable shock*. J. Comp. Physiol. Psychol. 66:402, 1968.
29. Brady, J., et al.: *Avoidance behavior and the development of gastroduodenal ulcers*. J. Exp. Anal. Behav. 1:69, 1958.
30. Weiss, J.: *Effects of coping behavior in different warning signal conditions on stress psychology in rats*. J. Comp. Physiol. Psychol. 77:1, 1971.
31. Seligman, M. and Meyer, B.: *Chronic fear and ulcers as a function of the unpredictability of safety*. J. Comp. Physiol. Psychol. 73:202, 1970.
32. Staub, E., Tursky, B., and Schwartz, G.: *Self-control and predictability: Their effects on reactions to aversive stimulation*. J. Pers. Soc. Psychol. 18:157, 1971.
33. Ball, T. and Vogler, R.: *Uncertain pain and the pain of uncertainty*. Percept. Motor Skills 33:1195, 1971.
34. Pervin, L. A.: *The need to predict and control under conditions of threat*. J. Pers. 31:570, 1963.
35. Haggard, E. A.: *Experimental studies in affective processes: I. Some effects of cognitive structure and active participation on certain autonomic reactions during and following experimentally induced stress*. J. Exp. Psychol. 33:257, 1943.
36. Glass, D., Singer, J., and Friedman, L.: *Psychic cost of adaptation to environmental stressor*. J. Pers. Soc. Psychol. 12:200, 1969.
37. Kanfer, F. and Seidner, M.: *Self-control: Factors enhancing tolerance of noxious stimulation*. J. Pers. Soc. Psychol. 25:381, 1973.
38. Thornton, J. W. and Jacobs, P. D.: *Learned helplessness in human subjects*. J. Exp. Psychol. 87:369, 1971.

39. Miller, W. and Seligman, M.: *Depression and the perception of reinforcement.* J. Abnorm. Psychol. 82:62, 1973.
40. Miller, W. and Seligman, M.: *Depression and learned helplessness in man.* J. Abnorm. Psychol. 84:228, 1975.
41. Seligman, M.: *Helplessness: On Depression, Development, and Death.* Freeman & Co., San Francisco, 1975, p. 82.
42. Hiroto, D. and Seligman, M.: *Generality of learned helplessness in man.* J. Pers. Soc. Psychol. 31:311, 1975.
43. Gatchel, R., McKinney, M., and Koebernick, L.: *Learned helplessness, depression, and psychological responding.* Psychophysiology 14:25, 1977.
44. Johnson, B. and Kilmann, P.: *Locus of control and perceived confidence in problem-solving abilities.* J. Clin. Psychol. 31:54, 1975.
45. Anderson, C.: *Locus of control, coping behaviors, and performance in a stress setting: A longitudinal study.* J. Appl. Psychol. 62:446, 1977.
46. Kahn, R., et al.: *Organizational Stress: Studies in Role Conflict and Ambiguity.* John Wiley & Sons, New York, 1964.
47. Seligman 1975, op. cit., entire work.
48. MacDonald, A. and Hall, J.: *Internal-external locus of control and perceptions of disability.* J. Consult. Clin. Psychol. 36:338, 1971.
49. Watson, D.: *Relationship between locus of control and anxiety.* J. Pers. Soc. Psychol. 6:91, 1967.
50. Donovan, D., et al.: *Relationships among locus of control, self-concept, and anxiety.* J. Clin. Psychol. 31:682, 1975.
51. Lowery, B., Jacobsen, B., and Keane, A.: *Relationship of locus of control to preoperative anxiety.* Psychol. Rep. 37:1115, 1975.
52. Kirscht, J.: *Perceptions of control and health belief.* Canadian Journal of Behavioral Science 4:225, 1972.
53. Andrew, J.: *Delay of surgery.* Psychosom. Med. 34:345, 1972.
54. Williams, R., Poon, L., and Burdette, L.: *Locus of control and vasomotor response to sensory processing.* Psychosom. Med. 39:127, March-April 1977.
55. Wallston, B., et al.: *Development and validation of the health locus of control (HLC) scale.* J. Consult. Clin. Psychol. 44:580, 1976.
56. Wallston, K., Wallston, B., and DeVellis, R.: *Development of the multidimensional health locus of control (MHLC) scales.* Health Educ. Monogr. 6:160, Spring 1978.
57. Rokeach, M.: *The Nature of Human Values.* Free Press, New York, 1973.
58. Craig, K. and Best, A.: *Perceived control over pain: Individual differences and situational determinants.* Pain 3:127, 1977.
59. Richter, C. P.: *The phenomenon of unexplained sudden death in animals and man.* In Feifel, H. (ed.): *The Meaning of Death.* McGraw-Hill, New York, 1959.
60. Engel, G.: *A life setting conducive to illness: The giving up-given up complex.* Ann. Intern. Med. 69:293, 1968.
61. Engel, G.: *Sudden and rapid death during psychological stress, folklore or folkwisdom?* Ann. Intern. Med. 74:771, 1971.
62. Kastenbaum, R. and Kastenbaum, B.: *Hope, survival and the caring environment.* In Palmore, E. and Jerrers, F. (eds.): *Prediction of Life Span.* Lexington Books, Division of D. C. Heath, Lexington, Mass., 1971, pp. 249-271.
63. Lefcourt, op. cit. p. 417.
64. Ibid. p. 422.
65. Ferrari, N. A.: *Institutionalization and Attitude Change in an Aged Population: A Field Study on Dissidence Theory.* Unpublished doctoral dissertation, Case Western Reserve University, Cleveland, 1962.
66. Engel, G.: *Psychological Development in Health and Disease.* W. B. Saunders, Philadelphia, 1962.
67. Schmale, A.: *A genetic view of affects.* Psychoanal. Stud. Child 19:287, 1964.
68. Engel 1968, op. cit. p. 296.
69. Pattison, E. M.: *Psychological predictors of death prognosis.* Omega 5:145, 1974.

70. Averill, J.: *Personal control over aversive stimuli and its relationship to stress.* Psychol. Bull. 80:286, 1973.

# SELECTED READINGS

Arakelian, M.: *An assessment and nursing application of the concept of locus control.* Advances in Nursing Science 3:25 October 1980.

Lowery, B.: *Misconceptions and limitations of locus of control and the I-E scale.* Nurs. Res. 30:294, September/October 1981.

Miller, W. R. and Seligman, M. E. P.: *Learned helplessness, depression and the perception of reinforcement.* Behav. Res. Ther. 14:7, 1976.

Wilson, J.: *Thinking with Concepts.* Cambridge University Press, London, 1970.

# 2

# POWERLESSNESS—DEVELOPMENTAL VULNERABILITIES

Individuals are vulnerable to powerlessness at different times throughout the life cycle. In Part 2, behavioral manifestations of powerlessness, coping behaviors, and some nursing approaches are discussed for each of three developmental groups: children, middle-aged women, and elderly persons.

The child's reactions to situations of no control at a time when autonomy had been well established are unique reactions for the child. Nurses must understand and interpret these reactions to parents. The child's coping behaviors are also unique to childhood. Coping behaviors of chronically ill adults (Chapter 2) can be contrasted with those of children (Chapter 4).

A prevalent chronic health problem of middlescent women is obesity. The relationship of obesity to powerlessness is discussed in Chapter 5. Empowerment strategies for women coping with the stressors of middle years and struggling with weight control are presented.

The relationship of long-standing, uncontrolled powerlessness and hopelessness is uncovered in the detailed case-study analyses of elderly patients (Chapter 6). The serious consequence of giving up is that the ill elderly person may invite death. Nursing care of elderly patients who are experiencing powerlessness is included.

# 4

# COPING BEHAVIOR
# OF CHILDREN
# EXPERIENCING POWERLESSNESS
# FROM LOSS OF MOBILITY

## DIANN RECKER BAUMANN

The physical and psychologic crises of illness in children are compounded when the confronting health problem causes immobility. Children bring their total developmental accomplishments and past experiences to each new situation that affects their ability to cope with new stresses encountered. Expected or normal development is a progression of children's gaining power and control through developmental achievements.

The purpose of this chapter is to identify coping behaviors of children experiencing powerlessness resulting from immobility. Detailed case studies of immobilized children at two developmental stages—toddler and preadolescent—are included, with specific nursing strategies to enhance children's feeling of control. A review of literature on coping and mobility reveals the importance of both for the child's normal development.

## COPING

Coping encompasses the problem-solving efforts that individuals make when faced with the demands that are relevant to their well-being. Murphy defines coping strategies as "the child's individual patternings and timings of his resources for dealing with specific problems or needs or challenges."[1] This often involves both the methods of dealing with the environment and the devices and mechanisms for tension aroused by the stimulus. Learning is necessary for children to develop their own coping strategies. Reality testing involves learning and promotes development of coping strategies. Reality testing is both a cognitive and a manipulative function and proceeds by creative restructuring in order to test potentialities. Murphy refers to coping as a synthesizing or integrative concept: ". . . it deals not only with techniques but with *strategy.*"[1]

Encountering some new or not yet mastered situation (a novel situation, an obstacle, or a conflict) initiates the process of coping. These situations may be gratifying, threatening, challenging, or frustrating. Murphy identifies how the child might act when faced with a threatening situation. The various directions for acting might be reduction of the threat, control of the threat by setting limits, destruction of the threat, or balancing of the threat with security measures.

Once the child learns methods of coping successfully in certain situations, the child integrates these methods for use in other situations. Patterns developed in one situation are drawn upon for use in new situations. The individual child displays variations in coping methods depending on problems encountered (degree of perceived threat), previous experiences, maternal involvement, and the child's unique coping repertoire.

# THE ROLE OF MOBILITY IN THE EMOTIONAL LIFE OF THE CHILD

On the biologic level, Adams and Lindemann identified movement as the first mechanism necessary for biologic coping: "Virtually all response to environmental challenge involves purposeful movement, either of the total organism or its appropriate parts."[2] Rank's study of aggression indicates: "The tension and/or anxiety finds its primary expression in motor-expressive discharge."[4] "The blocking of the normal emotional discharge channel of motor activity taxes the adaptive capacities of the child to the utmost."[4] Mobility is thus identified as significant for both biologic and psychologic reasons.

Mobility plays a particular psychodynamic role in the lives of children and adults. Mittlemann's study of mobility identifies a "motor urge" present in all age periods. This becomes the dominant urge in the second year of life. The motor urge is seen as one of the most important avenues of exercising such functions as mastery, integration, reality testing, and control of impulses. It is "significantly connected with nearly every other motivational striving, both of physiological (oral, excretory, genital) and more general emotional nature (love, dependency, etc.) and particularly self-preservation."[5]

Muscular maturation in the second year of life provides the child with the facility for locomotion. It is the time in development when the sense of autonomy makes significant growth. Mobility for the toddler is important in the development of autonomy, as well as for discharging of tension, reality testing, integration, and mastery. The toddler's sense of autonomy is facilitated by the drive and energy to move. Mittlemann describes the second year of life as including ". . . increase in self-assertion, and independence alternating with continued dependence on the environment, increase in aggression, fear of motor retribution, motor (imitative) identification, the readiness to translate impulses into activity, predominance of motor language in communication with the environment."[6]

In a similar fashion, the young adolescent strives to achieve a mature sense of self. Gallatine states:

The youngster elaborates upon the basic sense of autonomy that emerged during the second crisis of childhood. There is an echo of self-awareness of the adolescent of the toddler's dim recognition that he is an autonomous being.[7]

Mahler suggests that the child's sense of identity may be traced back to the first 2 years of life. She defines this feeling of identity as "the cohesive cathexes of our securely individuated and differentiated self-image."[8] In other words, "normal separation—individuation, is the first crucial prerequisite for the development and maintenance of the 'sense of identity.' "[8] In the toddler stage, the child develops the realization of being a separate body from that of the object (mother) in the symbiotic union of infancy.

Erikson writes about the stages of child development in terms of accruing a sense of ego strength. He identifies the potential outcome of the second stage, the stage of autonomy:

A sense of self-control without loss of self-esteem is the ontogenetic source of the sense of free will. From an avoidable sense of loss of self-control and of parental over-control comes a lasting propensity for *doubt* and *shame*."[9]

Mobility plays a particularly important role in both the toddler's life and the young adolescent's life. Motion and activity become significant as outlets and means to work through adolescent energies. The "craving for locomotion" expressed by Erikson[10] relates to the discontent and searching of youth. Vehicles of motion such as the automobile offer what Erikson calls "passive locomotion with an intoxicating delusion of being intensely active."[10] The young adolescent's nature keeps the youth on the go, seeking adventure and excitement in life.

Blos identifies the adolescent's forceful turning to the outside world to action and bodily motion as a form of resistance against regression.[11] Deutsch suggests that there is a "thrust of activity" before the sudden increase of passivity that inaugurates the young girl's development into womanhood. "The thrust of activity represents not an increase of aggression but rather an intensive process of adaptation to reality and of mastery of the environment made possible by the development of the ego."[12]

The child's motor system and how the child uses it have a significant relation to perceptions of, and feelings about, self. The intact motor system and the guidance to use it in socially acceptable ways contribute to the development of a healthy self-image and body image.[13]

Schilder describes the role of mobility in the development of body image. He states that what he calls the "postural model" of the body ". . . is in perpetual inner self-construction and self-destruction. It is living in its continued differentiation and integration."[14] He also states that motility is an outstanding factor in the differentiation of the postural model of the body. "In the care of total paralysis, there would still be impulses to move as long as life is present. Perceptions are only formed on the basis of the motility and its impulses."[15]

This brief literature review shows that mobility significantly influences normal child development. Mobility is important for the child in terms of exploring the environment, gaining a sense of autonomy, and expressing tension and anxiety. The motor urge plays a role in achieving mastery, integration, and reality testing. A healthy self-identity and body image are influenced by the child's mobility—particularly in the toddler and preadolescent stages, when the process of separation and individuation is underway. An appreciation for the child's need for mobility clearly provides an understanding of how the restriction of freedom of mobility can predispose a child to severe anxiety and frustration.

Two children coping with radical threats of powerlessness resulting from immobility will be described. The first discussion focuses on a toddler coping with the powerlessness of traction. The second discussion relates an analytic study of one preadolescent girl's coping behavior during the loss of control from a paralytic illness. The assessments and interventions are presented in terms of Johnson's model of nursing.

# JOHNSON'S BEHAVIORAL SYSTEMS MODEL OF NURSING

Johnson's behavioral systems model of nursing[16] identifies the nurse as a person who provides protection, nurturance, and stimulation so that the highest level of behavioral functioning in the child's eight subsystems can occur. These subsystems interact to make the person whole: achievement, affiliative, aggressive/protective, dependency, eliminative, ingestive, restorative, and sexual subsystems. When the goal of one subsystem is not met, an imbalance in one or more of the other subsystems may occur. Consequently, this imbalance might manifest itself in maladaptive behavior.

There is a need to regulate and control behavioral systems in order to maintain balance and stability and to achieve the highest behavioral goals appropriate for the child's individual developmental level. A wide variety of variables are taken into account when the nurse assesses the behavior and the environment of the child, such as the child's state of biologic functioning (maturation and growth) and psychologic functioning, nature of the family network, pathology, culture, and so forth.

When the child's supply of the functional requirements of protection, nuturance, and stimulation is lacking and the child's ability to adapt to stress is weakened by the illness, the nurse intervenes to become the external regulator of the child's environment. The overall objective of any nursing intervention is to establish regularities in the patient's behavior so that the goal of each subsystem will be met at the highest possible level.

# CLINICAL DATA AND NURSING STRATEGIES

## One Toddler Coping with the Restraint of Traction

Larry is a 34-month-old black boy who sustained a spiral fracture of his left femur resulting from a fall at home while playing with his 8-year-old sister. He is the youngest of an intact family of five children. He is described by his mother as a "talkative and outgoing, friendly" child. He has not been noted to have significant shyness with new people. His mother was proud of his ability to sing solos in front of a large group of people in the church.

Larry was placed in Russell's leg traction after his admission to a children's hospital. The primary nurse became involved with his care 1 week after the admission. The staff nurses reported that his mother visited only "a couple times a week." They reported that Larry had prolonged (more than a half hour) screaming and crying spells when his mother left. The staff identified Larry as a child who "fussed, screamed, and cried a great deal." One person described him as "spoiled." The staff had difficulty in dealing with Larry's coping behaviors; there was a noted "disturbed staff-family relationship." It was an apparent stress for the parents to cope with the child's hospitalization and injury.

The primary nurse began her care of Larry when he was free of the acute fracture pain. Circulatory and neurologic functions of the left leg were observed and found intact. Skin integrity was maintained in excellent condition. Skeletal alignment was maintained, as verified by follow-up x-ray.

The goal of the nurse-child relationship was to foster the child's highest possible level of behavior. Restricted mobility of traction and separation from his family were the paramount stressors in the child's altered environment. The nursing process was directed toward assessment of the function of each behavioral subsystem, identification of the primary sources of imbalance, and prescription of the methods of regulation of the external environment. The intervention was directed toward improving the child's ability to cope in general and specifically to cope with immobility.

The assessment was based on the knowledge of biologic and behavioral sciences, developmental research, and the interrelationships of the child's behavioral subsystems. Larry had the extraordinarily strong impinging forces of his restricted mobility in traction and the separation from his family. Because of his developmental stage, he was especially vulnerable to these impinging forces. As a result, Larry's behavioral systems were in an imbalance, and his ego integrity was threatened.

The child's efforts to cope with immobility may be successful or unsuccessful. If the child is not successful, there will be further tensions. If the method of coping does not reduce the strain, the external threatening forces and added internal upheavals rapidly become intermingled and reinforce one another. Nursing is to be directed toward assisting the child to cope—to find some tension-releasing activity—in order to stabilize behavioral subsystems and maintain equilibrium.

Maternal separation can result in specific phases of child behavior: protest, despair, and denial. Robertson and Robertson[17] found that if toddlers were separated from their mothers for 10 to 27 days in an adequate setting with a substitute mother, they did not respond in the protest-and-despair cycle. Another child, who was separated from his mother and subjected to the inadequacies of the residential nursery care, displayed acute distress and despair commonly exhibited by institutionalized children. Larry's screaming and crying episodes were in protest of the separation from his mother. Prolonged separation from the mother can affect the toddler profoundly and can potentially cause physiologic and depressive emotional disturbances.

The major stressors related to Larry's hospitalization were centered on the affiliative, achievement, and aggressive subsystems. The following subsystem assessment illustrates how these imbalances placed stress on the other subsystems. The behaviors noted were observable and, to some degree, functional in Larry's attempt to cope with the pressures of immobilization and separation. Through prescribed nursing intervention, Larry was moving toward improved coping behaviors and was releasing some of his inner tensions while dealing with the feelings of powerlessness.

## ACHIEVEMENT SUBSYSTEM

Larry's achievement subsystem was interrupted as noted by his regression to lack of bowel and bladder control. The variables in this subsystem related to his developmental stage of autonomy versus shame and doubt. His restricted mobility and autonomy caused frustration. His previous control and powers were lost.

Larry's negativistic expressions, his loud crying and screaming, and his refusal to eat or poor eating were identified as his striving to gain some control or power. The primary nurse focused on sustaining Larry's available facets of autonomy. Larry was guided to direct his aggressive behavior in compatible ways in an effort to gain some feeling of control and power. Alternative modes of aggressive behavior were supplied through the following nursing directives:

1. Provide choices (for toys and play).
2. Avoid reprimand for his temporary loss of toilet control. Do not shame this regressive behavior.
3. Accentuate positive reinforcement when he successfully manages bowel and bladder control. Assist his ability to do so by offering the bedpan frequently.
4. Utilize manipulative play activities with toys and artwork.
5. Encourage partial self-care (brushing teeth, bathing, and eating).

The short-term goal was to help Larry use acceptable modes of control and give him a feeling of having some power, some sense of autonomy. The long-term goal was the eventual return of his prehospitalization level of autonomy.

## AFFILIATIVE SUBSYSTEM

The affiliative subsystem was significantly altered as Larry perceived a loss of his primary love object in the separation from his mother. The experience and fear of separation created anxiety. Larry protested by screaming at each separation from his mother. His avoidance of new caretakers was observed in shy, negativistic, turning-away behavior.

Larry's developmental stage calls for understanding that he is highly vulnerable to fear of abandonment. Cognitively, he has no concept of time. Having a concept of time may have helped him cope with separation. Knowing when he would see his mother again, as well as go home, could facilitate mastery over feelings of abandonment. Larry apparently came from an intact family with evidence of good interrelations before the hospitalization. This positive variable was radically interrupted by the hospitalization. The family's lack of a telephone and inability to provide a daily visit hindered family communication.

Nursing focused on maintenance of the mother-child tie and a surrogate relationship to alter the fear of abandonment. The mode was to provide a consistent protective and nurturing relationship with the primary nurse. Directives to maintain mother-child ties include:

1. Encourage parents to visit despite difficulty in leaving.
2. Maintain daily visits and interaction with the primary nurse to provide a surrogate relationship.
3. Supply items to help the child feel ties with home:
   —Leave toys from home with the child.
   —Leave a family photo album with the child.
   —Talk with the child about his family.
   —Encourage mother and father to leave an article of clothing with the child to signify a plan to return.
   —Bring siblings' gifts of artwork to the child.
4. Cooperatively use the peek-a-boo game to assist in working through separation anxiety.
5. Interpret and defend the child's behavior to staff members who may appear to misunderstand.

The short-term affiliative goal was to maintain the mother-child relationship, and the long-term goal was toward the incorporation of the hospital experience without residual instability.

## AGGRESSIVE SUBSYSTEM

The aggressive subsystem was interrupted by his confinement and immobilization in traction. Larry's behavior was silence and withdrawal at times, as well as negativism, screaming, and tantrums. He would often assume an angry facial expression and throw items out of the crib. In Larry's toddler developmental stage, the aggressive system to express frustrations is active. Mobility and expressions in aggressive play would normally provide a toddler with healthy expression of frustrations.

Nursing care focused on guiding Larry to rechannel aggression in supportive presence of the caring nurse. Alternative modes of play activity utilizing some of the following toys and techniques for aggressive expression included:

1. Pounding bench toy.
2. Punching bag.
3. Pounding on a toy drum.
4. Manipulation via drawing and scribbling.
5. Motion of playing with cars.
6. Manipulation with hanging and pull-push toys.
7. Manipulation of wash cloth and water play at bath time.
8. Synergistic effect of being in the playroom with others.

The short-term goal was to support multiple acceptable aggressive activities as outlets for his internal frustration. The long-term goal was to have Larry readapt aggressive behavior to a moderate level appropriate for his age and in nondisruptive modes after hospitalization.

At the completion of treatment for the fractured leg, Larry was able to walk happily into his mother's arms, ready to return home. The primary nurse visited Larry's home 1 month later. He apparently was reintegrating well into the home environment, as evidenced by his outgoing and talkative behavior, playfulness, and returned motor ability. His behavioral subsystems balance had returned.

# DEVELOPMENTAL VULNERABILITY

Mobility plays an especially important role for the adolescent. Specific coping responses of an immobile adolescent experiencing the threat of paralysis are examined.

# A Preadolescent Girl Coping With Paralysis

Paralysis is identified as a "severe narcissistic wound."[18] The inability to function independently as a result of a sudden onset of flaccid motor paralysis is psychologically traumatizing. This is a crisis that places a significant stress on the individual's adaptive processes.

The hospitalized, paralyzed child is faced with normal developmental challenges compounded by both the physical and the psychologic crises of illness. The professional nurse is called upon to assist the child in coping with these stresses. The nursing approach is based on knowledge of preadolescent development and on understanding gained from the scant research on paralysis of children.

## PREADOLESCENT DEVELOPMENT

The "young adolescent" is referred to as the child between ages 10 and 14. This time span includes variations in sexual development. Individual tempos and styles of maturation are noted in young adolescents.

Attainments during the latency period represent the essential precondition for advancement to adolescence. Intellectual development is in transition from the state of concrete operations to one of abstract reasoning through the use of judgment, generalization, and logic. Socially, the child's empathy, understanding, and altruistic feelings have acquired significant stability. The child's physical stature allows for independence and mastery of the environment. Ego functions must have developed an increased resistance to regression and to disintegration under the stresses of the normal, everyday critical situations. Blos states:

. . . the synthesizing capacity of the ego must have become effective and complex; and finally, the ego must be sufficiently able to defend its integrity with progressively less assistance from the outside world. These latency achievements have to yield to the prepubertal increase in drive energy.[19]

The prepubertal hormonal alterations elevate the level of drive tension; such intensification becomes apparent both in mental content and in behavior. These matters alert nurses that the initial advances in preadolescent psychic restructuring are underway. The tentativeness of these processes instills in the preadolescent both the fear of losing familiar ground and the desire to go ahead to the unknown.[20]

Blos describes the psychic development in adolescence as the process of disengagement of libidinal aggressive cathexes from the internalized infantile love and hate objects. This creates ambivalence and emotional lability, which are characteristic of adolescents. Blos states that individuation cannot be accomplished without some regression. This type of regression constitutes an integral part of development at puberty. "The relentless striving toward increased autonomy through regression forces us to view this kind of regression in adolescence as regression in the service of development, rather than service of defense."[21]

In terms of Erikson's epigenetic stages, young adolescents should have some mastery of basic trust, autonomy, initiative, and industry in their psychosocial development. The young adolescent then is coming to the stage of "identity versus role confusion" in which the question "who am I?" takes on significant meaning. During puberty and adolescence, the previous stabilities are more or less questioned again. Rapid body growth and the addition of genital maturity present a psychologic revolution within the youth. Adolescents' primary concerns now are with both what they appear to be in the eyes of others and what they feel they are.[22]

The young adolescent is at a stage of life between a saddening farewell to childhood and a gradual transition through barriers toward the still-unknown adulthood. One major conflict relating to this "betweenness" stage of preadolescent development is the struggle between the desire to be dependent and the wish to be independent.

Preadolescent development displays a strong drive for growth and independence. There is a need to grow up, to achieve on one's own, and to experience and learn from the world. Descriptive of the adolescent attitude and quality are terms such as enthusiasm, an assortment of interests, a passion for adventure, readiness to be inspired, and eagerness to go all-out for a purpose.

The subjective and objective experience of instability in the adolescent years is explained by the many inner and outer bodily changes that occur in puberty. This demands a new orientation of the body ego, which most significantly interferes with the prepuberty concept of the self and the sense of identity. Adolescence is a time of life when the youth has a heightened awareness of what goes on in the body. The rapid changes in the bodily structure create stress for adolescents seeking their own identity and control. Adolescents must develop a sense of awareness of self and control of self. They must adapt to becoming physically and psychologically different.

The preadolescent cognitive developmental stage is an integrated picture constituting a natural culmination of the sensorimotor structures and of the grouping of concrete operations.[23] Young adolescents are building upon and expanding their capabilities.

They become capable of reasoning about propositions they do not believe yet, by means of differentiation of form and content. They become capable of drawing the necessary conclusions from concepts that are merely possible. This constitutes the beginning of hypothetic-deductive, or formal, thought. There is interest oriented toward the future, which adds futuristic dimensions to the child's thought process.

The preadolescent is seen as an active agent striving to master the situations of life by the use of various coping strategies. This struggle for mastery depends upon available energy and also upon expectations and trust in future gratification.[24] The total adolescent phase is a critical period of both turbulence and potentiality. Early adolescence is intrinsically a period of great stress and weakened coping skills; consequently, it is a time of high vulnerability.

During adolescence, a variety of coping strategies and behaviors are utilized in an effort to protect the integrity of the ego organization. There are years of struggle toward establishing new psychic equilibrium, which is recognized in the attainment of a personal and autonomous life-style.

There is much turmoil and searching in the lives of adolescents as they seek identity. During the whole gamut of preadolescence and adolescence, fluctuations between extreme opposites in feelings are deemed normal. This is a time of psychologic turmoil even without the complication of a physical impairment.


## THE PSYCHOLOGIC THREAT OF PARALYSIS

Langford studied children's adaptation to illness and hospitalization and identified that preadolescent youngsters "tend to express fears of permanent disability."[4] Paralysis, then, might be viewed as an internal deterioration of the body resulting in a powerful restraint of mobility.

Guillain-Barré syndrome is a distinct clinical entity characterized by a subacute development of symmetric paresis or paralysis in subjects of all ages. Weakness is identified as the major presenting complaint. The severity of motor weakness covers a wide spectrum, from a mild ataxia to a total paralysis of every motor and cranial nerve.[25] The etiology of this disease remains imperfectly defined. Although reversibility is characteristic of this syndrome, respiratory failure without compensation may present a fatal complication. The presence of complicating factors has been known to alter the usual progression of the syndrome.[26]

Reversibility of this disease varies in respect to the time for complete recovery. Low, Schneider, and Carter found that the period of complete recovery varied from 2 to 18 months. About one third of the 30 patients in their study recovered after 2 months; another third recovered after 6 months; and the final third recovered after 9 to 18 months.[27] Guillain-Barré syndrome presents a potentially fatal threat to the physiologic well-being and a potentially long-term course of rehabilitation for the patient. Consequently, the patient is presented with severe threats to self-preservation and psychic equilibrium. Bernabeu studied eight paralytic children and identified the "rage" response in reaction to the restraint of paralysis:

The core reactions to the crippling are frustration, anxiety, and rage . . . a major complicating factor in this situation arises from the fact that motor discharge, a major element in a child's normal economy of handling aggression, is either eliminated or seriously curtailed . . . .[28]

The crippled motor system, ". . . interfered with in its expressive, performance, and locomotor aspects, *fails in its function of serving ego development.*"[29] The significant function of motility is inhibited by the force of paralysis.

Bernabeu summarized the types of fears identified in the paralyzed children to include:

fear of death and suffocation, separation anxiety, fear of fragmentation, the castration anxiety—including the feelings of "difference" and inferiority linked to these. Fear of loss of love is reinforced by fear of physical relapse, since progress always depends on the attention of others. The fear of punishment is related to the fear of their own aggression as well as the onset of the disease.[30]

The victim of paralysis experiences a forced dependence on nursing care, which arouses a basic independence-dependence conflict. The child's level of mastery and autonomy is restrained. The paralyzed preadolescent, initiating the developmental task of identity, faces an adaptation crisis.

Carter and Chess studied the adaptations of organically handicapped children and stated that "the most predominant common symptom seen in the children was anxiety about attempting new experiences or facing new situations."[31] Seidenfeld had a similar finding in his study of the psychologic implications of breathing difficulties in poliomyelitis:

. . . the patient suffers withdrawal symptoms. Part of this is due to an internalized resistance to change, part to a profound sense of insecurity in an altered environmental situation, and a final part to a loss of confidence in the automatic control mechanism for respiration.[32]

Coyle and Miller cautioned nurses caring for patients with Guillain-Barré syndrome to consider the patients' possible residual disabilities and emotional reactions. Patients may react by becoming apathetic, irritable, and depressed. Their moods frequently range from impatience to overt expressions of hostility and resentment.[33]

Blake's empirical study identified immobilization as a crisis. She hypothesized specific tasks related to the immobilization of young persons. The child must learn new ways to cope with frustrations, change in body image, and loss of pleasure from activity. New patterns of interaction are sought to provide control over the child's feelings of helplessness and to promote the restoration of self-esteem and the feelings of self-direction and independence.[34]

Dadich[35] studied an 11-year-old girl's use of control while immobilized in halo-femoral traction and found that she coped with the anxiety by controlling herself as well as controlling others involved in her care. Mastery of overwhelming feelings was attained only if she had some power to control.

Seeley also found that an 8-year-old immobilized girl used similar coping behaviors. The subject concentrated on the reachievement of motility, control over people, and control over the situation.

# CLINICAL DATA AND NURSING STRATEGIES

## Loss of Control in a Preadolescent

The behavioral responses of an 11-year-old girl coping with loss of control during the reversible paralytic illness of Guillain-Barré were observed during the intensive-care and recovery phases of a 3-month hospitalization. The primary nurse assumed the role of participant-observer and described the girl's behavioral responses in the form of process recordings.

Joanne is an 11-year-old white girl. She ranks number seven in an intact family of nine children. Joanne's growth and development were reported as normal; she had been healthy during her childhood; she was a high scholastic achiever; and she led a socially active life before the onset of illness.

Four days before hospitalization, Joanne complained of weakness, vomiting, and feelings of numbness and tingling in her feet and hands. She had difficulty controlling her feet while walking. She experienced progressive weakness and paralysis.

On the day of hospitalization, Joanne experienced dyspnea and was transferred to the intermediate-care unit by ambulance. Four hours later, she was transferred to the intensive-care unit and was totally dependent on a mechanical respirator. A tracheotomy was performed on the fourth day of hospitalization to facilitate ventilation.

Joanne's respiratory-dependent state was but one of her symptoms of paralysis. She was unable to move from her neck downward, and she had lost both bladder and bowel control. She experienced dysphagia, aphonia, distortion of facial expression, and diplopia. She underwent a multitude of diagnostic and treatment procedures. Joanne was referred to the primary nurse on the fourth day of hospitalization. The referring staff nurse described Joanne as "scared to death."

### DATA COLLECTION

The primary nurse assumed the role of participant-observer during 32 sessions of recorded observations. These observations were made at varying times of the day and evening during 51 days of Joanne's 3-month hospitalization. The length of the observations averaged 1½ hours.

Immediately after the observations, process recordings were written describing both the verbal and the nonverbal behaviors of the child. Verbal behaviors of the child include the content and manner in which words and/or sounds were communicated. Nonverbal behaviors included aphonic mouthed words, facial expressions, body movements, and gestures. Verbal and nonverbal behaviors were observed in relation to the events at the time.

Content analysis of the 32 process recordings was utilized to identify the major coping behaviors manifested by the child. The behaviors were tabulated by frequency of occurrence in relation to the significant events of the illness and its treatment. Behaviors were then analyzed to identify both the modes and the pattern of responses observed over time in relation to the significant events of the illness and of its treatment.

Joanne's methods of coping with the degrees of loss of control and the feelings of powerlessness can be divided into two distinct phases. Phase 1, *the acute phase*, was the period when she experienced a complete loss of control. The predominant behavioral responses manifested during this phase were responses to control powerlessness and focused on activities of daily living. The controlling responses were categorized and will be discussed in the following order of frequency: directive, resistive, and compliant responses.

—*Directive* responses were those in which the child attempted to direct what was to be done to her, how it was to be done, and by whom.
—*Resistive* responses were those in which the child opposed the care of caretakers by refusal, postponement, or limitation of action. Grimacing, crying, and clicking of her tongue were classified as resistive. Refusal to participate was considered resistive in an effort to control or in resistive submission when there was no alternative means of control.
—*Compliant* responses included those indicative of yielding, consenting, or conforming to the caretakers and the caretaking activity.

Three modes of behavior—motion, breathing, and grooming and diversion—were observed in which controlling responses were used. These are specific behaviors within select subsystems of the Johnson framework in that motion is a behavior within the aggressive/protective subsystem, breathing is included in the ingestive subsystem, and grooming and diversion are included within the restorative subsystem. Because only the select components of the subsystem were observed and to enable the reader to more easily follow the data presented, the mode titles of motion, breathing, and grooming and diversion will be utilized instead of the entire Johnson subsystem headings.

Phase 2, *the recovery phase*, included the period when the child gradually regained control of body functions. The predominant behavioral responses manifested in the recovery phase were responses to control powerlessness and focused on activities of daily living. Although the order of frequency of controlling responses is different from the order in the acute phase, the definitions of these categories remain the same in both phases.

## PHASE 1: ACUTE PHASE

The raw data of the acute phase consist of 16 process recordings. This acute phase included the first 25 days of hospitalization. To cope with this paralytic illness and the multiple treatments and caretakers, Joanne attempted to maintain a sense of control. The directive (113), resistive (57), and compliant (34) responses appeared to aid her in maintaining some autonomy.

## Directive Responses

The frequency of 113 directive responses ranged from 0 to 25 per interaction during the acute phase. Directive responses were related to activities of daily living and occurred in the following order of frequency: motion (59), breathing (37), and grooming and diversional activities (17).

Examples of directive responses related to motion included Joanne's verbal orders regarding range-of-motion exercises, repositioning, and chest clapping, for example, "Turn my neck first," and, "Don't clap so hard." Directive responses within the breathing mode while Joanne was respirator dependent included, "Suction my tube," and, "Bag me faster, harder."

Grooming was considered an important part of Joanne's care in an effort to maintain her intact body image. Not only was Joanne unable to control body motion, she also experienced significant edema of her hands, feet, and face secondary to adrenocorticotropic hormone (ACTH) therapy. This edema may have presented a threat to Joanne's body image. Diversional activities were methods offered to stimulate her interests in things other than the illness and its treatments. Her directive responses included, "Lip gloss my lips," and, "Read some more."

Mail from Joanne's peers seemed to give her support. Fewer controlling responses were noted after she received communications from peers.

The most frequent directive responses in the acute phase were directives relative to motion (52.2%), and the majority (69.0%) of those related to motion were recorded during the first half of the acute phase. Directive responses related to breathing (32.8%) were evenly distributed throughout the acute phase. Grooming and diversional activity directive responses (15%) were observed less frequently and were distributed throughout the acute phase.

An increase in directive control measures was related to an increase in powerlessness-provoking events such as removal and reinsertion of a nasogastric tube, assignment of an unfamiliar nurse to her care, diarrhea, and performance of x-ray procedures. Directive responses related to breathing were evenly distributed throughout the acute phase.

## Resistive Responses

During the acute phase, Joanne communicated a total of 69 resistive responses. The frequency of resistive responses ranged from 0 to 11 during each observation in the acute phase. The resistive responses were related to activities of daily living in the following order of frequency: motion (42), breathing (11), and grooming and diversional activities (4).

Ten of the 11 resistive responses related to breathing (90.9%) occurred during the first half of the acute phase. Joanne's pattern of resistive responses may indicate that her anxiety related to the vital function of breathing was at its highest level during the first portion of the acute phase. More resistive responses were noted when her powerlessness was heightened, as on days when invasive procedures (manual removal of impacted stool, replacement of the nasogastric tube) were performed.

Only four resistive responses were observed related to grooming and diversional activities during the acute phase. It is significant to note that the activities in this category involve things done *with* rather than *to* Joanne and are of a more pleasurable nature. Perhaps this accounts for her absent or minimal resistance to grooming and diversional activities.

The most frequent resistive responses in the acute phase were related to motion (73.7%), and the majority (64%) of these were recorded during the first half of the acute phase. The resistive responses related to breathing (19.3%) occurred most often (91%) during the first half of the acute phase. Resistive responses to grooming and diversional activities (7.0%) were less frequent and were evenly distributed throughout the acute phase.

## Compliant Responses

During the acute phase, Joanne responded to treatments by caretakers with compliant responses a total of 35 times. Although compliant responses are perhaps less controlling responses, they are, however, chosen responses. The frequency of compliant responses ranged from 0 to 5 during individual observations. The compliant responses related to activities of daily living in the following order of frequency: motion (21), breathing (8), and grooming and diversional activities (5).

## Acute Phase Summary

Controlling responses in the modalities of motion, breathing, and grooming and diversion during the acute phase are summarized in Table 4-1. Joanne manifested a high frequency of controlling responses while coping with loss of control during the acute phase. Three types of controlling responses were identified: directive, resistive, and compliant. These controlling responses varied in frequency throughout the acute phase. Directive responses were the most frequently observed during this phase, and resistive responses were the second most frequently deserved. The most frequent directive and resistive responses were related to motion. The second most frequent directive and resistive responses were related to breathing. Compliance was the least frequent response observed during the acute phase. The least frequent of all the controlling responses were those related to grooming and diversional activities. Most days of high frequency of directive responses were also days of high frequency of resistive responses.

## PHASE 2: RECOVERY PHASE

The raw data of the recovery phase consist of 16 process recordings. Days 26 to 51 of hospitalization were identified as the recovery phase. The recovery phase is comprised of events that signify the initial regain of Joanne's body functions. Joanne's tidal volume increased; weaning from the respirator began in the middle of the recovery phase and was completed within 10 days. Bladder control was regained after the removal of the

**TABLE 4-1. Summary of Controlling Responses Observed During the Acute Phase**

| | Coping Responses Observed | Motion | | Breathing | | Grooming and Diversion | |
|---|---|---|---|---|---|---|---|
| | N | N | % | N | % | N | % |
| *Directive* | 113 | 59 | 52.2 | 37 | 32.8 | 17 | 15.0 |
| *Resistive* | 57 | 42 | 73.7 | 11 | 19.3 | 4 | 7.0 |
| *Compliant* | 34 | 21 | 61.8 | 8 | 23.5 | 5 | 14.7 |

urinary catheter. The nasogastric tube was removed 2 days later, and Joanne was able to eat. Near the end of the recovery phase, she could manage gross arm, hand, and finger movements.

To cope with the multiple treatments and caretakers during this gradual regain of control, Joanne continued to manifest controlling responses in her struggle for autonomy. The frequency of responses is different from that of phase 1 and is as follows: resistive (108), directive (98), and compliant (64). These controlling responses were used in relation to eating (ingestive subsystem), motion (aggressive/protective subsystem), breathing (ingestive subsystem), and grooming and diversion (restorative subsystem).

### Resistive Responses

During the recovery phase, Joanne communicated 108 resistive responses. The number of resistive responses ranged from 0 to 24 during individual observations. The resistive responses related to activities of daily living in the following order of frequency: eating (37), grooming and diversional activities (26), motion (25), and breathing (20).

Eating became a function Joanne was capable of controlling, and consequently a high frequency of resistive responses was observed in relation to eating. One observation contained 11 resistive responses related to eating. This observation noted the 12th new nurse Joanne encountered during the 41 days of hospitalization. During the first 10 minutes of the observation, this staff nurse repeatedly attempted to get Joanne to eat. ("Come on, you've got to eat.") Joanne responded, "No. Why does everybody have to stuff food down my throat? I'm not hungry!," and, "I wish I had some different food and a different nurse."

Within 20 minutes, and after Joanne's caretakers agreed to her request for a ride on the cart, her mood seemed to change to a more agreeable one (five compliant responses), and no further resistive responses were noted.

Joanne expressed more resistive responses related to grooming and diversional activities in the recovery phase (26) than in the acute phase (14). This seemed indicative of her concern about, and her desire to gain control over, her appearance. Her beginning of physical recovery gave her "hope," and she expressed ego strength through expressing her opinion and exerting resistance. A greater interest in diversional activities was noted in the recovery phase because of her decreased struggle over the more vital functions of breathing and so forth.

Joanne's recovery of motion of her body was gradual and progressed from her ability to move her head to minor motion of her shoulders and arms by the middle of the recovery phase. Toward the end of this phase, Joanne was able to perform gross arm, hand, and finger movements. She gained the ability to move her feet to a small degree. Both the gradual gains in motion and the ability to be moved in and out of her room on a cart afforded Joanne a sense of mobility by the middle of the recovery phase. It is speculated that this motion acted to decrease the frustration of her motor urge and to decrease her need to utilize responses related to motion during the last half of the recovery phase.

The same day that Joanne was completely weaned from the respirator, the decreased size of the tracheostomy tube enabled her to speak audibly. The gradual return of significant body functions apparently facilitated Joanne's feeling of autonomy.

In the recovery phase, 20 resistive responses were related to breathing. During the weaning from the respirator, Joanne selected resistive responses to maintain some control: "No, I'm tired," and, "Wait."

During the last half of the recovery phase, there were only four resistive responses related to breathing. It is speculated that the regain of respiratory functioning decreased her need to control through her resistant mode of behavior. There was no longer a struggle for physical control of this most vital bodily function and, consequently, no longer a need for manipulative control related to breathing.

In summary of resistive responses, Joanne manifested significantly more resistive responses during the recovery phase (108) than during the acute phase (57). Her most frequent resistive responses in the recovery phase were related to eating (34.3%). The resistive responses related to grooming and diversional activities (24.1%) were evenly distributed throughout this phase. Those related to motion (23.1%) occurred most often (92%) in the first half of the recovery phase. The resistive responses related to breathing (18.5%) occurred most often (80%) during the first half of the recovery phase.

## Directive Responses

During the recovery phase, Joanne's directive communications totaled 98. The range of frequency for the individual observations in this phase was 0 to 28. These directives related to activities of daily living in the following order of frequency: motion (73), breathing (15), and grooming and diversional activities (10).

All 15 of Joanne's directive responses related to breathing occurred during the first half of the recovery phase. The gradual regain of respiratory function increased her feeling of autonomy. As her feeling of autonomy increased, her need to use directive responses decreased.

Joanne manifested a similar number of directive responses in the recovery phase (98) as in the acute phase (113). Her most frequent directive responses were related to motion (74.5%), and the majority (78%) of these occurred in the last half of the recovery phase. All directives related to breathing (15.3%) occurred in the first half of this phase while she was still on the respirator. Directive responses to grooming and diversional activities (10.2%) were distributed evenly throughout this recovery phase.

## Compliant Responses

Joanne responded to treatments and progressive rehabilitative efforts with 66 compliant responses. The frequency range for compliant responses was 1 to 13 in the individual observations during the recovery phase. These compliant responses related to activities of daily living in the following order of frequency: grooming and diversional activities (28), motion (24), and breathing (12).

Participation in the weaning from the respirator was evidenced by Joanne's compliant responses. Initially, her progress was visualized with a graphic chart showing the increases in her tidal volume. Later, a chart was utilized to illustrate graphically the length of time Joanne breathed on her own power. She appeared to be proud of her achievements. Joanne's affect included smiles when progress was evident. "Yesterday I was off (the respirator) for 45 minutes," she reported one day. Joanne initially resisted being off the respirator; however, when she was given some signs of progress and when her readiness was considered, Joanne became involved with the effort to be weaned from the respirator. The graphic charts helped her increase control. These charts may have assisted her by offering a competitive and rewarding aspect to her efforts.

Joanne manifested a greater number of compliant responses during the recovery phase (64) than during the acute phase (34). Her most frequent compliant responses related to grooming and diversional activities (43.8%). The frequency of compliant responses related to motion (37.5%) and those related to breathing (18.8%) varied throughout the recovery phase. The greatest increase of compliant responses from the acute phase (8) to the recovery phase (24) was related to motion.

## Recovery Phase Summary

The controlling responses in the modalities of eating, motion, breathing, and grooming and diversion for the recovery phase are summarized in Table 4-2. Joanne manifested a high frequency of controlling responses while coping with the loss and gradual regain of control during the recovery phase. Resistive responses were the most frequently observed controlling responses during the recovery phase (108) as compared with the acute phase (57). Eating was the activity of daily living that related most frequently (34.3%) to these resistive responses. The focus of Joanne's resistive behavior changed. The frequency of resistive responses to breathing and motion decreased after she was able to breathe on her own and to experience a modified form of mobility (rides on a cart). The height of Joanne's resistive responses to all activities appeared to coincide; that is, on the day that she expressed a high resistance to eating, she also expressed a high resistance to motion, breathing, and grooming. The majority of all resistive responses occurred in the first half of the recovery phase.

Directive responses were the second most frequent controlling response observed during the recovery phase. The highest frequency (74.5%) of these directives was related to motion, and the majority (78%) of these occurred in the last half of the recovery phase after she had been given a modified form of mobility. The frequency of directive responses expressed during the recovery phase (98) was similar to the frequency expressed during the acute phase (113). The total number of compliant responses during

**TABLE 4-2. Summary of Controlling Responses Observed During the Recovery Phase**

| | Coping Responses Observed | Eating | | Motion | | Breathing | | Grooming and Diversion | |
|---|---|---|---|---|---|---|---|---|---|
| | N | N | % | N | % | N | % | N | % |
| Resistive | 108 | 37 | 34.3 | 25 | 23.1 | 20 | 18.5 | 26 | 24.1 |
| Directive | 98 | 0 | 0.0 | 73 | 74.5 | 15 | 15.3 | 10 | 10.2 |
| Compliant | 64 | 0 | 0.0 | 24 | 37.5 | 12 | 18.8 | 28 | 43.8 |

the recovery phase (64) was almost double the total of the acute phase (34). The greatest number of compliant responses during both phases related to grooming and diversional activities.

## CASE STUDY SUMMARY

This study described the behavior of an 11-year-old girl coping with loss of control accompanying a reversible paralytic illness during the acute and recovery phases of a 3-month hospitalization. Her behaviors were analyzed and categorized for the two distinct phases. Phase 1, the acute phase, was the period of complete loss of control of body functions. Phase 2, the recovery phase, included the period of gradual regain of control of body functions.

The predominant behaviors identified were controlling responses and focused on activities of daily living. The three types of controlling responses were directive, resistive, and compliant. The events or activities of daily living were motion, breathing, eating, and grooming and diversional activities.

In the acute phase, the most frequent directive and resistive behaviors were related to motion. The second most frequent directive and resistive behaviors were related to breathing. Most of the compliant behaviors were related to grooming and diversional activities.

In contrast, during the recovery phase, the most frequent resistive behaviors were related to eating. The most frequent directive behaviors in this phase were related to motion, and the most frequent compliant behaviors were related to grooming and diversional activities.

The pattern of controlling behavior during the recovery phase was characterized by a significant increase in resistive responses. The resistive responses related to motion and breathing during the recovery phase occurred most often during the first half of this phase while the subject was dependent upon the respirator. In contrast, most of the directive behaviors were related to motion, and the majority of these occurred during the last half of the recovery phase after she had been provided with a modified form of mobility (rides on a cart). Although the compliant responses were again the least frequently observed controlling behaviors, the frequency almost doubled during the recovery phase. As a result of this study, specific conclusions can be drawn.

Paralysis presented this preadolescent girl with a severe narcissistic wound involving several threats to her sense of autonomous and trusting behaviors. The child coped with threats related to loss of control of her autonomous respiratory, motor, eating, and bladder functions over which she had achieved control since toddlerhood. This child's vulnerability increased since these functions became the foci of intrusions by others. Furthermore, it was necessary for the child to cope with threats due to multiple caretakers who presented a variety of approaches.

Predominant strategies that the child manifested for coping with the major threats were identified. During the acute phase, directive behavior was the predominant coping strategy. This strategy was most evident in relation to motion. The strategy of resistive behavior was demonstrated with respiratory function. Related to grooming and diversional activities (the least painful and most pleasurable activities) was the strategy of compliant behavior.

During the recovery phase, resistive behavior was the predominant coping strategy, and this was related to eating. The child's predominant coping strategy related to motor function was directive behavior. Related to grooming and diversional activities was the strategy of compliant behavior.

There were changes in the coping behaviors over a period of time. After the child gained partial control of her eating function, she was provided a new avenue for expressing resistance as a means of controlling her environment. After the child gained respiratory autonomy, partial motor function, and a modified form of mobility, she utilized directive coping strategies as a mode of control.

This child's coping strategies varied in relation to what was being done to her and by whom. There was an increased frequency of controlling behaviors when new caretakers were introduced. There was a significant increase in controlling behaviors when new or different treatments (e.g., being placed on the Circ-O-Lectric bed or being weaned from the respirator) were introduced.

Recommendations evolving from this study focus on the approaches to the nursing care of the paralyzed child and on the need for further study. It was observed that this child expressed both the need and demand for control. Based on this observation, it is recommended that nurses who care for children suffering from paralytic illness plan for and devise approaches that allow for the child's exercise of control. These approaches include preparation for controlling events, participation, provision of emotional outlets, and development of a satisfactory mode of communication.

Each new caretaker presented a new threat to the child's sense of control. Based on this finding, it is recommended that nurses caring for children who are experiencing the threat of loss of control negotiate a plan for consistency of caretakers.

The findings also revealed that the subject had difficulty coping with the change related to weaning from the respirator. It is recommended that further study be conducted to identify clues indicating the readiness of a child for weaning from the respirator. Specific strategies to enhance control during the weaning could be tested, such as use of graphs as visual signs of improvement and reinforcement regarding ability to be off the respirator for lengthening periods.

## SUMMARY OF NURSING PRACTICE STRATEGIES FOR DEALING WITH POWERLESSNESS IN CHILDREN

The study and appreciation of the child's ability to cope with restricted mobility provide some understanding of the crisis of powerlessness in childhood. Both the toddler and the young adolescent suffered powerlessness, which accompanied the loss of mobility. Larry and Joanne were in critical stages of development during which mobility normally facilitates the sense of autonomy. Both patients exhibited controlling behaviors in an effort to maintain their autonomy.

The nursing approach in assisting children during the crisis of powerlessness or loss of control must be considered specifically for each child. Certain general speculative approaches are suggested in terms of preparation, participation, outlets for emotional responses, and communication.

# Preparation

Give children "time to get ready." They may feel they have some control if they have a moment to prepare and then can signal the nurse when they are ready.

Let them know that you are prepared and confident to treat them. Telling a child that you have helped other children with certain illnesses and treatments like this may give that child a feeling of confidence.

# Participation

Have children help choose time of treatment and the order in which they would like it given. Providing some method of working together gives children a sense of control. Methods can be used such as counting the repetitive motions (i.e., exercises), holding onto something related to the treatment, and allowing children to cry or scream if it helps them have a perceived sense of control.

# Outlets for Emotional Responses

Knowing that the restraint of mobilization causes anger and an aggressive response, the nurse should provide games and toys to act as outlets for these emotions.

There may be days of withdrawal and uncooperative attitudes in children coping with the impinging force of powerlessness, and the nurse might tell the child, "It's okay to feel that way right now."

# Communication

Children are special people who communicate in a variety of ways. The toddler was not always able to verbalize what he needed, and the preadolescent could only mouth her words. Children need interpretation for understanding of their special needs.

Multiple caretakers present a threatening aspect to the child's care. Any method to provide consistency in nursing care might decrease the child's anxiety and powerlessness. The primary-nurse approach provided some consistency and some evidenced trusting behavior in both the toddler and the preadolescent after much effort was expended by the nurse to earn trust.

Johnson's model for nursing provides a framework for caring for the immobilized child. The powerlessness of immobility will cause behavioral subsystem imbalance in all subsystems: affiliation, aggression/protection, dependency, elimination, ingestion, restoration, and sexuality. Specific manifestations of subsystem imbalance are influenced by the unique situational, environmental, cultural, and family stressors impinging on the child, as well as by the child's particular stage of development.

Nursing of children coping with powerlessness related to any illness or treatment can be a challenging and rewarding experience. The coping behaviors used by both children described in this chapter were viewed as controlling behaviors and were varied. For example, although Larry was in traction, he was able to use some motion—throwing toys out of the crib and playing. Joanne was not able to use motion, but she commanded motion and used controlling behaviors of resistance, direction, and compliance. Nurses need to identify each child's needs and unique efforts to control situations. Creative methods of nursing for the sake of providing control will facilitate the child's recovery.

# REFERENCES

1. Murphy, L. B.: *The Widening World of Childhood.* Basic Books, New York, 1962, p. 274.
2. Adams, J. E. and Lindemann, E.: *Coping with long term disability.* In Coelho, G. V., Hamburg, D. A., and Adams, J. E. (eds): *Coping and Adaptation.* Basic Books, New York, 1974, p. 132.
3. Rank, B.: *Aggression.* Psychoanal. Stud. Child. 3-4:43, 1949.
4. Langford, W. S.: *The child in the pediatric hospital: Adaptation to illness and hospitalization.* Am. J. Orthopsychiatry 31:673, 1961.
5. Mittlemann, B.: *Motility in infants, children, and adults.* Psychoanal. Stud. Child 9:142, 1954.
6. Mittlemann, B.: *Motility in the therapy of children and adults.* Psychoanal. Stud. Child 12:284, 1967.
7. Gallatin, J. E.: *Adolescence and Individuality: A Conceptual Approach to Adolescent Psychology.* Harper & Row, New York, 1975, p. 178.
8. Mahler, M. S.: *Thoughts about development and individuation.* Psychoanal. Stud. Child 18:309, 1963.
9. Erikson, E. H.: *Identity: Youth and Crisis.* W. W. Norton & Co., New York, 1968, pp. 109-110.
10. Erikson, E. H.: *The Challenge of Youth.* Doubleday & Co., Garden City, N.Y., 1961, p. 11.
11. Blos, P.: *The second individuation process of adolescence.* Psychoanal. Stud. Child. 22:183, 1967.
12. Deutsch, H.: *The Psychology of Women, Vol. 1.* Grune & Stratton, New York, 1944, p. 4.
13. Blake, F.: *Immobilized youth.* Am. J. Nurs. 69:2366, November 1969.
14. Schilder, P. *The Image and the Appearance of the Body.* John Wiley & Sons, New York, 1958, pp. 15-16.
15. Ibid. p. 15.
16. Johnson, D.: *One conceptual model of nursing.* Unpublished paper.
17. Robertson, J. and Robertson, J.: *Young children in brief separation: A fresh look.* Psychoanal. Stud. Child 26:264, 1971.
18. Bernabeu, E. A.: *The effects of severe crippling on the development of a group of children.* Psychiatry 21:176, 1958.
19. Blos, P.: *On Adolescence.* Free Press, New York, 1962, p. 57.
20. Blos, P.: *The Young Adolescent.* Free Press, New York, 1970, p. xii.
21. Blos 1967, op. cit. p. 173.
22. Erikson, E.: *Childhood and Society,* ed. 2. W. W. Norton & Co., New York, 1963, p. 261.
23. Baldwin, A.: *Theories of Child Development.* John Wiley & Sons, New York, 1967.
24. Murphy L.: *Vulnerability, Coping and Growth: From Infancy through Adolescence.* University Press, New Haven, Conn., 1976.
25. Arnason, B. G. W.: *Inflammatory polyradiculoneuropathies.* In Dyck, P. J., Thomas, P. K., and Lambert, E. H. (eds.): *Peripheral Neuropathy.* W. B. Saunders, Philadelphia, 1975, p. 1121.

26. Sodaro, E. and Perlick, Sister Nancy: *Gullain-Barré: The syndrome, patient care and some case findings.* Journal of Neurosurgical Nursing 6:102, December 1974.
27. Low, N. L., Schneider, J., and Carter, S.: *Polyneuritis in children.* Pediatrics 22:974, 1958.
28. Bernabeu, op. cit. pp. 176-177.
29. Ibid. p. 177.
30. Ibid. p. 179.
31. Carter, V. and Chess, S.: *Factors influencing the adaptations of organically handicapped children.* Am. J. Orthopsychiatry 21:837, 1951.
32. Seidenfeld, M. A.: *Psychological implications of breathing difficulties in poliomyelitis.* Am. J. Orthopsychiatry 25:796, 1955.
33. Coyle, N. and Miller, B.: *Guillain-Barré syndrome: Nursing care.* Am. J. Nurs. 66:2224, October 1966.
34. Blake, op. cit. pp. 2367-2368.
35. Dadich, K. S.: *An eleven year old girl's use of control while immobilized in halo-femoral traction.* Maternal-Child Nursing Journal 1:74, 1972.

# SELECTED READINGS

Bierman, J. S., Silverstein, A. B., and Finesinger, J. E.: *A depression in a six-year-old boy with acute poliomyelitis.* Psychoanal. Stud. Child 13:430, 1958.
Blaesing, S. and Brockhaus, J.: *The development of body image in the child.* Nurs. Clin. North Am. 7:597, December 1972.
Blau, A., et al.: *The collaboration of nursing and child psychiatry in a general hospital.* Am. J. Orthopsychiatry 29:77, 1959.
Blos, P.: *Character formation in adolescence.* Psychoanal. Stud. Child 23:245, 1968.
Brody, S.: *Some aspects of transference resistance in prepuberty.* Psychoanal. Stud. Child 16:251, 1961.
Campbell, J.: *Illness is a point of view: The development of children's concepts of illness.* Child Dev. 46:92, 1975.
Chodoff, P., Friedman, S. B., and Hamburg, D. *Stress, defenses, and coping behavior: Observations in parents of children with malignant disease.* Am. J. Psychiatry 120:743, 1964.
Clipper, M.: *Nursing care of patients in a neurologic I.C.U.* Nurs. Clin. North Am. 4:211, 1969.
Elkind, D. *Egocentrism in adolescence.* Child Dev. 4:1025, 1967.
Erickson, F. *Nursing care based on nursing assessment. Current Concepts in Clinical Nursing.* C. V. Mosby, St. Louis, 1965, pp. 171-177.
Erickson, F.: *When 6 to 12 year olds are ill.* Nurs. Outlook 8:48, July 1965.
Erickson, F.: *Helping the sick child maintain behavioral control.* Nurs. Clin. North Am. 2:695, December 1967.
Freud, A.: *The role of bodily illness in the mental life of children.* Psychoanal. Stud. Child 7:69, 1952.
Freud, A.: *Adolescence.* Psychoanal. Stud. Child 13:255, 1958.
Freud, A.: *The concept of developmental lines.* Psychoanal. Stud. Child 18:245, 1963.
Friedenberg, E. Z.: *The Vanishing Adolescent.* Dell Publishing, New York, 1962.
Fujita, M.: *The impact of illness or surgery on the body image of the child.* Nurs. Clin. North Am. 7:641, December 1972.
Furman, E.: *A contribution of assessing the role of infantile separation-individuation in adolescent development.* Psychanal. Stud. Child 28:193, 1973.
Gallatin, J. E.: *A Conceptual Approach to Adolescent Psychology.* Harper & Row, New York, 1975.
Geleerd, E. R.: *Some aspects of ego vicissitudes in adolescence.* J. Am. Psychoanal. Assoc. 9:394, 1961.
Glass, J.: *Nursing care of the paralyzed patient.* Journal of Neurosurgical Nursing 2:25, July 1970.
Greenberg, H. A.: *The management of the emotional problems of crippled children in a new type of institution.* Am. J. Orthopsychiatry 19:253, 1949.
Hamburg, B. A.: *Early adolescence: A specific and stressful stage of the life cycle.* In Coelho, G. V., Hamburg, D. A., and Adams, J. E.: *Coping and Adaptation.* Basic Books, New York, 1974, pp. 101-124.

Holmes, S.: *The use of control by a hospitalized five year old girl.* Maternal-Child Nursing Journal 5:189, 1976.

Hulbert, R.: *Acute polyneuritis.* Nurs. Times 72:257, February 1976.

Issner, N.: *The family of the hospitalized child.* Nurs. Clin. North Am. 7:5, March 1972.

Jacobson, E.: *Adolescent moods and the remodeling of psychic structures in adolescence.* Psychoanal. Stud. Child 16:164, 1961.

Josselyn, I. M.: *Emotional implications of rheumatic heart disease in children.* Am. J. Orthopsychiatry 19:87, 1949.

Josselyn, I. M.: *The Adolescent and His World.* Family Service Association of America, New York, 1952.

Josselyn, I.: *The ego in adolescence.* Am. J. Orthopsychiatry 24:223, 1954.

Josselyn, I. M.: *The Happy Child.* Random House, New York, 1955.

Josselyn, I. M., Simon, A. J., Eells, E.: *Anxiety in children convalescing from rheumatic fever.* Am. J. Orthopsychiatry 5:109, 1955.

Kaplan, S., Achtel, R. A., and Callison, C. B.: *Psychiatric complications following open-heart surgery.* Heart Lung 3:423, 1974.

Kimball, C. P.: *Psychosocial aspects of cardiac disease in children and adolescents.* Heart Lung 2:394, 1973.

Langford, W. S.: *Psychologic aspects of pediatrics.* J. Pediatr. 33:242, 1948.

Lazarus, R. S.: *Psychological Stress and the Coping Process.* McGraw-Hill, New York, 1966.

Lowman, C. L. and Seidenfeld, M. A.: *A preliminary report of the psychosocial effects of poliomyelitis.* J. Consult. Psychol. 11:30, 1947.

Murphy, L. B.: *Coping devices and defense mechanisms in relation to autonomous ego functions.* Menninger Clinic Bulletin 24:144, 1960.

Mushatt, M. D.: *Mind-body-environment: Toward understanding the impact of loss on psyche and soma.* Psychoanal. Q. 44:81, 1975.

Newton, K.: III: *The nurse in poliomyelitis care.* Am. J. Nurs. 47:370, June 1947.

Opie, J.: *Over My Dead Body.* E. P. Dutton & Co., New York, 1957.

Peters, B. M.: *Threat appraisal by an adolescent girl undergoing surgical correction of scoliosis.* Maternal-Child Nursing Journal 5:167, 1976.

Pfaiffer, E. and Stevens, M.: *Weaning the respirator patient.* Am. J. Nurs. 56:454, April 1966.

Piaget, J. and Inhelder, B.: *The Psychology of the Child.* Basic Books, New York, 1969.

Porter, L. S.: *On the importance of activity.* Maternal-Child Nursing Journal 2:85, 1973.

Prugh, D. G., et al.: A study of the emotional reactions of children and families to hospitalization and illness. Am. J. Orthopsychiatry 23:70, 1953.

Riddle, I.: *Nursing intervention to promote body image integrity in children.* Nurs. Clin. North Am. 7:651, December 1972.

Schilder, L.: *The Image and the Appearance of the Body.* John Wiley & Sons, New York, 1958.

Seeley, E. F.: *Coping behavior of an immobilized eight year old.* Maternal-Child Nursing Journal 2:15, 1973.

Seidenfeld, M. A.: *II Psychological considerations in poliomyelitis care.* Am. J. Nurs. 47:369, June 1947.

Seidenfeld, M.: *Rehabilitation of the patient with poliomyelitis.* In Soden, W. H. (ed.): *Rehabilitation of the Handicapped.* Ronald Press, New York, 1949.

Spiegel, L.: *Comments on the psychoanalytic psychology of adolescence.* Psychoanal. Stud. Child 13:296, 1958.

Sutton, H. A., Falstein, E., and Judas, I.: *Emotional reactions to medical procedures and illness in a hospital child psychiatry unit.* Am. J. Orthopsychiatry 28:180-187, 1958.

Walters, A. and Marugg, J.: *Beyond Endurance.* Harper & Bros., New York, 1954.

Wessell, Sister Mary Louise: *Use of humor by an immobilized adolescent girl during hospitalization.* Maternal-Child Nursing Journal 4:35, 1975.

Winder, A. E.: *Normal adolescence: Psychological factors.* In Winder, A. E. (ed.): *Adolescence: Contemporary Studies,* ed. 2. D. Van Nostrand, New York, 1974.

# 5
# MIDDLESCENT OBESE WOMEN: OVERCOMING POWERLESSNESS

## JUDITH FITZGERALD MILLER

Middlescent individuals who have never been concerned about controlling food intake and balancing dietary discretion with adequate energy expenditure are likely to be either obese (weighing 20 percent more than their ideal body weight) or overweight (weighing more than ideal body weight but less than 20 percent more than ideal body weight). One third of middle-aged Americans are 20 percent overweight,[1] and the majority of these are women. At least one of every five Americans is overweight.[1] It is a discouraging fact that "most obese persons will not remain in treatment. Of those who remain in treatment, most will not lose much weight and of those who do lose weight, most will regain it."[3] In a well-known literature review, Stunkard and McLaren-Hume[4] found only eight significant obesity studies. The samples of the eight studies provided a population of 1368 subjects. Only 16 percent of the subjects lost between 10 and 20 lb; 12 percent lost between 20 and 40 lb; and 5 percent lost more than 40 lb. The efficient health professional is frustrated in not having fast, accurate answers to a problem that seems to be treated simply enough—by having patients stop putting excessive food into their mouths. However, this problem with a seemingly simple treatment is complex.

Very little is known about self-control and eating behaviors. Theories by both obese subjects and scientists have been proposed, such as a carbohydrate intolerance; the belief that when some persons eat a carbohydrate, they cannot stop[5]; appestat dysfunction, in which the satiety center that acts like a thermostat may be set higher than normal; underactivity[6]; obese eating behaviors learned as a child from obese or non-obese parents; and parents' possible use of food with children as a reward, a means of comfort during anxiety, or a relief from feeling blue.

This chapter will examine yet another combination of factors that influence obesity in middle-aged women: powerlessness and a developmental vulnerability to obesity. The main thrust is to present a variety of strategies that may be used to enable obese women to control food intake. Assessing obesity is a first consideration.

Obesity is determined in a number of ways. A simple measure is to look at the patient's physical appearance. A woman 5 ft 3 in tall who weighs 180 lb will *look* obese. An approximate ideal body weight can be calculated by using the following formula[7]:

$$\text{Approximate ideal weight for women} = (\text{Height in inches} \times 3.5) - 110.$$
$$\text{Approximate ideal weight for men} = (\text{Height in inches} \times 4) - 130.$$

Factors not considered in this formula include whether the body frame is large, medium, or small, and the muscle content of the body. (Athletes weigh more but have increased muscle mass.) Measuring skinfold thickness is an accurate determination of body fat. The triceps skinfold is measured at a midpoint between the elbow and shoulder. A man aged 35 to 50 should have a triceps skinfold of less than 23 mm and a woman aged 35 to 40 should have a measurement of less than 30 mm.[6] Any larger measurement indicates that the body mass contains more than 39 percent fat. Height and age charts according to body frame (Table 5-1) are also used as an ideal weight index.

# DEVELOPMENTAL VULNERABILITY

## Obesity in Women

There are specific developmental vulnerabilities to obesity that occur during infancy, adolescence, pregnancy, the middle years, and menopause. During these phases, the individual or parent must be aware of the tendency to gain weight and must exercise restraint in overeating or overfeeding.

During infancy, the number of adipose cells increases (hyperplasia) owing to overeating. The increased number of cells stays with the individual for life, causing an extreme lifelong risk of obesity. Obesity that occurs during adolescence and adulthood results in hypertrophy of existing cells and is a less resistant form of obesity. After infancy, the developmental hazards are unique to women.

During adolescence, the growth spurt stops; however, the estrogen level in girls continues and promotes fat formation. Fat is laid down in the breasts and hips and will continue unchecked if eating is not controlled. Girls gain weight during adolescence, and boys lose weight during this time.

Pregnancy is the most vulnerable time for permanent weight gain.[5] One third of obese women became obese in relation to pregnancy.[8] The increased appetite may remain with the woman after delivery, and breast-feeding mothers may overindulge during a time when excess calories are allowed. Once a woman is 10 percent heavier than her ideal body weight, she has the lifelong potential for becoming obese and must be constantly on guard against that predicament.[5]

During middle age, ages 35 to 55, physiologic changes occur. Muscle tone and skin tone diminish, and basal metabolic rate decreases. Two thirds of the obese men become

## TABLE 5-1. Desirable Weights (in Pounds)*

| Height with Shoes 1" heel | Men of Ages 25 and Over Small Frame | Medium Frame | Large Frame |
|---|---|---|---|
| 5 ft 2 in | 112–120 | 118–129 | 126–141 |
| 5 ft 3 in | 115–123 | 121–133 | 129–144 |
| 5 ft 4 in | 118–126 | 124–136 | 132–148 |
| 5 ft 5 in | 121–129 | 127–139 | 135–152 |
| 5 ft 6 in | 124–133 | 130–143 | 138–156 |
| 5 ft 7 in | 128–137 | 134–147 | 142–161 |
| 5 ft 8 in | 132–141 | 138–152 | 147–166 |
| 5 ft 9 in | 136–145 | 142–156 | 151–170 |
| 5 ft 10 in | 140–150 | 146–160 | 155–174 |
| 5 ft 11 in | 144–154 | 150–165 | 159–179 |
| 6 ft 0 in | 148–158 | 154–170 | 164–184 |
| 6 ft 1 in | 152–162 | 158–175 | 168–189 |
| 6 ft 2 in | 156–167 | 162–180 | 173–194 |
| 6 ft 3 in | 160–171 | 167–185 | 178–199 |
| 6 ft 4 in | 164–175 | 172–190 | 182–204 |

| Height with Shoes 2" heel | Women of Ages 25 and Over Small Frame | Medium Frame | Large Frame |
|---|---|---|---|
| 4 ft 10 in | 92–98 | 96–107 | 104–119 |
| 4 ft 11 in | 94–101 | 98–110 | 106–122 |
| 5 ft 0 in | 96–104 | 101–113 | 109–125 |
| 5 ft 1 in | 99–107 | 104–116 | 112–128 |
| 5 ft 2 in | 102–110 | 107–119 | 115–131 |
| 5 ft 3 in | 105–113 | 110–122 | 118–134 |
| 5 ft 4 in | 108–116 | 113–126 | 121–138 |
| 5 ft 5 in | 111–119 | 116–130 | 125–142 |
| 5 ft 6 in | 114–123 | 120–135 | 129–146 |
| 5 ft 7 in | 118–127 | 124–139 | 133–150 |
| 5 ft 8 in | 122–131 | 128–143 | 137–154 |
| 5 ft 9 in | 126–135 | 132–147 | 141–158 |
| 5 ft 10 in | 130–140 | 136–151 | 145–163 |
| 5 ft 11 in | 134–144 | 140–155 | 149–168 |
| 6 ft 0 in | 138–148 | 144–159 | 153–173 |

*Derived from Metropolitan Life Insurance Co. Build and Blood Pressure Study, Society of Actuaries, 1959, and from Bray, G.: *Obesity: Comparative Methods of Weight Control.* Technomic Publishing, Westport, Conn., 1980, p. 3.

obese during the middle years, whereas only one fourth of the women become obese during that time.[8] Aging causes the basal metabolic rate to decrease approximately 5 percent; so for every 10 years after age 25, the caloric intake should be decreased by 7.5 percent.[9]

During the middle years, life events that were previously controlled and that provided security and comfort may now be a source of anxiety and grief, for example, role reversal (middle-aged child caring for elderly, dying parents), young adult children leaving home and entering life-styles disapproved by parents, adolescent children experiencing developmental crises, marital strain, uncertainty of future, and feeling of unproductivity. Overeating may be the individual's means of coping with these stressors of middle years.

Weight gain from overeating may be insidious. Increasing food intake by 100 calories a day without increasing exercise will result in a 10-lb weight gain in 1 year.[10] The woman's attitude may be, "I've had three children; what do you expect my figure to look like?" This passive resistance blocks success in a weight-control program.

Weight gain may increase in women at menopause. At this phase of development, the obesity has been attributed to hormonal changes and decreased activity, as well as to depression.[11]

In addition to developmental vulnerability to weight gain, powerlessness is a factor in obesity.

# POWERLESSNESS AND OBESITY

Powerlessness (the perception that individual behavior will not affect outcomes) is a prevalent theme in obesity in two dimensions:

1. Powerlessness results when weight loss does not occur after attempts at dieting, and
2. Powerlessness is a factor that contributes to overeating.

Considering the first dimension, powerlessness is a perception that is confirmed in obese individuals after binging on "forbidden foods" or having lost no weight after a week without desserts. The lack of positive reinforcement of immediate weight loss as a result of what the obese person perceives to be a drastic change in eating behaviors contributes to powerlessness. The feeling that nothing the individual does will result in weight loss causes helplessness (powerlessness). The prevailing feeling of powerlessness causes the individual to give up trying and to return to overeating, feeling guilt and a sense of no control. Thus the cycle (Fig. 5-1) has been completed.

The key in breaking the cycle may lie in the nurse providing reinforcement for slightly altered behavior patterns and not focusing on weight loss. The patient needs to set realistic weight loss goals—no more than an *average* of a 2.5-lb loss per week. Helping the patient feel some sense of accomplishment in having changed the bedtime snack from an ice cream sundae to a more acceptable, lower-calorie treat is an example of positive feedback without anxiously waiting for the scale to record a 2-lb loss after 2 days of slight diet modification.

Powerlessness may not only result from weight loss failure but may also contribute to obesity in the first place. Individuals may have a lifelong pattern of behaviors resulting from powerlessness contingencies. "Powerlessness contingencies" refers to those psychosocial states that stem from a long-term perception of being unable to influence outcomes (being powerless). The psychosocial states prompt a behavior pattern that may result in overeating and little energy expenditure through exercise. These powerlessness contingencies may be categorized as self-induced and other-induced. Select contingencies of powerlessness and the resulting behavior pattern related to obesity are presented in Table 5-2. The self-induced contingencies are low tension tolerance, inabil-

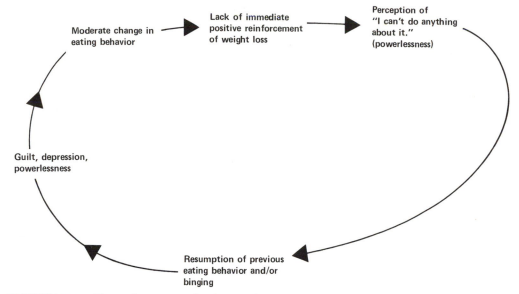

FIGURE 5-1.   Powerlessness obesity cycle.

ity to increase activity, inability to accurately identify and express emotions, self-depreciation, unconscious positive meanings of fatness, lack of insight into eating behavior, uninvolvement in caring for self, and lack of self-confidence. Examples of other-induced powerlessness contingencies are family interactions, parents' use of food as a reward, and stigmatizing reactions of persons in the social network. Although each powerlessness contingency results in a unique behavior pattern, the consequence is the same—overeating and underexercising. Powerlessness contingencies contribute to maladaptive behavior patterns that are so ingrained that changing them may be difficult, if not impossible. The ultimate consequence is obesity.

Some research findings reinforce the fact that powerlessness is a problem in obesity. McCall[12] noted that 169 refractorily obese women differed on the Minnesota Multiphasic Personality Inventory (MMPI) from the 181 Take Off Pounds Sensibly (TOPS) members who were successful with their weight-reduction program and who kept their weight within 5 percent of ideal body weight for 6 months. Women who were resistive to weight loss were found to have more:

—feminine dependence.
—touchiness.
—body overconcern.
—psychic hurting.
—somatization.
—rebelliousness.
—compulsive and ruminative tendencies.
—bizarre or confused thinking.

## TABLE 5-2. Powerlessness Contingencies and Consequences

| Powerlessness Contingencies | Behavior Pattern | Consequence |
|---|---|---|
| **Self-induced** | | |
| Low tension tolerance. | Recognizes or develops few or no alternatives for tension release. | Overeating. |
| Lacks ability to mobilize self to exercise. | Moves as little as possible in daily activities. No exercise routine. | Imbalance of energy intake and expenditure. |
| Lacks ability to identify and express emotions (anger, unhappiness, frustration). | Short circuiting vague feelings without clear identification of feelings. Interprets as a need for food.[32] | Overeating. |
| Self-depreciation. | Feelings of low self-esteem, depression. | Overeating. |
| Perceptions of fat as positive. | Feeling comfort in being obese as a protection from sexual exploitation; keeping part of their mother; and/or protection of husband's fears and jealousy of slimmer shapely wife.[26] | Overeating. |
| Lacks self-insight, awareness. | Unaware of eating behavior—quantity consumed, internal cues of hunger and satiation. Unaware of mood states. | Overeating. |
| Uninvolved in caring for self. | Detaches own behavior from outcomes —can do nothing about it attitude. "Whatever happens is beyond my control." | Overeating. |
| Lacks self-confidence. | Unusual dependence on other persons or things for self-satisfaction. | Overeating. |
| **Other-induced** | | |
| Family and society influences. | Use of food as rewards, overfeeding children, clean-the-plate syndrome from childhood. Use of alcohol and food to provide an unguarded, comfortable milieu in social encounters. | Overeating. |
| Stigmatizing reaction of persons in social network. | Withdrawal, reinforcement of poor self-concept. | Overeating. |

Although the findings of dependence lend some support to the powerlessness theory proposed in this chapter, McCall is quick to point out that we cannot determine whether the degrees of psychologic disturbance present in refractorily obese persons are antecedent or consequent to the obesity.

Powerlessness in obese individuals is reinforced by the stigmatizing behaviors of others. Obese people are automatically categorized as sloppy, weak willed,[13] nonproductive, lazy, slow paced, easygoing, jolly, and obsessed with oral gratification. Employers may view obese employees as a liability due to health risks (missed work days, insurance payments) as well as portrayal of a poor company image. In the American culture, obese persons are characterized as immature, passive, dependent, low in self-esteem, and responsible for their fatness. At the same time, obese persons do not appear to be assuming responsibility for adherence to prescribed weight-reduction programs. Physicians were found to have negative attitudes toward obese individuals,[14] which contributed to the dropout rate in weight-reduction programs. The obese subjects suffer shame and self-derogation when returning to the physician after failing to lose weight.[15] Thin people generally do not like obese people, and obese people do not like other obese persons.[13]

Reactions to condemnation by others lead the obese subject to conclude, "No one would want to be associated with me or seen in public with me." This negative self-talk reinforces individuals' perceptions that they are powerless even in maintaining close personal relationships. Stunkard and Mendelson[16] found through interviews with 74 obese subjects that obese persons experienced two behavior disorders. First, they overate; second, they experienced a disturbance in body image, that is, they felt their bodies were grotesque, loathsome, and viewed by others with contempt.

Eating behaviors of obese individuals may indicate no control. The fact that the obese have particular vulnerabilities and eating style has been supported[17-21] and refuted.[23,24] Because eating behavior may be drastically altered both in experimental conditions and when the subjects are eating in public, eating-style studies must be evaluated carefully. Obese persons overeat in privacy but seldom do so in public.[13] The obese person's susceptibility to food cues includes environmental stimuli of food sights, smells, familiar binging places, and time of day without regard to internal cues of hunger and satiety as signaled by blood sugar levels, gastric motility, and gastric stretch receptors.

Binge eating is sporadic, seemingly uncontrolled eating of large quantities of food associated with agitation and self-condemnation.[25] Orbach[26] describes compulsive (binge) eating by obese persons as eating when not physically hungry, feeling out of control around food, feeling awful about self as someone who is out of control, spending time thinking and worrying about food and fatness, scouring latest diets for new information, and feeling awful about their bodies. Eating is done quickly and usually furtively during binging.

Bruch[21] describes obese individuals not only as being unable to control eating but as having the feeling that other forces are in control of their life situation. Bruch goes on to state that obese persons do not correctly identify hunger and differentiate emotional feelings from hunger. A significant relationship between control and social responsibility and weight loss was found by Hartz and coworkers.[27] Women with low control and low social responsibility scores were less successful in weight control than were women with high control and high social responsibility. Rodin[28] found obese persons were more dependent on others and more persuadable than were persons of normal weight.

Persons who believed that they, rather than fate or others, were responsible for what happened to them lost weight at a significantly faster rate than did those who did not hold this belief.[29]

Eating styles of thin persons do not have characteristics of no control. Thin persons generally do not eat very quickly, nor do they take large bites, without stopping to taste the food. Life-styles and eating behaviors of thin persons need careful scrutiny so that the skills they have used to remain thin can be utilized in therapy for obese persons. Sundberg[13] determined that thin persons' skills included ability to balance exercise with energy intake, to discriminate between adequate and excessive food intake, to adhere to regular meal patterns and control snacking (keeping frequency and type of snack food controlled), to adapt to negative emotions by means other than using food, to accurately perceive how others view them, to obtain sexual satisfaction, and to make a conscious successful effort to control weight through understanding the impact of indiscriminate eating and drinking.

## Summary of Powerlessness and Obesity

Powerlessness is a factor in causing obesity, and powerlessness is a problem that results when individuals feel they have failed in a weight-loss program. Lack of control is also evident in the obese individual's eating style (vulnerability to food cues and so forth). The powerlessness contingencies presented provide an analysis of the etiology of over-eating. The research base on powerlessness and obesity is almost nonexistent. Studies need to be done to develop the nursing diagnostic category of powerlessness and to determine the relationship between powerlessness and obesity.

The terms obese, fat, and corpulent all have negative connotations and prompt a reaction of reproach from others. Bruch[21] describes obese persons as being under the influence of others and not in control of their bodies. Fat people talk about their bodies as being external to themselves; some do not feel identified with the bothersome ugly physical thing. The litany of excuses obese people use for not being able to lose weight also point to their perception of being powerless, not only in having gotten that way but also in recovering from obesity.

## MIDDLESCENT OBESE WOMEN

### Stressors Confronting Middle-aged Women

Most middlescent obese women became obese before reaching their middle years. The woman's obese state is either maintained or escalated during the middle years. The stresses of middle years* (ages 35 to 55 years) contribute to maladaptive behavior or successful coping. One example of maladaptation is overeating (Fig. 5-2). Stressors are those stimuli requiring adaptation. In middle-aged women, stressors may include caring for aging parents and parents-in-law; dealing with children becoming independent; having to resolve that previous nurturing patterns are no longer needed; feeling unproductive—handling new freedom without learning new skills; experiencing role conflicts from various factors such as social pressures for liberation; dealing with changing marital intimacy; managing physical changes that result in worry and preoccupation with health; and grieving over loss of youth. Each stressor will be discussed briefly.

The role reversal of middle-aged daughter now having to assume responsibility for care of aging parents creates stress, affects family harmony, and may cause feelings of resentment, guilt, or despair. In some instances, an ill single parent is displaced into the

---

*For a thorough analysis of the middle years, see Stevenson, J.: *Issues and Crises During Middl-escence.* Appleton-Century-Crofts, New York, 1977.

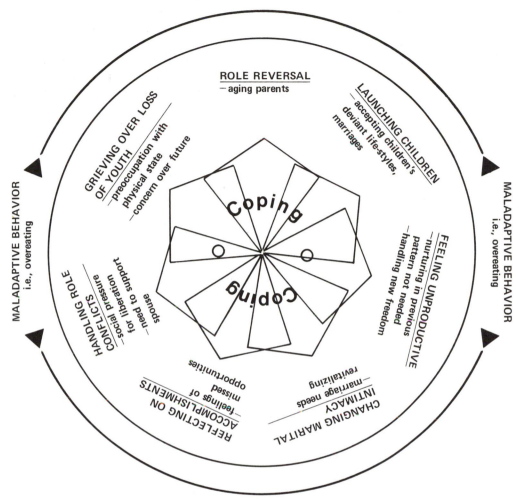

**FIGURE 5-2.  Stressors of middle-aged women.**

daughter's home or into a nursing home. Disrupted family systems, conflicts, and emotional energy expenditure take place in either instance.

At the same time, young adult children may be leaving home and beginning marriages, careers, and life-styles that the parents may oppose. The mother fully realizes that previous patterns of nurturing not only are no longer needed but also may be shunned by her offspring. New ways of finding satisfaction for mothering need to be learned. Obese middle-aged women who had no children *may* need to resolve a sense of loss over a missed opportunity to bear children.

Unless a woman has planned for and developed productive skills throughout her life, she may find herself feeling unneeded, unproductive, and unsure of her identity. Prock[30] describes the need for women to develop multiple anchors so that when one anchor (e.g., a dependent child) is gone, other anchors still provide a sense of stability and self-worth. These anchors prevent women from feeling adrift without direction. Examples of anchors may include having a job, maintaining developed social activities, and doing volunteer work.

Marital intimacy and the source of strength to each other that was once present in that marital bond *may* be waning during the middle years. As a result of routine, communication between husband and wife may be decreasing. Husbands may have well-established patterns of confiding in business associates or fellow workers, while wives may be caught up in activities they consider of no particular interest to men—PTA, household management, and the desire to talk about returning to school. Feelings are not shared, and sexual relationships become dull. New sources of conflict may arise, such as disagreement over each other's goals. Confirmation of affection may have disappeared from a humdrum marriage. Unless time and effort are spent to develop and share interests, few common interests will remain. The full-blown feeling of disenchantment after 20 years of marriage, although insidious in coming, has arrived. Eating may soothe the need for affection.

Coping with physical changes may precipitate a preoccupation with health. The changes may be anything from changes in the oral cavity (receding gum line), to graying of the hair, to pathologic conditions such as hypertension. These changes emphasize the realization that youth is lost.

The liberation of women in our society creates new pressures for women. Women may no longer reap self-satisfaction from supporting husbands in their successful careers. Women no longer move from school to higher education to home for child rearing, and then to low-paying jobs reserved for women when they are a stable work force (after childbearing years). Now women move from higher education to professions and child rearing, and remain in the productive work force. Multiple role expectations—children, career, spouse needs, and so forth—all create role strain. Women who have not been engaged in professions may feel a more intense pressure to be productive without having developed skills.

Although there may be a wide variety of responses to these stressors, one response is overeating. Obese individuals respond to stress by overeating, whereas thin people do not; on the contrary, a thin person's behavior during stress may be to eat less.

Being fat is a stressor in and of itself. Orbach[26] recorded her observations resulting from leading a therapeutic diet group with various women participants for 5 years. Some of the connotations fat had for these obese women included:

To be fat means to compare yourself to every other woman looking for the ones whose own fat can make you relax.
To be fat means to be excluded from contemporary mass culture, fashion, sports, and the outdoor life.
To be fat means to worry every time a camera is in view.
To be fat means having to feel ashamed for existing.
To be fat means having to wait until you are thin to live.
To be fat means to have no needs.
To be fat means to be constantly trying to lose weight.

To be fat means never saying "no."

To be fat means to have an excuse for failure.

To be fat means to wait for the man who will love you despite the fat—the man who will fight through the layers.[31]

Other life circumstances of middle-aged women may influence eating. There may be a change in exercise, with little physical energy expenditure taking place. The physical demands of a young family are gone. Boredom may be a result, with concomitant overeating. In a routinized marriage, there may be little motivation to maintain a sexually attractive appearance. There may also be misconceptions that interfere with weight loss, such as believing that losing weight may increase vulnerability to cancer and communicable diseases. A healthy appetite may be equated with general health, and quick complete satisfaction of appetite is needed to stay healthy. Frank rationalizations for overeating are used by some obese persons. Such rationalizations are described by Orbach[26] and include:

—fear that food will not be available later so must overeat now to tide me over.

—need to have something in my mouth.

—had a bad day so need to cheer up with noshing a pan of brownies.

—had a great day so I deserve one lemon pie.

—eating because it is the only way I know to give myself pleasure.

—there's nothing else to do in the evening.

Themes of using food to alleviate boredom, and as a tranquilizer, reward, and means of oral gratification are noted in the patient comments above.

## Uniqueness of Obesity in Women

Women are the fatter sex. Edelstein[5] explains that men burn twice as many calories as women do for the same amount of exertion. A man's body contains more muscle mass than a woman's body. Muscle requires five more calories per pound to maintain itself than fat or connective tissue. However, even though the woman's body requires half as many calories as a man's, the woman's appetite is the same as a man's.[5] The fat pad is necessary as a mechanism for food storage and heat protection during pregnancy for the fetus. Unfortunately, the extra fat is always with the woman, pregnant or not. Female hormones, estrogen and progesterone, are fat-producing, fat-hoarding hormones.

Generally, women have more exposure to food stimuli than men. In most households, women are responsible for planning appealing menus and spend a good deal of their time preparing food and "cleaning up" leftovers.

Obese women are more stigmatized than obese men. Fat men may be viewed as having authority and substance, whereas fat women are viewed as undisciplined slobs.[5]

In Orbach's[26] feminist viewpoint on obesity, she proposes three explanations for overeating in women: (1) Women with children are constantly giving to others, feeding the world, and feeling everyone else's needs are to be met first. The mother uses food as a means of replenishing herself. (2) Becoming fat is a rebellion against pressure to look and act shapely, and be sexually attractive to men. Fat is a protection from sexual exploitation. (3) Conflicts and ambivalences in mother-daughter relationships express themselves in fat. Eating serves as a source of love, comfort, and warmth, which may have been missing in the mother-daughter relationship. Fat may be viewed by some women as taking part of their mothers with them.

In our society, it may be more difficult for women than men to express anger in socially acceptable ways.[32] Women have also been socialized to be less assertive.[26] Women feel safer using their mouths to feed themselves rather than to talk assertively and thus satisfy internal frustration.

Some women equate their "good mothering" role with ability to provide delicious baked goodies ready to satisfy an adolescent's never-ending appetite. Efforts to maintain good communication with adolescents takes place, and mother's sharing the goodies is an example of spending time trying to show interest in, understand, and communicate with the child; at the same time, this extra effort is deleterious to ideal body weight.

The yo-yo effect of losing weight, gaining it back, losing, and gaining leads to giving up trying. The giving up phenomenon can be avoided if the refractory nature of weight loss is understood by patients and health workers. The basal metabolic rate (BMR) decreases by as much as 20 percent after a month of dieting.[25] Fewer calories are used to maintain the body's metabolic function. For example, an obese woman whose daily calorie intake is 2000 calories and whose BMR is 1400 calories with 600 calories activity expenditure is maintaining her obese state. If she goes on a 1000-calorie diet, she will have lost approximately 1 kg a week. The BMR adapts to a change in calorie intake and decreases by 20 percent, so that after 1 month the BMR is not 1400 calories but 1100. If the woman's activity level decreases, despite strict adherence to the 1000-calorie diet, weight loss will not continue.[25]

Still another reason for failure of dieting may be the patient's lack of understanding that a relatively unorthodox eating style is the cause of obesity. For example, night eaters consume excessive calories from dinner time until bedtime and have morning anorexia. They take pride in not eating throughout the day but eat excessively at night. The sudden glucose load is quickly absorbed and converted to fat. Calorie intake should remain moderate and spread throughout the day. A daily exercise routine is of paramount importance. Consuming all 1400 calories at once most likely will result in weight gain.

Whatever the underlying etiology, middle-aged obese women must struggle against weight gain and fight for control to maintain any weight loss achieved. This struggle for weight control must continue for the rest of their lives.

Powerlessness has been described as one component of obesity that both contributes to becoming obese and results from aborted attempts at weight reduction. The first goal should be to help the obese individual feel less powerless. Empowerment strategies nurses can use to help obese women will be discussed in terms of behavior therapy, physical activity, dietary counseling, assertiveness, and rational emotive therapy to handle the stressors of middle years.

# NURSING STRATEGIES—EMPOWERMENT OF THE OBESE

## Behavior Therapy

Behavior therapy means involving the individual to change an undesirable behavior to a desirable behavior. In obese persons, the undesirable behavior is overeating. There is no emphasis on uncovering intrapsychic conflicts or changing the personality structure. The focus is on changing the maladaptive behavior. Teaching the client self-application of techniques to change behavior enables the client to be in control.

Behavior is influenced by its consequences. Brightwell, Lemon, and Sloan[2] summarize the learning of specific behaviors through the sequence of stimulus, behavior, event, or reward reinforcement. The sequence of eating behavior is summarized in Figure 5-3.

The components of behavior therapy proposed for obesity control include obtaining an obesity profile; patient self-monitoring; environmental management; self-reinforcement; and contracts.

### OBESITY PROFILE

Obtaining a comprehensive understanding of the individual's eating behaviors, including the stimuli that prompt eating, is the first step in developing client and nurse insight into the unique patient situation. An obesity profile contains the following components: history of obesity, eating style, patient's social network, patient's knowledge, motivation, developmental stressors present, concept of self, need satisfaction and appropriate reward system, and analysis of assigned patient tasks (Fig. 5-4).

### SELF-MONITORING

The obese individual needs to be involved in analyzing the data gathered in the obesity profile. The goal is to begin to sensitize the client to her eating style. The client should develop an awareness of amounts and types of foods eaten, how food is eaten and in response to what stimuli, and the time of the day when the client is increasingly vulnerable to food cues and has an excessive appetite. When the appetite becomes excessive, as during the afternoon and evening, a plan for engaging in substitute activities needs to be made. For example, food preparation can take place in the early afternoon so that the woman is not exposed to food cues during the vulnerable time of day. An exercise routine can be employed during the vulnerable time. In discussing this with the woman, various substitute activities that are meaningful to her can be determined, for example, practicing the piano, doing the correspondence, gardening, and doing library work. Physical activity decreases appetite, so substituting such an activity would be beneficial.

Teaching the client record keeping is a good means of self-monitoring. The record, or diet diary, helps clients become aware of their behavior; it also helps control food intake because whatever clients put into their mouths is recorded on paper for themselves and

| Stimulus ———————➤ | Behavior ———➤ | Response |
|---|---|---|
| Desire to eat | Eating | Relief of hunger |
| Boredom, anger, anxiety | Eating | Relief of negative emotions |
| Depression | Eating | Alleviation of depression |
| Joy, elation | Eating | Continued pleasure |
| Food cues, sights, smells, environment | Eating | Relief of desire to eat |

FIGURE 5-3.   Sequence of learning eating behavior.

others to review. A variety of diary formats can be used. An example is given in Figure 5-5.

## ENVIRONMENT MANAGEMENT

Restricting food cues that signal eating is another aspect of behavior therapy.[20] This includes avoidance of fast foods, potato chips, candy, and ice cream by not having them in the house or easily accessible. Whenever possible, places and situations contiguous with eating are to be avoided. For example, the client should be advised not to take a coffee break in the snack room where workers share home-baked treats daily.

Having the client examine what prompts eating is helpful for developing insight. This includes becoming aware of whether eating occurs in response to the time of day, seeing other people eat, smells, low blood sugar, or increased peristalsis. Clients also need to know what prompts them to stop eating, such as extreme full feeling, having eaten all food, or seeing that eating companions have finished.

Other environmental management techniques, called cue elimination, include eating in the same room at home, using the same dishes and placemats, doing nothing else while eating, shopping from a list, and shopping only after a meal. Eating slowly, concentrating on what is eaten, setting the fork down between bites, using a smaller plate, eating with someone, and saving one item from a meal to eat later are all cue-suppression techniques.[33] Eating with the nondominant hand and swallowing each bite before eating another are techniques to help the overeater slow down.

The goals of environmental management are to increase cues that support discretionary eating patterns and to decrease cues that lead to overeating.

Mahoney and Mahoney[10] include responding to friends and family as social environment management. Significant others may be the obese person's worst support. Mahoney and Mahoney[10] describe four harmful patterns of reactions from loved ones.

1. Teasing about weight and size, and severely criticizing eating.
2. Open sabotage by offering high-calorie foods.

A. History
1. When did you become overweight (obese)?
2. Can you recall gaining weight associated with any particular event or period of development?
3. Family history of obesity—parents, sibilings, children, spouse?
4. Health problems present (thyroid disfunction, diabetes, hypertension, coronary artery disease).

B. Eating style
1. At what time/times during the 24-hour day are you more likely to overeat?
   When is your appetite the strongest?
   When is your temptation tolerance to food cues the lowest?
2. What types of stimuli prompt eating?
3. Are you aware of your own eating behaviors:
   Amounts of food consumed, size of bites, speed of eating; automatically take seconds?
4. Do you eat until you feel full?
5. Where are you located when eating your meals?

C. Social network
1. Who prepares meals?
2. Number of family members eating meals together or separately in the same home?
3. Are your significant others a help or deterrent to weight control?
4. Relationship with spouse?

D. Knowledge
1. What are the basic food groups?
2. What are your dietary excesses and deficits?
3. Do you understand the calorie restriction according to food exchange lists?
4. Awareness of caloric value of foods routinely and occasionally consumed?
5. What are the health hazards due to obesity?

E. Motivation
1. Whose idea was it to begin a weight-control program?
2. What has been your previous involvement with weight-control programs?

3. How long did you persist in trying to be successful in previous weight-control programs?
4. OBSERVATION—Does the client present a package of excuses for not losing weight in the past as well as how any new approach will not work?
5. What do you expect to accomplish in this weight-reduction program?

F. Developmental and life stressors
1. What have been your most stressful events during the past year?
2. How do you respond, cope with stress?
3. Developmental needs—adjustment.

G. Concept of self
1. Does the client use negative self-talk?
2. How would you describe your physical appearance?
3. Do you see yourself as being fat, slightly overweight, grossly overweight, obese?
4. Do you feel you are able to influence what happens to your weight?
5. OBSERVATION—Client behavior indicate high or low self-esteem?

H. Need satisfaction and reward system
1. Do you have a need for immediate satisfaction of needs and desires in all facets of life?
2. Do you find it necessary to satisfy hunger immediately?
3. What would be a positive reward for yourself when you have done a good job? (Preferably not food.)

I. Analyses of assigned client tasks
1. Explain self-monitoring and record keeping.
2. At later sessions review diet dairy (food intake, moods, times, places) for each 24-hour period. The number of days of self-recording depends upon how beneficial this direct feedback is to the client.
3. Provide appropriate feedback on analyses of client self-monitoring.

**FIGURE 5-4.  Obesity profile.**

3. Ignoring dieter's efforts.
4. Giving verbal support, yet demanding high-calorie treats to be on hand in the house.

Another harmful reaction is hypervigilant scale watching by a domineering spouse.

Nurses can help family members become sensitive to their influence on the obese loved ones. Because their behavior can facilitate success or failure, family members must cooperate. The assistance may include avoidance of any jokes and derogatory comments such as, "Not another diet." Family members must not offer food and eat empty calories (to be avoided by the dieter) in front of the overweight person. In some instances, open communication needs to be promoted so that food is not viewed as a display of affection. (I show my love for my husband by concocting luscious desserts!) The husband who is anxiety ridden about his wife's weight, expecting reports of foods consumed and daily weigh-in quotas while levying much critique and verbal abuse, is

| Date | Time | Food eaten, amounts | Calories | Place | Stimulus prompted eating | Related feelings before eating | Feelings after eating | Type and duration of exercise |
|------|------|---------------------|----------|-------|--------------------------|--------------------------------|-----------------------|-------------------------------|
|      |      |                     |          |       |                          |                                |                       |                               |

FIGURE 5-5.  Diet and activity diary.

supporting weight gain and may be the cause of overeating in the first place. The efforts of his behavior need to be reviewed by the nurse. His perceptions and anxiety state need attention as well.

## SELF-REINFORCEMENT

To maintain accurate monitoring and changes in behavior, a method of self-rewards should be determined. Types of rewards are endless, including enjoying solitude while listening to a favorite symphony, making a phone call to a friend, spending time at a hobby, or spending extra time relaxing in a bubble bath before dinner. One client who was very poor would walk to the newsstand and buy an evening paper on the days she was exceptionally good with her prescribed diet and exercise routine. Involving significant others in other types of rewards may be very helpful. For example, a husband may participate more in unpleasant household chores, such as scrubbing floors, when his wife has been successful in changing her eating behavior. Another self-reinforcement technique is having clients list adverse consequences of overeating and review this list. Reviewing the adverse outcomes helps counteract the pleasure of eating.[34]

## CONTRACTS

For some, reinforcement that is formally specified in a written contract is effective. An example of using a contract is described by Harris and Hallbauer.[34] Subjects were to decide on a reasonable amount of weight they would lose in 12 weeks and deposit a sum of money for each pound lost. Whatever amount the subject determined was acceptable. The money was refunded to the subject the week after the weight loss, providing the weight loss was maintained. The contract specified that any money remaining for failure to lose weight or dropping from the program was automatically forfeited. The forfeited money was equally divided among remaining group participants at the end of 12 weeks. Three groups with three conditions for weight control were compared after 12 weeks. Group 1 used a contract and was given information regarding diet; group 2 was given a contract and was counseled on diet and exercise; group 3 was a control group and met to discuss dieting problems. Group 2 experienced the most weight loss. The nonparticipants (dropouts) achieved significantly less weight loss than all three types of participants.[34] The contract approach weeds out obese persons who are not seriously motivated to lose weight.

# Physical Activity

Routine physical activities need to be reviewed by the obese woman, and a means of increasing calorie expenditure through daily exercise needs to be adopted. Obese individuals tend to expend less energy than thin persons during routine activities, that is, they move as little as possible. The mother may become aware that she is requesting the children to change the channel on the TV, bring a glass of water to her in the living room, walk to the mailbox, and so forth. The first step to increase activity is to simply move about more in daily routines. The next is to deliberately park two blocks away from the destination, walk the stairs instead of using the elevator, and incorporate some enjoyable physical outlet into the daily routine. Unless the new exercise is viewed as pleasurable, it will not be continued. The exercise must not be contradictory to the person's health state. The routine may become more firmly established if the exercise is combined with performing other roles, such as bike riding with the children to spend time with them and get exercise at the same time. Other examples include walking, running the dog, and renewing or establishing mutual interests with a spouse by taking up tennis or some other form of exercise of common interest. This may be the beginning of a whole new communication pattern for the couple and may help resolve one of the stressors of middle-aged women as identified in Figure 5-2. Estimated energy expenditure for selected physical activities is presented in Table 5-3 and also in Chapter 11, Table 11-2.

# Dietary Counseling

Clients need a basic understanding of nutritional values of foods, for example, how fats, proteins, and carbohydrates differ in caloric values. One gram of protein equals 4 calories, 1 gram of carbohydrate equals 4 calories, and 1 gram of fat equals 9 calories. One gram of alcohol contains 7 calories. Realizing how their own diets have deviated from required nutritional intake provides an initial insight. Edelstein[5] suggests the following dietary changes: (1) Obese women without other pathology need to eat 1000 calories a day to lose weight. (2) Spreading calories throughout the day is important because more weight is gained if 800 calories are consumed at dinner and 200 calories are eaten in the morning. Edelstein gives the following suggested breakdown: Breakfast—250 calories, lunch—250 calories, and dinner—500 calories. (3) Approximately 40 percent to 50 percent of the caloric intake should be protein.

Some clients tolerate dietary change and are more adherent in the long run when changes occur gradually. One major problem may have to be eliminated each week, such as omitting the ice cream at bedtime and substituting a lower-calorie carbohydrate such as a graham cracker.

The prescribed diet and environmental management techniques need to be given to the client in writing. The American Dietetic Association exchange list is a most effective means of teaching diet and ensuring variety in the diet. Consultation with a dietitian is needed so that an individual's calorie-restricted diet will incorporate nutritional requirements of the basic four food groups and will be individually tailored to the client's likes and dislikes.

**TABLE 5-3. Energy Equivalents of Food Calories Expressed in Minutes of Activity\***

| Food | Calories | Walking† | Riding bicycle‡ | Swimming§ | Running¶ | Reclining** |
|------|----------|----------|-----------------|-----------|----------|-------------|
| Apple, large | 101 | 19 | 12 | 9 | 5 | 78 |
| Bacon, 2 strips | 96 | 18 | 12 | 9 | 5 | 74 |
| Banana, small | 88 | 17 | 11 | 8 | 4 | 68 |
| Beans, green, 1 c | 27 | 5 | 3 | 2 | 1 | 21 |
| Beer, 1 glass | 114 | 22 | 14 | 10 | 6 | 88 |
| Bread and butter | 78 | 15 | 10 | 7 | 4 | 60 |
| Cake, 2-layer, 1/12 | 356 | 68 | 43 | 32 | 18 | 274 |
| Carbonated beverage, 1 glass | 106 | 20 | 13 | 9 | 5 | 82 |
| Carrot, raw | 42 | 8 | 5 | 4 | 2 | 32 |
| Cereal, dry, 1/2 c with milk, sugar | 200 | 38 | 24 | 18 | 10 | 154 |
| Cheese, cottage, 1 tbsp | 27 | 5 | 3 | 2 | 1 | 21 |
| Cheese, cheddar, 1 oz | 111 | 21 | 14 | 10 | 6 | 85 |
| Chicken, fried, 1/2 breast | 232 | 45 | 28 | 21 | 12 | 178 |
| Chicken, TV dinner | 542 | 104 | 66 | 48 | 28 | 417 |
| Cookie, plain | 15 | 3 | 2 | 1 | 1 | 12 |
| Cookie, chocolate chip | 51 | 10 | 6 | 5 | 3 | 39 |
| Doughnut | 151 | 29 | 18 | 13 | 8 | 116 |
| Egg, fried | 110 | 21 | 13 | 10 | 6 | 85 |
| Egg, boiled | 77 | 15 | 9 | 7 | 4 | 59 |
| French dressing, 1 tbsp | 59 | 11 | 7 | 5 | 3 | 45 |
| Halibut steak, 1/4 lb | 205 | 39 | 25 | 18 | 11 | 158 |
| Ham, 2 slices | 167 | 32 | 20 | 15 | 9 | 128 |
| Ice cream, 1/6 qt | 193 | 37 | 24 | 17 | 10 | 148 |
| Ice cream soda | 255 | 49 | 31 | 23 | 13 | 196 |
| Ice milk, 1/6 qt | 144 | 28 | 18 | 13 | 7 | 111 |
| Gelatin, with cream | 117 | 23 | 14 | 10 | 6 | 90 |
| Malted milk shake | 502 | 97 | 61 | 45 | 26 | 386 |
| Mayonnaise, 1 tbsp | 92 | 18 | 11 | 8 | 5 | 71 |
| Milk, 1 glass | 166 | 32 | 20 | 15 | 9 | 128 |
| Milk, skim, 1 glass | 81 | 16 | 10 | 7 | 4 | 62 |
| Milk shake | 421 | 81 | 51 | 38 | 22 | 324 |
| Orange, medium | 68 | 13 | 8 | 6 | 4 | 52 |
| Orange juice, 1 glass | 120 | 23 | 15 | 11 | 6 | 92 |
| Pancake with syrup | 124 | 24 | 15 | 11 | 6 | 95 |
| Peach, medium | 46 | 9 | 6 | 4 | 2 | 35 |
| Peas, green, 1/2 c | 56 | 11 | 7 | 5 | 3 | 43 |
| Pie, apple, 1/6 | 377 | 73 | 46 | 34 | 19 | 290 |
| Pie, raisin, 1/6 | 437 | 84 | 53 | 39 | 23 | 336 |
| Pizza, cheese, 1/8 | 180 | 35 | 22 | 16 | 9 | 138 |
| Pork chop, loin | 314 | 60 | 38 | 28 | 16 | 242 |
| Potato chips, 1 serving | 108 | 21 | 13 | 10 | 6 | 83 |
| Sandwiches: Club | 590 | 113 | 72 | 53 | 30 | 454 |

**TABLE 5-3.** *Continued*

| Food | Calories | Minutes of Activity | | | | |
|---|---|---|---|---|---|---|
| | | Walking† | Riding bicycle‡ | Swimming§ | Running¶ | Reclining** |
| Hamburger | 350 | 67 | 43 | 31 | 18 | 269 |
| Roast beef with gravy | 430 | 83 | 52 | 38 | 22 | 331 |
| Tuna fish salad | 278 | 53 | 34 | 25 | 14 | 214 |
| Sherbert, ⅙ qt | 177 | 34 | 22 | 16 | 9 | 136 |
| Shrimp, French fried | 180 | 35 | 22 | 16 | 9 | 138 |
| Spaghetti, 1 serving | 396 | 76 | 48 | 35 | 20 | 305 |
| Steak, T-bone | 235 | 45 | 29 | 21 | 12 | 181 |
| Strawberry shortcake | 400 | 77 | 49 | 36 | 21 | 308 |

*Reprinted with permission from Konishi, F.: *Food energy equivalents of various activities.* J. Am. Diet. Assoc. 46:186, 1965.
†Energy cost of walking for 150-lb individual = 5.2 calories per minute at 3.5 mph.
‡Energy cost of riding bicycle = 8.2 calories per minute.
§Energy cost of swimming = 11.2 calories per minute.
¶Energy cost of running = 19.4 calories per minute.
**Energy cost of reclining = 1.3 calories per minute.

Consuming preloads of food works for some people to decrease volume of food consumed at a subsequent meal. The preload, taken approximately 30 minutes before eating, should be low in calories and high in volume, for example, two or three glasses of water or diet soda or raw vegetables.[10]

Other strategies to control food intake may be helpful to some individuals. Have the obese client eat in front of a full-view mirror, paying attention to body size, double chins, rotund appearance, and so forth. Frustration tolerance needs to be developed so that the need for *immediate* need satisfaction is eliminated. Teach the client that instead of gratifying a perceived need for between-meal snacks by eating, she should set a timer for 10 or 15 minutes. When the timer rings, if the snack is absolutely necessary, have it—ideally, a food permitted on the diet and preferably something saved from a previous meal. Creating a different response to the stimulus to eat is helpful. In response to a need to have baked goodies, bake a favorite dessert and give it away.[17] Leaving a bit of each type of food on the plate helps to eliminate the clean plate signal to stop eating. However, this strategy is unacceptable to individuals conscious of food costs.

## Assertiveness

Assertiveness can be developed and used as a means of achieving control over life situations in general, thereby enhancing control over eating. "Assertion is any open expression in word or deed that leads others to consider seriously your desires. Assertive behavior is emotionally honest, direct, self-enhancing, and expressive."[35] Assertive behavior leads to self-respect and respect from others. Open, genuine, direct means of expressing self are characteristics of assertiveness. A goal of developing assertiveness is to enhance self-worth[36] to eliminate indirect, self-denying, and dishonest communication. The emotional reactions concomitant with low self-assertion are destructive to self-worth. Feelings of anxiety, anger, frustration, and guilt lead to generalized powerlessness, and the behavioral consequence may be overeating. Quereshi and Soat[37] found that persons addicted to alcohol were low in self-assertiveness. Self-assertion needs to be studied in persons addicted to food. Obese individuals cannot afford to be passive when others are suggesting and offering forbidden foods.

The four components of teaching assertiveness as identified by Lange and Jakubowski[38] are a useful guide in developing assertiveness in the obese individual. The components include:

1. Helping individuals identify needs, and their rights as well as the rights of others.
2. Helping individuals differentiate among assertive, aggressive, and passive behaviors.
3. Decreasing obstacles to assertive behavior—previous communication patterns learned throughout development, anxiety, guilt, low self-worth.
4. Trying out assertive behaviors in controlled-environment group practice.

In order to be successful with these components, individuals need to begin to think and talk positively about themselves. "When nonassertive behavior is practiced, high anxiety and low self-esteem are the result for all participants in the interaction."[39] It is hoped that obese individuals will cope with life situations by self-assertion and not by overeating.

## Rational Emotive Therapy and Stressors of Middle Age

Being able to accurately recognize thoughts related to events helps one to be able to control feelings resulting from the event. The identified stressors of middle years stimulate thoughts, feelings, and coping behaviors. Rational emotive therapy (RET) is effective in dealing with the stressors of middle years. If each stressor is rationally analyzed, the overeater's maladaptive behavior may be avoided.

The basis for RET is that control of emotions lies in the individual's thoughts about the precipitating event.[40] A goal of RET is to help clients think rationally, developing a realistic but not self-defeating outlook regarding the event; subsequently, coping behaviors will not be self-destructive or maladaptive as in overeating. Consider a stressor of middle years as an example:

A. (Event) Children leaving home.
B. (Thoughts) Isn't this awful?
C. (Feelings) Anxious, depressed, guilty over missed opportunities while children were home and dependent.

The cycle continues with the symptoms being the event:

A. (Event) Anxiety, depression, guilt.
B. (Thoughts) This is awful; I can't stand these feelings. This must stop.
C. (Feelings) Deepened depression, increased anxiety, and increased guilt.

The cycle may seem to be made temporarily tolerable to the individual by overeating (or using some other maladaptive behavior). Ellis[41] has added two more stages to RET with which the nurse can instrumentally help the client (1) disputing the irrational thoughts and (2) analyzing effects of the disputed thoughts.

D. Disputing or challenging irrational thoughts and beliefs. Continuing with the above example: Why is this awful? Why can't I stand this change? In what way does this normal developmental progression affect my own growth?
E. Analyzing the effects of disputing the thoughts and beliefs.
   1. It is not awful for young adult children to move out on their own.
   2. This change is a mark of maturity and independence in normal young adults.
   3. Love bonds are maintained and continue to be expressed.
   4. "This developmental progression marks new opportunities for me." This is the substituted self-talk.

Each stressor of middle-aged women can be confronted using RET. The desired end is abatement of overeating, a maladaptation to the stressors of middle years.

# SUMMARY

Physiologic hazards of obesity have been well documented in the literature, as have some psychosocial characteristics of obese individuals. This chapter proposed another variable—powerlessness—to be considered in analyzing the etiology and response pattern of obese persons. It is also proposed that a plan of empowerment strategies be designed and implemented as a weight-control program. The dimensions of this empowerment program for obese individuals include behavior therapy (use of obesity profile, self-monitoring, environment management, self-reinforcement, and contracts), physical activity prescriptions, dietary counseling, assertiveness training, and rational emotive therapy (RET). Because the impact of this program is being tested, the results are not yet available. The goal is to have clients realize they are their own best therapists. They have the ability to control food intake and exercise (weight), as well as many other aspects of their lives. Rodin and coworkers[29] state that believing that the individual is in control has proven beneficial in achieving significant weight loss.

# REFERENCES

1. Howard, L.: *Obesity: A feasible approach to a formidable problem.* Nursing Digest 4:86, Winter 1976.
2. Brightwell, D., Lemon, F., and Sloan, C.: *New Eating Behavior: Practical Management of Obesity.* Pennwalt Corp., Rochester, N.Y., 1975.
3. Stunkard, A.: Preface. In Stuart, R. and Davis, B.: *Slim Chance in a Fat World.* Research Press, Champaign, Ill., 1972.

4. Stunkard, A. and McLaren-Hume, M.: *The results of treatment for obesity.* Arch. Intern. Med. 103:79, 1959.
5. Edelstein, B.: *The Woman Doctor's Diet for Women.* Ballantine Books, New York, 1977.
6. Mayer, J.: *Overweight: Causes, Cost and Control.* Prentice-Hall, Englewood Cliffs, N.J., 1968.
7. Mahoney, M. and Mahoney, K.: *Permanent Weight Control: A Total Solution to the Dieter's Dilemma.* W. W. Norton & Co., New York, 1976, p. 13.
8. Kemp, R.: *The over-all picture of obesity.* Practitioner 209:654, 1972.
9. Williams, S.: *Nutrition and Diet Therapy.* C. V. Mosby, St. Louis, 1970.
10. Mahoney, M. and Mahoney, K.: *Permanent Weight Control: A Total Solution to the Dieter's Dilemma.* W. W. Norton & Co., New York, 1976.
11. Diekelmann, N.: *Primary Health Care of the Well Adult.* McGraw-Hill, New York, 1977.
12. McCall, R.: *MMPI factors that differentiate remediably from irremediably obese women.* Journal of Community Psychology 1:34, 1973.
13. Sundberg, M.: *Framework for nursing intervention in the treatment of obesity.* Issues in Mental Health Nursing 1:25, Fall 1978.
14. Maddox, G. L. and Liederman, V. R.: *Overweight as a social disability with medical implications.* J. Med. Educ. 44:214, 1969.
15. Stunkard, A. and Mendelson, M.: *Obesity and the body image: Characteristics of disturbances in the body image of some obese persons.* Am. J. Psychiatry 123:1296, 1967.
16. Ibid.
17. Bruno, F. J.: *Think Yourself Thin.* Nash Publishing, Los Angeles, 1972.
18. McDonald, M. D.: *Obesity: Why a losing fight?* Psychiatric News 12:27, 1977.
19. Stunkard, A. and Kaplan, D.: *Eating in public places: A review of reports of the direct observatin of eating behavior.* International Journal of Obesity 1:1, 1977.
20. Stunkard, A. and Penick, S.: *Behavior modification in the treatment of obesity.* Arch. Gen. Psychiatry 36:801, 1979.
21. Bruch, H.: *Eating Disorders.* Basic Books, New York, 1973.
22. Schacter, S.: *Some extraordinary facts about obese humans and rats.* Am. Psychol. 26:129, 1971.
23. Mahoney, M. J.: *Fat fiction.* Behavior Therapy 6:416, 1975.
24. Adams, N., et al.: *The eating behavior of obese and nonobese women.* Behav. Res. Ther. 16:225, 1978.
25. Straw, W. and Sonne, A.: *The obese patient.* J. Fam. Pract. 9:317, 1979.
26. Orbach, S.: *Fat is a Feminist Issue.* Berkley Publishing, New York, 1978.
27. Hartz, A., et al.: *A study of factors associated with the ability to maintain weight loss.* Prev. Med. 8:471, 1979.
28. Rodin, J.: *Research on eating behavior and obesity: Where does it fit in personality and social psychology?* Personality and Social Psychology Bulletin 3:333, 1977.
29. Rodin, J., et al.: *Predictors of successful weight loss in an outpatient obesity clinic.* International Journal of Obesity 1:1, 1977.
30. Prock, V.: *The mid-stage woman.* Am. J. Nurs. 75:1019, June 1975.
31. Orbach, op. cit. pp. 32-33.
32. McCall, R. and Siderits, M. A.: *Becoming a Graceful Loser: Psychological Factors in Weight Control.* TOPS Club, Milwaukee, Wis., 1977.
33. Stuart, R.: *A three-dimensional program for the treatment of obesity.* Behav. Res. Ther. 9:177, 1971.
34. Harris, M. and Hallbauer, E.: *Self-directed weight control through eating and exercise.* Behav. Res. Ther. 11:523, 1973.
35. Stuart, R.: *Act Thin, Stay Thin.* W. W. Norton & Co., New York, 1978, pp. 126-127.
36. Gareri, E.: *Assertiveness training for alcoholics.* J. Psychiatr. Nurs. 17:31, January 1979.
37. Quereshi, M. and Soat, D.: *Perception of self and significant others by alcoholics and nonalcoholics.* J. Clin. Psychol. 32:189, 1976.
38. Lange, A. J. and Jakubowski, P.: *Responsible Assertive Behavior: Cognitive Behavioral Procedures for Trainers.* Research Press, Champaign, Ill., 1976.
39. Herman, S.: *Becoming Assertive.* D. Van Nostrand, New York, 1978, p. 129.

40. Ellis, A.: *Rational-emotive therapy.* In Corsini, R. (ed.): *Current Psychotherapies.* F. E. Peacock Publishers, Itasca, Ill., 1979, pp. 185-229.
41. Ellis, A.: *Humanistic Psychotherapy: The Rational Emotive Approach.* Julian Press, New York, 1973.

# SELECTED READINGS

Allon, N.: *The stigma of overweight in everyday life.* In Bray, G. (ed.): *Obesity in perspective, Vol. 2, Part 2.* Department of Health, Education and Welfare, Washington, D.C., 1973.

Bellack, A.: *Behavioral treatment for obesity appraisal and recommendations.* In Herson, M., Eisler, R., and Miller, P. (eds.): *Progress in Behavior Modification, Vol. 4.* Academic Press, New York, 1977, p. 38.

Mahan, K.: *Sensible approach to the obese patient.* Nurs. Clin. North Am. 14:229, June 1979.

Maiman, L., et al.: *Attitudes toward obesity and the obese among professionals.* J. Am. Diet. Assoc. 74:331, 1979.

Stevenson, J.: *Issues and Crises During Middlescence.* Appleton-Century-Crofts, New York, 1977.

# 6

# POWERLESSNESS IN THE ELDERLY: PREVENTING HOPELESSNESS

JUDITH FITZGERALD MILLER
CHRISTINE BOHM OERTEL

Aging is basic to the human experience. It is a process that begins at the moment of birth and continues until death. The losses and stresses experienced by the elderly make them vulnerable to powerlessness.[1] The increased vulnerability of the elderly is related to their having fewer intact resources than do individuals in the middle years or young adulthood. For example, the elderly may have less physical strength and reserve, decreased psychologic stamina (resiliency), and diminished social support network; lower self-esteem; decreased energy; and in some instances, less motivation to improve their health or adhere to medical prescriptions. (See patient power resources model, Fig. 1-1, Chapter 1.) Coping resources of the elderly are challenged by sociologic, physiologic, and psychologic stressors. For example, financial management is a stress because many elderly exist near poverty levels on fixed incomes during inflationary periods. Approximately 18 percent of persons over age 65 are living beneath the poverty level.[2] Maintaining adequate housing may be difficult. Other sociologic stressors include maintaining social contacts, getting to and depending on public transportation, gaining access to continuous health care, maintaining nutrition, and combating stereotypes and myths imposed by a youth-oriented society.[3,4]

Psychologic stressors include demands to adapt to rapid change inherent in our Western society.[5] In addition to the stress of living in a "fast-paced" society, the elderly have to deal with changes resulting from unexpected losses such as deaths, retirement, and relocation (a move to a different city, to retirement complexes, or to nursing homes). Decreased sensory acuity may lead to misinterpretation of stimuli, suspicion, and withdrawal,[3] especially after relocation to a strange environment. Maintaining protection from victimization of crime[6] and dealing with other fears, such as personal injury from falls or accidents, are other examples of psychologic threats.

Physiologic stressors include adapting to multiple structural and functional losses. Physiologic changes of aging will be highlighted later as a cause of perceived powerlessness in the elderly.

The purpose of this chapter is to examine powerlessness as a behavioral variable in the aging person threatened by chronic illness and hospitalization. Case studies are included to depict situational powerlessness in the elderly and to portray the devastating consequence of uncontrolled powerlessness. When powerlessness is not contained, a self-destructive cycle of powerlessness-depression-hopelessness occurs, which may hasten death.[7] The powerlessness-hopelessness cycle is illustrated in Chapter 16, Figure 16-3. Identifying powerlessness in the elderly in order to intervene and prevent hopelessness is of critical importance for nurses. Being able to identify patients' perceived situational powerlessness is the first step. The initial development of a behavioral assessment tool to identify powerlessness in the hospitalized elderly is included in this chapter. It is beyond the scope of this chapter to present analyses of biologic, psychologic, and sociologic theories of aging.

# DEVELOPMENTAL VULNERABILITY

## Powerlessness in the Elderly

Various factors cause powerlessness in the elderly. Langer and Benevento[8] classified contextual events that may render a person "helpless." These contextual events include (1) being assigned a label that connotes inferiority in relation to other persons, (2) engaging in a consensually demeaning task, and (3) no longer engaging in a previously reinforcing, valued task. When applied to the elderly, examples of each contextual event easily come to mind. Elderly persons are the targets of many false labels, myths, and stereotypes. They are characterized as being rigid, inflexible, intolerant, and senile.[9]* Other myths that aging is a decremental process rendering the victim unteachable, asexual, less than beautiful, and unable to actively participate in one's own health care,[11] as well as unable to grow emotionally,[3] destroy self-esteem, cause inferiority, and induce powerlessness. Many elderly persons internalize these beliefs imposed by others in their social spheres.[3]

When assigned a consensually demeaning task, as may occur when elderly persons live with offspring or in nursing homes, the elderly individual erroneously infers self-incompetence. If a task of sealing envelopes is viewed as unimportant, elderly persons could conclude that they are incapable of doing anything more important. If the elderly person who is living with a son, daughter-in-law, and family is included in household activities only by being asked to make his or her own bed but is capable of much more, the elderly individual feels self-incompetence and helplessness.

---

*Shanas and Maddox[10] point out that senility caused by organic brain disease occurs in only 2 percent of the population at age 65.

No longer engaging in tasks that are reinforcing to the individual may occur after retirement. That is, the individual may not be able to make a transition from a work-centered role to a leisure-centered role[12] and maintain a feeling of self-worth and importance to others.

Chronic illness in the elderly is another cause of powerlessness. Kalish[2] states that 85 percent of persons over age 65 report at least one chronic illness, and about 50 percent of these report limitation of desired activity because of chronic health problems.

Roy[13] describes the elderly as having a constricted sphere of influence and control that increases powerlessness. ''Independence, or the ability to provide for one's needs, is the most important aim of the majority of the elderly regardless of their state of health.''[14] When this goal is fulfilled, a sense of control, or powerfulness, can result. Frustration of this goal leads to powerlessness. Powerlessness is frequently experienced by aging persons in our culture and is a prominent nursing diagnosis of elderly persons admitted to acute-care facilities. The aging person is vulnerable to powerlessness because of physiologic and psychosocial changes inherent in the aging process.

## OVERVIEW OF PHYSIOLOGIC AND PSYCHOSOCIAL CHANGES OF AGING

Aging is a time marked by multiple losses and multiple changes. The onset of these losses varies from individual to individual and is not correlated with any specific chronologic age. There seems to be a reduction in the reserve capacity for the aged person to adapt to changes and to stress. This reduction occurs at a time when there is a corresponding increase in the number and intensity of stressors in the person's life. The changes accompanying aging demand an adaptive response and represent a potential source of powerlessness. Because the changes are multiple, only a limited overview is provided in this chapter.

As the human organism ages, sensory changes occur. Changes in vision include decreased peripheral vision, decreased color perception, increased threshold for light stimulation, increased intraocular pressure, and presbyopia. There is a decreased pupil accommodation and diminished pupil size. Changes in hearing include lessened ability to hear high tones and to differentiate sounds. Aging also results in a marked decrease in the sense of taste. By age 75, there is a 64 percent loss of taste buds.[15] Taste buds that detect bitter and sour remain intact.[16] This increased sensitivity to bitterness and decreased sensitivity to sweetness and saltiness may account for some dietary indiscretion in the elderly; however, further research is needed.[17] Although there are reports of a marked decrease in the sense of smell,[15] there is wide variation from person to person.[17] Olfactory acuity is influenced by environmental toxins and occupational odors that have been present throughout the individual's life. The sense of touch also becomes less acute, with a steady loss of peripheral pain perception.

The aging person must cope with an altered body image. The person in the mirror, as well as the person trying to fit into clothes, may not be the person the individual expects to see. It is not uncommon for older persons to remark about still feeling like 35 until they look in the mirror or attempt to do what they were able to do at age 35. The alteration of body image results from changes such as loss of subcutaneous tissues, atrophy of muscle, skin dryness, decreased skin elasticity and thickness, decreased number of sweat glands, atrophy of hair follicles with hair loss, loss of pigment in hair and skin, increased angularity of the body, degenerative joint changes, and a shortening or stooping posture related to the narrowing of the vertebral disks. The loss of subcutaneous fat accounts for the elderly person's sensitivity to cold.[18] If tooth loss occurs, it is usually due to change in supportive structures, that is, gingival recession and bone osteoporosis, not tooth decay.[18]

Important physiologic changes occur in the cardiovascular system. As aging occurs, there is a decrease in cardiac efficiency despite a lack of change in heart size. Heart valves become thick, rigid, and less effective. The cardiac rate at rest may be similar to that of a younger adult, but under stress it does not increase as much and takes longer to return to normal. Arterial changes include elongation, fibrosis, and calcification. There can be a decreased blood flow to organs such as the kidney, liver, heart, and brain because of arterial changes. Blood pressure may have a higher normal value resulting from increased arterial resistance.

The lung tissue of the older person becomes less elastic. This results in about 40 percent decline in the mechanical efficiency of air exchange.[19] There is also a decreased capacity for oxygen uptake by the red blood cells. Respirations are further compromised by limited lung expansion related to musculoskeletal changes and resulting posture change—stooping.

The reabsorptive and excretory abilities of the kidneys decrease. The kidneys are less able to concentrate urine and thus prevent dehydration. There is a slowed compensatory response to acid-base shifts and altered chemical composition of the blood.

The individual's homeostatic mechanisms become less effective with age. Imbalances tend to develop more easily. A longer period is needed to restore equilibrium. A greater degree of deviation can result from a much lesser provocation with less tolerance. There is a diminished reserve capacity of organs and tissues.

The accumulative effect of these physiologic changes can mean decreased functional ability, diminished energy stores, and an overall lessening of speed and efficiency. Because these changes occur gradually, the individual is usually able to adapt to them, maintaining a sense of powerfulness. When these changes are complicated by the presence of one or more chronic pathologic conditions, the individual's ability to adapt successfully may be impaired. Loss of control or an inadequate knowledge base regarding the changes increases the aging individual's vulnerability to powerlessness. One author describes old age as "a time for savoring life, the world, and all that is in it. It is a time for making peace with oneself and the universe."[20] In reality, for many, aging may not result in such a beautiful experience.

Aging can threaten one's self-concept. The restrictions imposed by the social and cultural environment may deny the individual prestige and authority. Security may be bought at the price of loneliness and inactivity. According to Rynerson,[21] who completed a review of literature on self-esteem and the elderly, lower-level needs for food and safety may be met, while higher needs for affection, social recogntion, and a role in society in which to maintain dignity, self-worth, and self-satisfaction may be neglected. Enhancing self-esteem would mean "generating attitudes that lead to one's feeling of being useful and necessary in the world."[21] Maintaining self-esteem in the elderly combats despair and promotes successful attainment of the developmental task of ego integrity versus despair.[22]

Psychosocial losses of aging may include loss of former roles and status, loss of family members and friends, loss of economic security, and loss of familiar surroundings. In addition, there may be loss of health and function. The number of significant others in the older person's life may be reduced, compromising the individual's loving support system. Diminished physiologic reserves may force the individual into social isolation. The elderly person may be forced to face fears, dependency, chronic illness, and death alone. The aging person may respond to these overwhelming odds with perceived powerlessness and eventual despair.

As persons become more dependent on outside agencies for assistance, the individual's decision-making role and personal control are usurped.[23] The stressors that alter the elderly person's perceived control are specifically pertinent for this chapter. The following research reviewed is limited to perceived control in elderly subjects.

## Research on Control and the Elderly

Schulz[24] studied the effect of increased predictability and control on physical and psychologic well-being of 40 elderly subjects living in a retirement home. Subjects were randomly assigned to one of four college student visit conditions: (1) subjects were in control of frequency and duration of visits; (2) subjects were informed when they would be visited and how long the visit would last (subjects in this group could predict this event); (3) subjects experienced a random visit schedule; and (4) subjects were not visited. Subjects in the predictable- and control-visit groups had significantly higher hope levels, less time lonely, less time bored, greater zest for life, and greater happiness, usefulness, and activity level than subjects in the no-treatment and random-visit groups. Schulz concluded that the decline in physical and psychologic status associated with aging may be inhibited or reversed by providing residents with predictable or controllable positive events. Schulz and Hanusa[25] did a follow-up study on these same subjects. Data on physical and psychologic status were collected 24, 30, and 42 months after completion of the 1976 study. No positive long-term effects attributable to the interventions were found. Instead, those persons who initially benefited from the interventions exhibited precipitous declines after the study was terminated, and those subjects who showed no improvement in the original study remained stable in physical and psychologic functioning over time. Schulz and Hanusa[25] warn other researchers engaged in similar field studies to provide substitute predictable and controllable events after treatment conditions of control are terminated.

The effects of enhanced personal responsibility and choice on alertness, activity participation, and overall sense of well-being were studied in 91 ambulatory nursing home residents.[26] Subjects were assigned to two treatment groups. The first group was given a communication by the nursing home director emphasizing self-responsibility and decision making regarding their environment and activities. Subjects in this group were given a plant they selected and were then responsible for the plant care. Subjects in the other treatment group were given a message that emphasized staff's responsibility for them. These subjects were given a plant the staff tended. Subjects in the responsibility-induced group were significantly more active, alert, happy, and generally improved. The improvement rating was determined by nurses' blind rating. No significant difference was found on the perceived-control measure between the two treatment groups.

Rodin and Langer[27] did an 18-month follow-up study on 26 of the subjects from Langer's 1976 study.[26] Those subjects in the control-induced group had sustained beneficial effects. Mortality showed a striking difference in that only 7 (15 percent) of the 47 subjects in the responsibility-induced group had died during the 18 months, whereas 13 (30 percent) of the 54 subjects of the comparison (staff-controlled) group died. Significant difference was noted at the 0.01 level.

A study of 50 residents in a home for the elderly was done to determine predictors of residents' self-reported morale. Variables considered were the resident's perceived degree of choice in moving to the home, perceived degree of choice currently existing in the home, and amount of time spent in social interactions weekly, as well as age, income, recent loss of a significant other, and length of time at the home. The only significant predictors of morale were perceived choice within the home and amount of time spent in social interactions each week. Those residents who perceived greater choice and who spent more time in social interactions reported higher levels of morale.[1] Fuller emphasized that current opportunity to make choices is predictive of well-being. Opportunities for resident decision making can be provided by nurses.

Chang[28] found that of 30 nursing home residents studied, those who perceived themselves in control of their immediate situations as determined by the Situational Control of Daily Activities scale[29] had higher morale scores regardless of their internal or external personality orientations. Self-determination (person's own control of daily activities) resulted in higher morale for subjects with both internal and external locus of control orientations. In a similar study, Chang[30] examined congruence of locus of control and the patient's perceived situational control with morale in 39 patients in skilled nursing facilities. All subjects completed a self-rating of their health. Internals who rated their health as "fair" and whose locus of control was congruent with their perception of having situational control had high morale compared with the incongruent group ($p=0.04$). No significant differences were found in subjects with health ratings other than "fair." Of the externals with "fair" health ratings, incongruent subjects had low morale more frequently than did the congruent subjects (0.03). No differences were found in terms of comparisons of race or sex. Chang also found a strong correlation between internality and high morale (0.05 level of significance).

In other studies of locus of control and the elderly, external locus of control correlated with depression,[31] and internal locus of control correlated with a positive self-concept.[32] Ziegler and Reid[33] confirmed that desired control is related to psychologic adjustment. Desired control was significantly negatively correlated with depression and positively correlated with health, knowledge of services for the elderly, and use of services for the elderly in 88 elderly community residents. The researchers also studied 77 elderly men in a chronic-care hospital ward. Desired control was significantly positively correlated with life satisfaction, self-concept, tranquility, and subject senescence.[33]

In studying 72 elderly retirees, Brodie[34] found that the greater the subject's fearfulness, the less social activity the individual had. In addition, it was surprising to find that the greater the internality of locus of control, the less social activity the person experienced.

Bradley[35] studied locus of control in 306 subjects whose ages ranged from 19 to 90. Locus of control in three areas of activity—intellectual, social, and physical—was studied. Bradley found that subjects over age 60 perceived themselves as having less control in the social area than did subjects in the 35-to-50 age-group.

## POWERLESSNESS-HOPELESSNESS-DEATH

Loss of hope can have catastrophic consequences by hastening death.[7] Seligman reviewed studies of death from helplessness in animals and anecdotes of death from to helplessness-hopelessness in humans. Death was documented to have occurred in humans soon after death of a spouse, parent, or loved one; after loss of status; and during times of extreme threat. In all instances, the subjects were described as helpless.[7] Seligman warns that loss of control that accompanies hospitalization further weakens a sick person and may cause death. "We should expect that when we remove the vestiges of control over the environment of an already weakened human being, we may well kill him."[36]

Rowland[37] completed a review of literature to determine the effect of three environmental events on death of the elderly. The three events were (1) death of significant others, (2) relocation, and (3) retirement. The research reports reviewed suggest that death of a significant other and relocation may predict death for the elderly under certain circumstances. Relocation predicted death for those elderly who were in poor physical health, which may or may not have been accompanied by poor mental health. Forced relocation may remove the last perceived control the elderly had over situations and events.[7] Death of a significant other seems to predict death under certain conditions. The risk of death is greatest during the first year of bereavement, and Rowland's summary suggests the risk is higher for men than for women. The suggestion that those elderly who have few contacts with others may be more likely to die needs investigation. No conclusive evidence existed regarding retirement as a predictor of death in the studies reviewed by Rowland.[37]

## NURSING IMPLICATIONS

Any action that promotes elderly persons' maximum control over their lives will maintain or improve overall well-being[1] and may have an effect on life expectancy. Simple measures to enhance perceived control in a nursing home include providing the resident with food selection alternatives, having the resident decide on the schedule for hair appointments, or enabling the resident to request specific works from an assortment of library offerings. Meaningful control measures can be assumed by residents of nursing homes according to their own desires but should not be of a temporary nature serving someone else's best interest. Meaningful activities could include:

—caring for plants.
—surveying residents for activity desires or other needs.

—providing scheduled companionship time with more disabled residents.
—delivering mail; reading it to visually impaired.
—organizing a monthly newsletter.
—recognizing residents' birthdays by planning specific events or surprises.
—sharing favorite recipes.
—conducting musical evenings (playing "old favorites" on records or piano).
—helping others with correspondence.
—organizing discussions after and about the national news on television.
—planning field trips.

The residents themselves could devise creative activity lists based on their own talents and interests.

The elderly person can be helped to realize retirement is a fulfilling, self-enriching time to "savor life." Without some specific preparation for retirement, the newly found freedom may fade into disenchantment and depression.[12] Nurses in all practice settings, especially community agencies, may have specific responsibilities for promoting elderly persons' health through satisfying use of leisure time, helping persons recognize leisure as a "personally significant" self-actualizing activity. Community health nurses also help the elderly take advantage of resources geared to them, for example, senior citizen centers, meal programs for the elderly, and special transportation services. The elderly are to be provided with the options for decision making for various needs, such as using resources, engaging in activities for the elderly, and relocating or modifying living environments. Emphasis is to be given that the elderly person can make the decision.

Aging persons may need to look beyond self to find meaning and order in their lives and to resolve fears of death. To meet this need, religion may take on new importance.[38] The nurse can discuss spiritual well-being and ways appropriate for individuals to attain this well-being (prayer, meditation, religious rituals, reading the Bible and/or religious writings, listening to tape recordings on faith, and so forth). Despair is incongruent with spiritual well-being. Feeling a relationship with God combats loneliness.[40]

Assessment of manifestations of powerlessness in the elderly is important so that early and accurate nursing diagnoses can be made and appropriate interventions can be implemented. Roy[13] states that the indicators of powerlessness include apathy, withdrawal, resignation, fatalism, malleability, anxiety, restlessness, sleeplessness, wandering, aimlessness, and lack of decision making. Because these behaviors could be indicative of many nursing diagnoses, validation of the nurses' clinical impressions by using a valid, reliable tool is desirable.

## PERCEIVED CONTROL ASSESSMENT TOOLS FOR THE ELDERLY

Specific tools to measure situational control in the elderly have been developed.[29,32] Chang's tool[29] was developed to measure elderly subjects' situational control in institutional settings. Situational control refers to the perception that either the individual or others determine the use of time, space, and resources in daily activities.[41] The Situational Control of Daily Activities (SCDA) scale has two factors: (1) control of socializing and privacy, and (2) control of physical care. Test-retest reliability was 0.96. Subjects respond to questions about eight activities in terms of whether they themselves or others control the activities. The activities include ambulating, dressing, eating, grooming, socializing in a group, socializing in a twosome, using the toilet, and performing solitary activities. This tool is a valuable contribution for nurses to use in validating the elderly's perceived situational control.

A General Health Status (GHS) scale for the elderly was developed by Haney and coworkers,[42] and its validity and reliability have been established. The tool was correlated with a detailed valid Physician Assessment of Health Status scale. The GHS is a simply constructed tool in which subjects respond to 27 questions indicating whether they have trouble with the item by marking "yes," "no," or "don't know." There are 11 items related to day-to-day activities, such as "putting on or tying shoes," "going up stairs," "remembering things," "bathing," "preparing meals," and so forth. There are 16 items dealing with health problems, for example, "cannot sleep through the night," "trouble seeing," "trouble starting or stopping urine," and "swollen feet." The 11 items about daily activities are helpful in alerting the nurse to problems of control for the elderly individual.

Reid, Haas, and Hawkings[43] developed a tool to measure locus of desire and expectancy for control in the elderly. The tool was situationally specific (instead of measuring an enduring personality trait of locus of control) and considered the immediate environment as well as desires and interests of the subjects. Subjects rated each of 14 items on a Likert-type scale. For example, "How desirable or important is it for you to be able to decide on your own daily activities?" is an item on the interest and/or desires component of the tool. Subjects rated the item as (1) not important/desirable, (2) somewhat important/desirable, (3) generally important/desirable, or (4) very important/desirable. The same question is rephrased on the expectancy component of the tool: "How often can you decide what your daily activities are going to be?" Subjects respond by answering (1) never, (2) sometimes, (3) quite often, or (4) always.

In studies of institutionalized elderly persons, positive self-concept as determined by the Schwartz and Tangri scale correlated positively with internal locus of control using the Reid, Haas, and Hawkings scale. Internality also correlated positively with nurses' ratings of subjects' happiness, and with subjects' self-ratings of contentment and happiness. Negative correlations were found between internality and length of residency in the nursing home and age.[32]

Ziegler and Reid,[33] using the desired-locus-of-control scale, confirmed that desired expectancy for control is related to psychologic adjustment in their studies of 88 elderly community residents and 77 elderly residents in a chronic-care hospital ward.

Many other health assessment tools can be modified for appropriate use with the elderly.[44] The following clinical examples further illustrate the impact of powerlessness. Patient behaviors and literature reviewed provide the base for developing a behavioral assessment tool for powerlessness in the elderly.

# CLINICAL DATA AND NURSING STRATEGIES

The effect of powerlessness in chronically ill, hospitalized elderly persons will be depicted by two clinical examples. The first case illustrates the outcome of ineffective intervention to counteract powerlessness in an 80-year-old woman. The second case illustrates the results of nursing interventions to counteract powerlessness in a 71-year-old woman.

Mrs. A. was an 80-year-old married woman with no children who was admitted to the hospital for arterial ulcers on both feet. Her husband was 86 years old but was unable to provide much support to Mrs. A., as he seemed to be coping with his own aging and had become accustomed to being dependent on his wife for care and household management. His normal coping behavior was to seek attention and support from his wife. Prior to admission, Mrs. A. was noted to be a warm, energetic, goal-oriented person. She expressed a perceived sense of being able to control most of the circumstances of her life in spite of her age. She boasted about being able to do all the housework, including washing, cleaning, and grocery shopping. She stated that these tasks were her responsibility and that she had no difficulty doing them.

Mrs. A.'s knowledge about her health problems was another sign of her control. She had a pacemaker and a 5-year history of non-insulin-dependent (diet-controlled) diabetes. She understood the necessity for pacemaker battery replacement every 2 years, stating that it did not alter her life-style in any way. She was aware of longer-lasting battery cells but felt that at her age it would be "foolish" to spend the extra money on one.

Mrs. A. was able to define diabetes and explain its effect on the human body in simple terms. She understood the relationship between her diabetes and the lack of healing in the skin lesions of her feet. She had been doing treatments at home under her physician's orders: soaking her feet in warm water, cleansing them with pHisoHex, applying antibiotic ointment, and redressing the lesions. She had difficulty understanding the reason for activity restrictions. She had been very determined not to be hospitalized for treatment of the necrotic lesions. She stated that hospitalization meant a loss of control over her own life. She said, "In the hospital you have to do things when they tell you to do them. At home I can do things when I decide to do them."

After 3 weeks of treatment at home with little improvement of the necrotic lesions and cellulitis, Mrs. A. was admitted. Mrs. A. had expected to remain in the hospital for about 1 week to treat the infection. Instead of 1 week, she was hospitalized for 1 month. She endured several episodes of hypoglycemia, survived an episode of acute tubular necrosis following arteriography, became progressively weaker, and died. At the time of her death, the cellulitis of her lower extremities had been resolved. Her diabetes was stabilized. The acute tubular necrosis had been reversed. Mrs. A. had suffered from intense lack of control. The prolonged powerlessness led to despair and eventual death.

Upon admission, Mrs. A. was placed on bed rest; oral antibiotics and chlorpropamide (Diabinese) were begun. Foot treatments were initiated; these consisted of warm-water soaks with pHisoHex and application of antibiotic ointment and dressing to the lesions three times a day.

Bed rest became an immediate source of conflict for Mrs. A. She expressed a lack of understanding of the reason for the activity restriction. She asked repeatedly to be allowed to sit up in a chair. Initially, she was given no rationale for being placed on bed rest. The nursing staff simply told her that she was not allowed out of bed. Mrs. A. perceived this direction as meaning that she was not allowed to move, so she moved very little in bed. When she began to express her desire to get up, the reason for the bed rest was explained more fully, and movement in bed was encouraged. The nursing staff, however, was not successful in obtaining an order for chair rest with her legs elevated during the day.

Although behavioral indicators of powerlessness were not manifested in the conflict over bed rest, Mrs. A. expressed that being in bed all the time made her feel weak and helpless. She maintained control over her environment by expressing her desire to be out of bed and by expressing her anger when that desire was thwarted. She also went to the bathroom on her own instead of using the bedpan despite the order for bed rest.

At the beginning of the conflict over bed rest, Mrs. A. remained a goal-oriented person. Her goal was to increase her activity in order to avoid becoming weak and helpless. Her appetite remained good. She took an active interest in her care. She would actively compare the treatment being done in the hospital to what she had done at home.

As the conflict over bed rest continued, subtle changes took place in Mrs. A.'s behavior. She became more quiet, making less reference to getting out of bed. Her appetite decreased; she began to pick at her food. She demonstrated less interest in the care being done for her.

At the same time, she began experiencing hypoglycemic episodes that increased her feeling of weakness. The decision was made to discontinue the chlorpropamide. Mrs. A. responded by stating that she knew "those pills had been no good for me." Her hypoglycemic episodes ceased, and her blood sugar stabilized within normal limits.

The necrotic lesions on her feet were showing improvement. Necrotic tissue was debrided. Some skin granulation was apparent. There was also a decrease in the extent of edema and inflammation. At this time, the medical staff decided to do an arteriogram of her lower extremities. After the arteriogram, Mrs. A. developed acute tubular necrosis in response to the dye used. Vigorous medical treatment (peritoneal dialysis) was instituted. Mrs. A. regained normal kidney function within 3 days. Her comments included, "I don't know why they insisted on doing all those tests in the first place." Her systemic response was one of extreme weakness and fatigue. Because of her age and lowered adaptation resources, the weakness and fatigue did not resolve quickly. Within 24 hours of her return to normal renal function, the medical staff decided to transfer Mrs. A. to the rehabilitation unit in the hospital. Mrs. A. protested that she was not ready for the transfer. The transfer was delayed another day, but the patient still felt that she was not ready for the transfer. Her protests were ignored.

## Giving Up

More changes were noted in Mrs. A.'s behavior during the acute tubular necrosis and immediately after her return to normal renal function. She no longer took interest in her care, demonstrating apathy and resignation toward all procedures that were initiated at this time. She expressed a sense of uselessness and a fear that she was becoming a burden to everyone. Her anorexia continued. Her depression and lowered sense of self-esteem increased. She began to verbalize her desire to die, stating that she wished the doctors would just put something into her veins that would do away with her. Her expressed desire to die was followed by the acknowledgment that she had no control over that either. She felt the assaults by the various treatments were so devastating that the staff who inflicted them could also voluntarily end her life.

After her transfer to the rehabilitation unit, Mrs. A. became more apathetic and withdrawn. She was placed on the standard rehabilitation therapeutic program. All patients were required to be out of bed by 8 A.M. and were to remain up, participating in scheduled activities until midafternoon. During the first days on the rehabilitation unit, Mrs. A. protested that she was too weak and too tired to remain up in a wheelchair for an extended period. The nursing staff was resistant to any adaptation of their routine in order to meet Mrs. A.'s request. Mrs. A. responded by withdrawing from further verbal communication. She failed to cooperate with efforts to mobilize her physically or to take an active part in her therapeutic regimen. She ceased to participate in activities of daily living, although she retained the functional capacity to perform these activities. Rapid physical deterioration began. Within 2 weeks after her transfer to the rehabilitation unit, Mrs. A. died.

The changes in behavior observed in Mrs. A. correlated with those behaviors that have been suggested as indicators of powerlessness. These behaviors include apathy, withdrawal, resignation, fatalism, malleability, anxiety, restlessness, sleeplessness, wandering, aimlessness, and lack of decision making.

Mrs. A. entered the cycle of powerlessness-hopelessness at the time of conflict over bed rest. When her attempts to control the situation failed, she felt immobilized. This sense of immobilization was reinforced by actions of the nursing and medical staffs that denied Mrs. A. control over her environment or decision-making responsibility about what was being done for her. Her perceived sense of powerlessness was exhibited by the ceasing verbal protests, decreased appetite, and apathy.

The powerlessness Mrs. A. had begun to perceive was further reinforced by the physical onslaught of acute tubular necrosis, which left her in a weakened physical condition. At this point, she began to refer to herself as "useless" and "something to be gotten rid of." Depression and hopelessness were manifested in her death wish. The perception that she would not recover was reinforced by the complications that had negated her original expectations related to her hospitalization. There was no recognition at this point by the medical staff or nursing staff that an elderly person needs more time to restore equilibrium within the body because of less effective homeostatic mechanisms.

Isolation developed when Mrs. A. was transferred to the rehabilitation unit. At this point, the dichotomy between her own perceived needs and the plan of care to which she was subjected was complete. Any effort on her part to achieve control over her environment had been thwarted. Figure 6-1 depicts the events with hypothetical degrees of power assigned. On the scale, 10 is maximum powerfulness, and 0 refers to complete powerlessness.

## Preventing Hopelessness

The second patient, Mrs. B., was a 71-year-old married woman with five children, two of whom lived in town. Her husband was an active man 77 years of age with no major

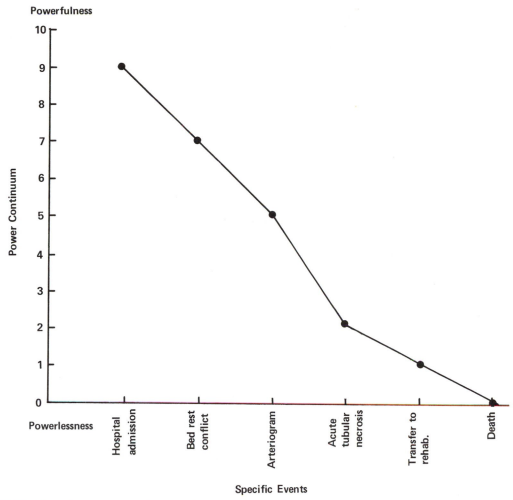

**Powerfulness**

**Power Continuum**

**Powerlessness**

Hospital admission

Bed rest conflict

Arteriogram

Acute tubular necrosis

Transfer to rehab.

Death

**Specific Events**

**FIGURE 6-1.   Degree of powerlessness and health-illness events of Mrs. A.**

health problems. The couple lived in a low-rent townhouse during the summer and spent their winters in Florida in a trailer home they owned. Before her hospitalization, Mrs. B. had managed to maintain a high level of independence, in spite of a progressive deterioration of her right hip joint.

About 3½ years before this hospitalization, Mrs. B. had sustained a subcapital fracture of her right leg, which had been pinned. Within 1½ years, she began experiencing progressive pain in her right hip joint, causing an ambulatory deficit that necessitated the use of a walker. Radiologic examination revealed deterioration of the right hip joint. After another 1½ years of pain and disability, Mrs. B. was admitted to the hospital for an elective total hip replacement. At the time of her admission, her health history revealed no significant findings. There was no evidence of any other chronic disease.

Upon admission Mrs. B. presented herself as an energetic person. She detailed how she and her husband were able to maintain their two homes. She did not seek outside help, expressing a perceived sense of control over most of the circumstances of her life. She demonstrated a high degree of knowledge related to the hip deterioration and the planned total hip replacement. She was able to describe the planned surgery in basic terms. Her expectation of her hospitalization was a stay of about 3 weeks.

Mrs. B. underwent surgery for the total hip replacement on May 21. For the first week, her postoperative course was uneventful. She maintained a positive, goal-oriented approach to her convalescence, participating in her care, seeking information, and complying with all that she perceived would enhance her return to health. On May 30, Mrs. B. became dyspneic and cyanotic and complained of chest pain. Diagnostic examination revealed multiple pulmonary emboli. She was transferred to the intensive-care unit and started on heparin therapy. The expected response to the heparin therapy was not achieved. Further testing revealed that Mrs. B. had a serum factor that caused platelets to aggregate in contact with heparin. On June 6, Mrs. B. developed a deep iliofemoral thrombosis of the right leg with marked edema and discoloration of the lower portion of the leg. A venous thrombectomy was performed the next day. Subsequently, gangrene of the right foot developed from the impairment of circulation with ischemic changes. The right foot was treated conservatively, using pHisoHex soaks. Pulmonary status returned to normal. Mrs. B. remained hospitalized for the treatment of her right foot. Most of this time was spent on the rehabilitation unit.

During the acute crisis, Mrs. B. became withdrawn, interacting less with the persons in her environment. Her appetite decreased. She expressed a sense of being overwhelmed by her circumstances, stating, "I'm not sure what is happening to me." She also expressed a lack of previous experience to provide her with needed coping mechanisms stating, "I've never been through anything like this before." Much of the time she was quiet.

Mrs. B. returned to the surgical unit on July 18, for debridement of the lesion on her right foot and a possible transmetatarsal amputation. When she returned to the surgical unit, Mrs. B. was in a state of depression, expressing resistance to the amputation and using denial. She stated that she did not know who she was anymore and desired to go home to "find herself." In contrast to her knowledge of the original surgery, Mrs. B. had a low level of knowledge about this surgery and expressed a lack of desire to know anything about it. A transmetatarsal amputation of the right foot was performed on July 19.

Her first postoperative day was uneventful. On her second postoperative day, Mrs. B. began to exhibit acute anxiety behavior. She referred to this as her "nerves being so uptight." In her interaction with her husband, she was slightly hostile and withdrawn. The focal stimulus of her anxious behavior was the pending dressing change on her foot that had been spoken of by the surgical team during morning rounds. There was a delay of several hours before the dressing change was actually done. She stated that she wished that she "could tell them what to do and when to do it." She referred to the surgical team as "the Gestapo" and felt that no matter what she did that she was "at their mercy." Her expectations of the dressing change were all negative. She perceived that it would be extremely painful, that she would not be medicated in time, and that the meperidine (Demerol) would not be effective. Mrs. B. also expressed concern that she would not be able to control her own reactions to the dressing change.

Mrs. B.'s behaviors at this point demonstrated a high degree of perceived powerlessness. The first step in intervention was to recognize the existing state of powerlessness. After the powerlessness was recognized by the nursing staff, the next intervention was to help Mrs. B. recognize her sense of powerlessness. This was done by identifying the behaviors and interpreting them to Mrs. B. An attempt was then made to reduce her global sense of helplessness to a more specific focus. This involved separating things Mrs. B. could control from things she could not control. For example, Mrs. B. could control the extent of the pain that occurred during the dressing change by requesting and receiving pain medication and by learning relaxation and refocusing techniques. She could also control the extent of the pain by using the presence of a support person in the environment. She could not control the fact that the procedure would involve pain. She also could not control the time that the surgical team would do the procedure.

As a result of these interventions, the patient became more relaxed. Her body position showed less tension. She was able to sleep for short intervals. Her verbalization was increasingly goal-directed in terms of stating that perhaps she could control the amount of pain she would experience. Although the actual dressing change was a difficult experience for Mrs. B., her sense of powerlessness was reduced. This was demonstrated in her comments the next day regarding further dressing changes: "I really screamed yesterday when they took that dressing off, but it wasn't so bad this morning when the nurses did it." Her other comments during the day revealed a much more positive, goal-oriented, hopeful approach to her circumstances. She stated that her foot was less painful, that she had decided to walk again, and that she felt like eating. She also had begun to take an active interest in herself, using part of her time in the morning to set her hair.

Because of the changes in her behavior, time was spent reinforcing her increased sense of powerfulness. Mrs. B. was helped to identify those events in her current situation that indicated improvement. These included the need for less pain medication, the discontinuation of IV therapy, and her increased interest in food. This nursing intervention was effective in increasing Mrs. B.'s level of hopefulness by refocusing her attention away from the series of complications that had induced the sense of powerlessness within her, and toward attending to signs of improvement.

Mrs. B. continued to move from powerlessness to powerfulness. She began to exert more control over her immediate environment, although she remained on bed rest. She began deciding where things should be kept and directed her care givers accordingly. The nursing staff reinforced this behavior by allowing Mrs. B. to decide when she wanted to have her bath or have a procedure done. She began to express future-oriented thinking, planning for things she would do after her discharge. Mrs. B. also began to seek information about the effects of the amputation on her ability to walk. Her anxiety was markedly decreased, and previous signs of withdrawal and depression were absent.

Mrs. B.'s return to powerfulness was threatened when she was informed that she would need a skin graft at the amputation site. Her perception of this proposed treatment was that she was not improving. This perception reinforced her former negative expectations. She began to express uncertainty about returning home, frustration over not receiving information from her attending physicians, and reluctance to have further anesthesia. Her perceived powerlessness increased, having a more global all-encompassing effect this time. She demonstrated anxiety toward trying something new, such as using the walker. She said, "Please don't let go of me. I can't walk alone with this thing." Despair was noted in Mrs. B.'s responses, "What's the use? There have been so many setbacks."

Mrs. B.'s increased sense of powerlessness was also due to her inability to obtain answers from the surgical team to her questions about the planned skin graft ("they don't stay long enough to ask questions"). She felt a perceived loss of control in the area of decision making related to her body. She had not received sufficient information to even agree to have the skin graft. She also felt perceived loss of control over persons making the decisions in that she could not keep them in her environment long enough to get the information she wanted.

Her increased powerlessness also resulted from a lack of knowledge about the procedure, the rationale for doing it, the time it would occur, and the expected outcome.

Again, nursing intervention began by recognizing that a state of powerlessness existed. Mrs. B. was helped to recognize her feelings of powerlessness. To increase her sense of powerfulness, the focus of her greatest concern regarding the skin graft was identified. Her identified concern was that the physicians would not give her needed information. Her right to ask questions was reinforced. A strategy was developed to obtain information from the surgical team. Mrs. B. identified specific questions she wanted answered. She then set a goal to get these questions answered. As she focused on this task, her anxiety behaviors decreased. Her verbal comments changed from fear and depression to references to specific things she could do. Mrs. B. was able to achieve her goal, which enhanced her sense of power.

During the days before the skin graft procedure, Mrs. B. vacillated between a sense of powerfulness and one of powerlessness. She demonstrated a heightened anxiety level but was more realistic in approaching the problem than she had been previously. Her anxiety was not accompanied by apathy, depression, withdrawal, or pessimism. She continued to maintain control over her immediate environment and directed nursing care. She also continued her goal of walking with the walker.

Nursing interventions at this time focused on reinforcing Mrs. B.'s sense of powerfulness by supplying her with needed realistic information and encouraging her to make decisions related to her care. Anxiety was kept within limits by means Mrs. B. determined, for example, planning for physician's rounds by writing down questions and using television soap operas as a distraction from her own plight. She expressed relief to know that it was all right to feel some anxiety.

Her powerlessness increased after the skin graft at the time of the first dressing change. This was manifested by a high degree of anxiety, a lack of goal orientation, and verbalization of negative expectations. She became very angry with the surgical team during the procedure. This anger seemed to indicate her growing realization that she had a right to have control over her circumstances. This right was being thwarted by the surgical team's actions. She expressed her sense of the discrepancy between the words and the actions of the surgical team: "You can't trust them at all. They said that they would soak the dressing off, but instead they rush in and rip it off. They lie to you every chance they get."

During the subsequent days of hospitalization, Mrs. B.'s physical status continued to improve. Nursing interventions were directed toward helping Mrs. B. identify specific indicators of physical improvement. These included the progressive healing of the skin graft and her increased ambulation. Mrs. B. responded with increased hopefulness and futuristic, goal-oriented thinking. She became involved in activities of daily living and in her dressing changes. Her anxiety level related to the dressing changes became markedly reduced. She no longer viewed these as potential complications but as routine procedures. She retained a sense of powerlessness in response to the surgical team, commenting on their tendency to do whatever they pleased.

At the time of her discharge, Mrs. B. was ambulating well with a walker. Her foot was healed. She was doing her own dressing changes with assistance from her husband. She had begun to plan how they would manage activities of daily living at home in spite of alterations in her health. She expressed confidence in her ability to work this out. Her increased self-esteem, goal-oriented behavior, and positive responses to her situation indicated that powerlessness had been resolved and she was returning to a functional state of powerfulness.

Mrs. B. entered the powerlessness cycle at the time when multiple complications to her recovery began to occur. Within her frame of reference, these complications were seen as being outside her control. This perception led to immobilization. Her growing sense of powerlessness was reinforced by the actions of medical and nursing staffs. Their lack of perception of Mrs. B.'s need to be incorporated into decision making enhanced her perception of powerlessness. Nursing interventions that recognized Mrs. B.'s state of powerlessness and assisted her to learn new methods of control proved effective in returning Mrs. B. to a state of powerfulness. The events, with hypothetical degrees of powerlessness for Mrs. B., are depicted in Figure 6-2. No quantitative powerlessness scores were used to validate the clinical impressions depicted in figures 6-1 and 6-2.

# Discussion

As demonstrated in these two case studies, powerlessness has serious nursing implications. Powerlessness affects a person's behavioral responses. In the individual experiencing powerlessness, learning or goal achievement is not seen as helpful in affecting an outcome. "Acquisition of knowledge or goal-directive behavior is simply irrelevant or unnecessary when the individual does not perceive that future events can be controlled by his own actions."[45] Knowledge or goal-directive behavior can mean the difference between successful or unsuccessful adaptation to illness. The aging patient is more vulnerable to powerlessness because of the aging process itself. In facing powerlessness, the elderly patient is less able to cope because of diminished psychosocial reserve capacity.

Powerlessness can be prevented. In the two case studies presented, there are some common factors that precipitated powerlessness. For both individuals, hospitalization meant some degree of loss of control, which they were able to limit through their

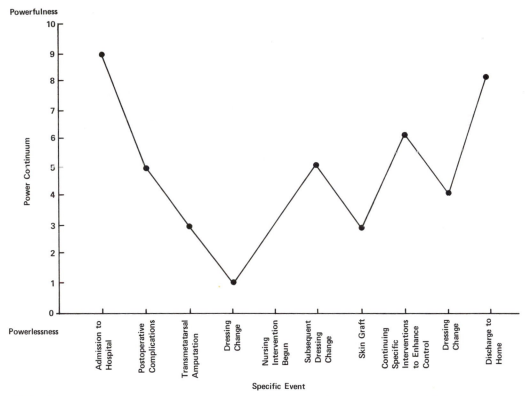

FIGURE 6-2.  Degree of powerlessness and health-illness events of Mrs. B.

expectations of a limited hospital stay. Complications in recovery precipitated a lack of fulfillment of these expectations, leading to some degree of immobilization in both patients. These complications also produced increased physical powerlessness in both patients. Both individuals viewed the complications as being outside their sphere of control.

A second factor that contributed to the development of powerlessness in both individuals was the tendency of both medical and nursing staffs to dehumanize. There was a failure to recognize the individual's right and need to be incorporated into the decision-making process, as well as failure to note special adaptive needs and limited coping capacity of the elderly. Information was not supplied fully to either individual. Decisions were made without consulting either individual. No alternatives were presented.

Because of these factors, nursing strategies for preventing powerlessness need to be aimed at preventing loss of involvement and supplying the patient with an adequate knowledge base. Preventive strategies would include involving aging individuals in planning their own care, enhancing their self-esteem by referring decisions directly to them, supplying them with cognitive control through helping them anticipate events and outcomes, and giving them time to adjust to changes. Strategies also need to be developed to help individuals understand complications that occur, bringing them into a framework that diminishes the sense of loss of control.

As a result of this clinical study and literature review, a powerlessness behavioral assessment tool (Fig. 6-3) was developed. The tool is an observational guide for nurses to use to diagnose powerlessness. The tool contains four categories of assessment data: verbal response, emotional response, participation in activities of daily living, and involvement in learning about care responsibilities. Nurses rate patient behaviors for each item on the tool using a 4-point scale: (1) patient never manifests this behavior; (2)

Patient Behaviors                                                        Nurse Rating of Behaviors

| | 1 Never | 2 Occasionally | 3 Frequently | 4 Always |
|---|---|---|---|---|
| **VERBAL RESPONSE** | | | | |
| Verbal expressions of lack of control over what is happening. | | | | |
| Verbal expressions of doubt that self-care measures can affect outcome. | | | | |
| Verbal expressions of giving up. | | | | |
| Verbal expressions of fatalism. | | | | |

| | | | | |
|---|---|---|---|---|
| **EMOTIONAL RESPONSE** | | | | |
| Withdrawal. | | | | |
| Pessimism. | | | | |
| Undifferentiated anger. | | | | |
| Diminished patient-initiated interaction. | | | | |
| Submissiveness. | | | | |

| | | | | |
|---|---|---|---|---|
| **PARTICIPATION IN ACTIVITIES OF DAILY LIVING** | | | | |
| Nonparticipation in daily personal hygiene. | | | | |
| Noninterest in treatments. | | | | |
| Refusal to take food or fluids. | | | | |
| Inability to set goals. | | | | |
| Lack of decision making when opportunities are provided. | | | | |
| Dependency on others for activities of daily living. | | | | |

| | | | | |
|---|---|---|---|---|
| **INVOLVEMENT IN LEARNING ABOUT CARE RESPONSIBILITIES** | | | | |
| Lack of questioning concerning illness. | | | | |
| Low level of knowledge of illness after being given information. | | | | |
| Lack of knowledge related to treatment. | | | | |
| Lack of motivation to learn. | | | | |

FIGURE 6-3.   Powerlessness behavioral assessment tool.

patient occasionally manifests this behavior; (3) patient frequently manifests this behavior; (4) patient always manifests this behavior. Although the tool was developed as a result of field work with the elderly, its application is appropriate for adults of all ages. In order for nurses caring for elderly to use the tool, careful in-service training would be needed.

Validity and reliability of the tool have not yet been established. Nurses can be alerted to potential or existing nursing diagnoses of powerlessness if patients' scores on items are 3 or more. Specific nursing interventions to alleviate powerlessness are needed for a cumulative score of 57 or more.

Altering an existing state of powerlessness requires taking into account the losses and changes the person has had to respond to and the individual's strengths in coping with these. Assessment of losses and changes experienced by patients is necessary so that the nurse detects the potential for powerlessness.

Patients can be assisted in recognizing that powerlessness is the state that may be underlying their behavior. The global effect of powerlessness—that is, the tendency for feelings of loss of control over a single sphere to be transferred to all spheres of an individual's life—must be decreased. Nursing interventions that assisted individuals to focus on what controls they still retained were effective in limiting powerlessness. Giving back to individuals the expectation that they are the decision makers also reduces powerlessness. Specifically, patients need to be consulted about scheduling of care. Patients need to be involved in learning the consequences of alternative major treatments. Powerless persons also need to relearn to set goals and expect to be successful in accomplishing their goals. The accomplishment of small daily goals reinforces the perception that the individuals' actions are effective in altering their circumstances. Altering an existing state of powerlessness requires patience and consistency.

Powerlessness, or the perceived loss of control over the outcome of events in one's life, poses a threat to the individual's ability to recover from illness. The problem of powerlessness is more severe for the elderly, who may have fewer intact power resources to use. The assessment tool presented in this chapter was designed to determine the presence and the degree of powerlessness in hospitalized elderly patients but can be applied to all adults. The case studies provided qualitative data about powerlessness and emphasized the critical need for intervention to prevent hopelessness and, in some instances, to prevent death.

# REFERENCES

1. Fuller, S.: *Inhibiting helplessness in elderly people.* Journal of Gerontological Nursing 4:18, July-August 1978.
2. Kalish, R.: *Late Adulthood: Perspectives on Human Development.* Brooks/Cole Publishing, Monterey, Calif., 1975.
3. Lancaster, J.: *Maximizing psychological adaptation in an aging population.* Topics in Clinical Nursing 3:31, April 1981.
4. Aguilera, D.: *Stressors in late adulthood.* Family and Community Health 2:61, February 1980.
5. Eisdorfer, C. and Wildie, R.: *Stress, disease, aging and behavior.* In Birren, J. E. and Shaie, J. W. (eds.): *Handbook of the Psychology of Aging.* Van Nostrand Reinhold, New York, 1977, pp. 251-275.

6. Robb, S.: *Resources in the environment of the aged.* In Yurick, A., et al. (eds.): *The Aged Person and the Nursing Process.* Appleton-Century-Crofts, New York, 1980.
7. Seligman, M.: *Helplessness: On Depression, Development and Death.* W. H. Freeman & Co., San Francisco, 1975.
8. Langer, E. and Benevento, A.: *Self-induced dependence.* J. Pers. Soc. Psychol. 36:869, 1978.
9. Butler, R. N.: *Why Survive?* Harper & Row, New York, 1975.
10. Shanas, F. and Maddox, G.: *Aging, health, and the organization of health resources.* In Binstock, R. H. and Shanas, E.: *Handbook of Aging and the Social Sciences.* Van Nostrand Reinhold, New York, 1976, p. 602.
11. Atchley, R.: *Common misconceptions about aging.* Health Values: Achieving High Level Wellness 5:7, 1981.
12. Robinson, F.: *Leisure well-being for longer living people.* Health Values: Achieving High Level Wellness 5:55, 1981.
13. Roy, Sister Callista: *Introduction to Nursing: An Adaptation Model.* Prentice-Hall, Englewood Cliffs, N.J., 1976.
14. Culbert, P. and Kos, B.: *Aging: Considerations for health teaching.* Nurs. Clin. North Am. 6:607, December 1971.
15. Hayter, J.: *Biologic changes of aging.* Nurs. Forum 13:289, 1974.
16. Shore, H.: *Designing a training program for understanding sensory loss in aging.* Gerontologist 16:157, 1976.
17. Yurick, A.: *Sensory experiences of the elderly person.* In Yurick, A., et al. (eds.): *The Aged Person and the Nursing Process.* Appleton-Century-Crofts, New York, 1980, pp. 291-310.
18. Rossman, I.: *Human aging changes.* In Burnside, I. M. (ed.): *Nursing and the Aged.* McGraw-Hill, New York, 1976, pp. 81-91.
19. Culbert and Kos, op. cit. pp. 604-613.
20. Hayter, op. cit. p. 307.
21. Rynerson, B.: *Need for self-esteem in the aged: A literature review.* J. Psychiatr. Nurs. 10:22, January-February 1972.
22. Erikson, E.: *Eight ages of man.* In Rebelsky, F. (ed.): *Life: The Continuous Process, Readings in Human Development.* Alfred A. Knopf, New York, 1975.
23. Angrosino, M.: *Anthropology and the aging: A preliminary community study.* Gerontologist 16:174, 1976.
24. Schulz, R.: *Effects of control and predictability on the physical and psychological well-being of the institutionalized aged.* J. Pers. Soc. Psychol. 33:563, 1976.
25. Schultz, R. and Hanusa, B.: *Long term effects of control and predictability-enhancing interventions: Findings and ethical issues.* J. Pers. Soc. Psychol. 36:1194, 1978.
26. Langer, E. and Rodin, J.: *The effects of choice and enhanced personal responsibility for the aged: A field experiment in an institutionalized setting.* J. Pers. Soc. Psychol. 34:191, 1976.
27. Rodin, J. and Langer, E.: *Long term effects of a control-relevant intervention with the institutionalized aged.* J. Pers. Soc. Psychol. 35:897, 1977.
28. Chang, B.: *Generalized expectancy, situational perception, and morale among the institutionalized aged.* Nurs. Res. 27:316, September-October 1978.
29. Chang, B.: *Perceived situational control of daily activities: A new tool.* Research in Nursing and Health 1:181, 1978.
30. Chang, B.: *Black and white elderly: Morale and perception of control.* Western Journal of Nursing Research 2:371, Winter 1980.
31. Hanes, C. and Wild, B.: *Locus of control and depression among noninstitutionalized elderly persons.* Psychol. Rep. 41:581, 1977.
32. Reid, D., Haas, G., and Hawkings, D.: *Locus of desired control and positive self-concept of the elderly.* J. Gerontol. 32:441, 1977.
33. Ziegler, M. and Reid, D.: *Correlates of locus of desired control in two samples of elderly persons: Community residents and hospitalized patients.* J. Consult. Clin. Psychol. 47:977, 1979.
34. Brodie, J.: *Social behavior of the elderly: Effects of fearfulness and perceived locus of control.* Issues in Mental Health Nursing 1:63, Spring 1978.

35. Bradley, R.: *Age-related differences in locus of control orientation in three behavior domains.* Hum. Dev. 19:49, 1976.
36. Seligman, op. cit. p. 186.
37. Rowland, K.: *Environmental events predicting death for the elderly.* Psychol. Bull. 84:349, 1977.
38. Brown, P.: *Religious needs of older persons.* In Thorson, J. and Cook, T. (eds.): *Spiritual Well-Being of the Elderly.* Charles C Thomas, Springfield, Ill., 1980, pp. 76-82.
39. Moberg, D.: *Social indicators of spiritual well-being in the elderly.* In Thorson, J. and Cook, T. (eds.): *Spiritual Well-Being of the Elderly.* Charles C Thomas, Springfield, Ill., 1980, pp. 20-37.
40. McCreary, W.: *Creative transformation and the theological resources for loneliness.* In Thorson, J. and Cook, T. (eds.): *Spiritual Well-Being of the Elderly.* Charles C Thomas, Springfield, Ill., 1980, pp. 108-112.
41. Chang: *Perceived situational control of daily activities,* op. cit. p. 183.
42. Haney, C. A., et al.: *A measure of health status in an elderly population.* Health Values: Achieving High Level Wellness 5:61, 1981.
43. Reid, Haas, and Hawkings, op. cit.
44. Moyer, N.: *Health promotion and the assessment of health habits in the elderly.* Topics in Clinical Nursing 3:51, April 1981.
45. Johnson, D.: *Powerlessness: A significant determinant in patient behaviors.* J. Nurs. Educ. 6:40, April 1967.

## SELECTED READINGS

Benson, E.: *Health promotion for the elderly: Clinical learning experiences in nontraditional settings.* Nurs. Clin. North Am. 14:577, December 1979.
Burnside, I. M., Ebersole, P., and Monea, H.: *Psychosocial Caring Throughout the Life Span.* McGraw-Hill, New York, 1979.
Dimond, M., King, K., and Burt, M.: *Forced relocation and the elderly: Identifying facilitators and barriers to adjustment.* In American Nurses' Association: *Clinical and Scientific Sessions.* American Nurses' Association, Kansas City, Mo., 1979.
Eliopoulos, C.: *Chronic care and the elderly: Impact of the client, the family and the nurse.* Topics in Clinical Nursing 3:71, April 1981.
German, P.: *Delivery of care to older people: Issues and outlooks.* Topics in Clinical Nursing 3:1, April 1981.
Goodell, H.: *Coming of age: A chronicle of personal growth.* Health Values: Achieving High Level Wellness 5:36, 1981.
Gubrium, J.: *The Myth of the Golden Years: A Socio-Environmental Theory of Aging.* Charles C Thomas, Springfield, Ill., 1973.
Gubrium, J.: *Time, Roles, and Self in Old Age.* Human Sciences Press, New York, 1976.
Hain, M. J. and Chen, S.-P.: *Health needs of the elderly.* Nurs. Res. 25:433, November-December 1976.
Hirschfeld, M.: *Research in nursing gerontology.* Journal of Advanced Nursing 4:621, 1979.
Kuypers, J.: *Internal-external locus of control, ego functioning, and personality characteristics in old age.* Gerontologist 12:168, 1972.
Lee, R.: *Self-images of the elderly.* Nurs. Clin. North Am. 11:119, March 1976.
Linn, M.: *Studies in rating the physical, mental, and social dysfunction of the chronically ill aged.* Med. Care 14 (Supplement No. 5):119, 1976.
Smith, D. and Bierman, E.: *The Biologic Ages of Man from Conception through Old Age.* W. B. Saunders, Philadelphia, 1973.
Spencer, M. and Dorr, C.: *Understanding Aging: A Multidisciplinary Approach.* Appleton-Century-Crofts, New York, 1975.
Thomas, E.: *Application of stress factors in gerontologic nursing.* Nurs. Clin. North Am. 14:607, December 1970.

Thomas, E.: *Morbidity patterns among recently relocated elderly.* In American Nurses' Association: *Clinical and Scientific Sessions.* American Nurses' Association, Kansas City, Mo., 1979.
Timiras, P. S.: *Developmental Physiology and Aging.* Macmillan, New York, 1972.

# 3

# POWERLESSNESS IN SPECIFIC
# CHRONIC HEALTH PROBLEMS

In Part 3, emphasis is given to analyzing powerlessness that occurs in specific health problems. Stressors are identified that promote powerlessness in patients with chronic renal failure (Chapter 7) and long-term infections (Chapter 10). Another dimension of an individual's perception, locus of control, is developed from two standpoints: (1) in a pure practice application, a qualitative study of patients with peripheral vascular disease (Chapter 8), and (2) in a controlled quantitative study of patients with diabetes (Chapter 9). Because of our commitment to use findings from the behavioral sciences that have relevance for nursing in day-to-day practice, a behavioral assessment tool for locus of control was devised. This empirical referent can be appropriately used instead of paper-and-pencil tests by practicing nurses to measure locus-of-control tendencies.

The research study by Gotch examined the relationship between diabetic patients' locus-of-control tendency and their ability to implement health regimens. Before nurses strive to influence the locus-of-control attribute—that is, develop patients' internality as suggested by Arakelian[1]—much more research needs to be conducted.

Compliance as a coping task of patients with diabetes and all chronically ill patients is discussed in Chapter 12. Health belief factors and the powerlessness dimension influencing compliance in black patients with diabetes are included.

Energy is a patient power resource and is compromised in chronically ill patients. This deficit is pronounced in patients with arthritis. Unique components of an energy-expenditure model for chronically ill patients are included in Chapter 11. Providing for energy needs is one measure in alleviating powerlessness.

# REFERENCE

1. Arakelian, M.: *An assessment and nursing application of the concept of locus of control.* Advances in Nursing Science 3:25, October 1980.

# 7

# RECOGNIZING POWERLESSNESS: CAUSES AND INDICATORS IN PATIENTS WITH CHRONIC RENAL FAILURE

## SUSAN STAPLETON

The multiple stressors confronting patients with chronic renal failure (CRF) can be interpreted as contributing to powerlessness in this particular patient group. Stressors identified in the literature can be categorized as physiologic, psychologic, role-disturbance, and life-change stressors. The purpose of this chapter is to present a summarized review of literature of these stressors, as well as to report observations of powerlessness in patients with CRF. Conclusions about patient responses to powerlessness will be made in order to help nurses be able to identify behavioral indicators of the nursing diagnostic category powerlessness in other chronically ill patients.

## LITERATURE REVIEW

### Physiologic Stressors

The toxic effects of uremia are manifested in virtually every body system. The pathophysiology described by Bailey[1] and by Harrington and Brenner[2] includes effects on the following: (1) body biochemistry—disturbance of body water homeostasis, metabolic acidosis, and elevation of serum potassium, sodium, phosphorus, calcium, magnesium, and uric acid; and (2) organ systems—hypertension, heart failure, anemia, gastrointestinal irritation, osteodystrophy, soft-tissue calcification, clotting deficiencies, altered endocrine function, and neuropathy.[1,2]

Wright, Sand, and Goodhue[3] also report body-function changes as a stressor in 12 patients on chronic dialysis. They cite weakness, decreased energy, impaired concentration, insomnia, weight loss, and restricted use of extremity with shunt or fistula as factors contributing to the stress. Cummings[4] reports that the mechanisms of attention and concentration are among the first cognitive skills affected by the azotemia of CRF, impairing the higher intellectual functions (e.g., abstraction, generalization).

The individual's lack of control over the physical changes and the course of the illness would seem to be a major factor resulting in powerlessness. Individuals cannot predict or control how they will feel and function from day to day.

## Psychologic Stressors

A psychologic stressor related to the changes in appearance and function of the body is alteration in self-concept (specifically, body image). Wittman[5] reported that 6 of the 15 subjects with CRF interviewed had poor self-concepts and questioned their usefulness to their families. DeNour and Czaczkes state, "It is not uncommon for body image distortions to occur in which the patient thinks of himself as part of the machine or endows the machine with human qualities."[6] Abram states, "The patients have seemingly incorporated into their body image the machines upon which they are so dependent for life. They unconsciously think of themselves as not entirely human and, therefore, freakish."[7] The individual experiences a temporary loss of body part each time he undergoes dialysis in that the patient attached to the dialysis machine views the blood flowing outside the body. This visual experience causes a disturbance in body image.[5]

It is important to note that the changes in body function are not completely alleviated by dialysis. Even with dialysis, the individual remains chronically ill and less able to function. As Abram, Moore, and Westervelt state, "Dialysis makes people feel better, but it does not make them feel well."[8] Body image, self-concept, and self-esteem are all closely related to how individuals perceive their ability to function. Roy[9] states that one of the behaviors indicating low self-esteem is an expression of feelings of helplessness.

A second psychologic stressor for patients with CRF reported in the literature is the frustration of basic drives, including aggression, satisfaction of hunger and thirst, and sexual expression. Halper discusses the limitations placed on normal outlets for the aggressive drive, particularly in men: "They cannot compete as successfully at work and their capacity to participate in athletics and other physical activities is limited."[10]

Another basic drive that is frustrated in the individual with CRF is the need to satisfy hunger. The difficulty that patients have in complying with the dietary restrictions is frequently discussed in the literature. Eating is a satisfying and pleasurable experience.[11] As a mode of oral gratification, eating is more than satisfying hunger.

The individual with CRF also frequently experiences frustration of basic sexual drive in that there is a marked deterioration in sexual interest and/or performance. Levy found that "hemodialysis patients of both sexes, but particularly men, as well as male transplant recipients, had substantial deterioration in sexual functioning."[12] Levy's study and one done by Abram and coworkers[13] showed a further decrease in sexual performance in about 35 percent of the patients after the initiation of dialysis. Finkelstein, Steele, and Shambaugh, in separate studies, report some degree of sexual dysfunction, which seemed to contribute to patient and spouse depression and marital discord in most couples.[14,15,16] This marital discord was judged to be moderate or severe in 53 percent of the couples studied by Finkelstein. Frustration of basic drives is beyond the individual's control and may be seen as contributing to powerlessness.

A third psychologic stressor reported by Beard[17] is what he refers to as "fear of death and fear of life." "It is essential to keep in mind that the prolongation of life involves not only adding to the length of life, but it also involves the matter of the quality and worthwhileness of the life that is prolonged."[17] Individuals with CRF fear that their lives will be cut short, yet at the same time they fear that their lives may not be acceptable. In a study of life satisfaction of patients on dialysis, Jackle reported that these patients rated their present lives as slightly less satisfactory than did the normative group. They rated their past lives, however, near the top of the life-satisfaction scale.[18] There is also a strong fear that something will go wrong during dialysis—events such as hypovolemic shock, ruptured dialyzer, or separation of tubing connections. Individuals frequently feel that they are at the mercy of the machine and are powerless to control it. Abram quotes one patient as saying that the machine "maintains a powerful hold on my life—I find it impossible to make friends with the monster."[19] Witmann reported that more than half the subjects interviewed experienced depression as the problems of living with dialysis became apparent.[5]

A dependence-independence conflict is a fourth psychologic stressor that has been reported as affecting the individual with CRF. The patient is expected to comply with the treatment regimen, which requires very dependent behavior; however, the patient is also told to remain independent and live a "normal" life, including meeting family, job, and social obligations. Reichsman and Levy[20] state that the major feeling experienced by patients is one of helplessness: "They feel trapped between the wish to be passive and dependent on one hand, and the expectation of health personnel that they be active and independent on the other."[20] Both Reichsman and Levy, and DeNour and Czaczkes[6] report that the degree of dependence-independence conflict experienced is related to the individual's predialysis personality in that subjects who were dependent before dialysis had fewer dependence/independence conflicts after beginning dialysis; those subjects who were independent had greater dependence/independence conflicts after beginning dialysis. Wittman reports that all 15 subjects interviewed exhibited a dependence-independence conflict.[5]

# Role Disturbances

Role disturbances are closely related to both physiologic and psychologic stressors. Because of the illness, the patient may be forced to eliminate social, family, and occupational roles that are important to the self-concept. Wright, Sand, and Goodhue[3] list loss of membership in groups and loss of job or occupation as two of the stressors described by individuals with CRF. Wittman[5] also reports loss of group membership and feelings of isolation and disengagement in almost 75 percent of the subjects. In a study of the family unit's response to dialysis, Maurin and Schenkel[21] described a withdrawal of the entire family from social life into an existence focused on the family and, in some instances, focused only on the patient.

There are also disturbances in family roles. Anger states, "Role reversal is a common occurrence, especially when the patient is the breadwinner of the family."[22] Cummings states, "Three aspects of the male role—breadwinner, disciplinarian, and decision maker—seem to be particularly vulnerable."[4]

The individual may experience guilt at being unable to fulfill role expectations. This inability to perform expected role behaviors is a great threat to the individual's self-esteem and may well contribute to powerlessness.

## Life-Style Changes

All the previously mentioned factors contribute to life-style changes in the individual with CRF. In addition, other stressors have been identified in this category. Loss of financial security is reported by Levy[12]; Anger[11]; Cummings[4]; Wright, Sand, and Goodhue[3]; Wittman[5]; and Brand and Komorita.[23] Financial insecurity was found to be a stressor even after the passage of the Social Security Act of 1973. Although the medical expenses are covered, there is still a loss of income if the breadwinner is unable to work full time. There may be a deep concern about decreasing living standards. Wittman found that financial adjustments caused a great alteration in life-styles for all the subjects interviewed.[3]

A second stressor related to life-style changes is failure of future plans. Wittman found that all patients planned on a day-to-day basis, with future planning being related to transplantation.[5] Wright, Sand, and Goodhue also report the stress of being unable to plan for vacations, a new home, or children's education because of uncertain outcomes of the illness.[3]

The time required for dialysis is also a stressor that affects life-style since the average patient spends 10 to 18 hours per week on dialysis. Comty, Leonard, and Shapiro[24] found that the average diabetic patient with CRF also spends 2.6 days per month in the hospital with complications of CRF or diabetes.

## Summary

Table 7-1 summarizes stressors of CRF that are reported in the literature. It is evident that the illness and its management have a widespread effect on the individual's life. Many of these stressors may be seen as contributing to a feeling of powerlessness. There are, in reality, many factors regarding this illness over which the patient has little or no control. In response to these stressors, the patient may manifest varying degrees of powerlessness.

## CLINICAL DATA

Six patients with CRF were studied using a participant-observer method for a period varying from 3 to 6 months. Factors causing powerlessness and the patients' responses were identified. General indicators of powerlessness manifested in the patients were lack of information seeking, failure to share relevant health information, decreased

**TABLE 7-1. Summary of Stressors in Chronic Renal Failure**

| Physiologic | Psychologic | Role Disturbances | Life-Style Changes |
|---|---|---|---|
| Body biochemistry changes | Alterations in body image: | Loss of group membership | Loss of financial security |
| Effects of uremia on organ systems | Inability to control body functioning | Loss of job or occupation | Forced acceptance of government assistance |
| Lack of control over symptoms | Body does not function normally | Role reversal with spouse | Time required for dialysis |
| Uncertain course of the illness | Incorporation of dialysis machine into body image | Decreased ability to fulfill role expectations | Limitation of activity |
| | Loss of body part, blood, kidneys | Marital discord and family tension | Failure of future plans |
| | Change in body structure—shunt or fistula | | |
| | Frustration of basic drives: | | |
| | Cannot express aggression | | |
| | Dietary and fluid restrictions | | |
| | Decreased sexual drive and/or performance | | |
| | Fear of death and fear of life: | | |
| | Uncertain life expectancy | | |
| | Fear of death due to illness | | |
| | Fear of death due to malfunction of dialysis machine | | |
| | Decreased life satisfaction | | |
| | Fear that life will not be acceptable | | |
| | Dependence-independence conflict: | | |
| | Expected compliance with treatment regimen | | |
| | Dependence on others and machine for satisfaction of needs | | |
| | Subconscious desire for dependence | | |
| | Societal expectations of independence | | |

willingness to make decisions, expression of loss of hope, crying and depression, and verbal expression of loss of control.

Specific factors that contributed to the powerlessness state in these patients were the disease process, hospitalization, relationship with health-care personnel, the dialysis procedure and medical regimen, changes in family relationships, and employment and financial concerns. Each factor contributing to powerlessness and examples of patient responses are included in the following discussion.

## Disease Process of Chronic Renal Failure

The disease process itself is a factor over which the individual feels little control. The symptoms of CRF are quite uncomfortable and have a marked impact on the individual's life-style. Fatigue and weakness are very disturbing symptoms and curtail the individual's activities a great deal. Comments such as "I'm always so tired—I can never get anything done" and "I'll never get this house painted if I can only do this much without getting exhausted" indicate how incapacitating the fatigue can be. The unpredictability of the energy level also contributes to feelings of powerlessness. Mrs. F. describes this, "Maybe the next day you'll have a good day and be able to get something done, and maybe not. You never know." This unpredictability makes it difficult for the individual to make plans for activities and may greatly decrease social life. Mrs. M. states, "After a while you just stop associating with other people. You lose a lot of friends. You just don't have the energy." Although the individual may desire to participate in certain activities, the physiologic status prevents the patient from doing so.

Other central nervous system manifestations of CRF include decreased alertness, memory loss, and impaired thought processes. Mrs. M. described the frustration of these symptoms: "People think you're crazy or something is wrong with you mentally. You feel so dull, aren't interested in others, and can't carry on a conversation. You forget what you wanted to say."

The general downward course of the illness causes many individuals with CRF to feel powerless. Mrs. F. stated, "It's like dying slowly when you're on dialysis. Every day you know that you're going downhill, but what can you do?" Mr. O. described himself as "feeling like I'm in a car going downhill and the brakes don't work."

The inability to control or predict the outcome of the kidney transplant is a real cause of feelings of powerlessness in the postoperative transplant patient. This is often expressed verbally with statements such as "It's really hard not knowing what's going to happen" and "I wish I could do something to be sure the kidney keeps working." The realization that the outcome of the surgery is out of one's control may cause severe depression. Mrs. B. cried, "It's not fair! I did everything just the way I was supposed to and I still rejected the kidney." Most patients finally resign themselves to this and make comments such as, "I guess you have to get used to the idea that you really don't have much control over what happens with the transplant."

Severe pain, which may occur postoperatively as a result of the surgery or complications, may cause feelings of powerlessness. Anxiety, depression, and prolonged pain often decrease the individual's ability to control the response to pain. Mr. F. experienced severe bladder spasms postoperatively and stated, "They come so suddenly that I don't have time to get ready for them. It's all I can do to keep from screaming." When the etiology of the pain is unknown, the feelings of powerlessness are even more acute. Mr. F. repeatedly asked me what might be causing his leg pain and stated, "This really has me scared. I don't know what it is, but it must be pretty serious if it hurts this bad."

# Hospitalization

Hospitalization automatically results in a tremendous loss of control for an individual. Decisions such as when to eat, sleep, exercise, and bathe are made for the patient, sometimes with little consultation. As a result of patient role expectations, individuals who are hospitalized may demonstrate passive behavior, follow staff directions without comment or question, and have difficulty making small decisions when given the opportunity to do so. These behaviors are all indicative of a feeling of loss of control, or powerlessness. Even individuals who have previously managed their medical regimens alone without difficulty suddenly have them managed by others. Nurses administer medications, which the patient may take without knowing or asking what they are. The dietitian calculates the patient's diet, while other staff members weigh the patient and record intake and output.

One aspect of this management by others that contributed to feelings of powerlessness in Mrs. M. was her dependence on the nurses for pain medication. She often had to wait longer than she felt was necessary, and she expressed the feeling that the staff was "taking advantage of me because I'm so helpless." This feeling was strengthened when Mrs. M. was told by a nurse, "Your imagination can make you think that you're having pain."

Frequently, hospital routines and efficiency are given higher priority than patient needs, resulting in patient feelings of powerlessness. A nurse on the renal transplant unit told Mr. F., "You'll have to eat breakfast and wash up later. Radiation Therapy is ready to do your treatment now." Mr. F. started to protest, "But I'm hungry . . .," then shrugged his shoulders and walked over to the wheelchair. When Mrs. Z. was told that she had to move to a different room because her private room was needed for another patient, she said, "I'm low man on the totem pole, so I don't have anything to say about whether or not I move." She was told to hurry her packing so the room could be cleaned, then she sat in the lounge for 6 hours because no one was available to clean rooms. Mrs. Z. merely accepted this passively and said, "I'm being evicted."

Because of a malfunctioning machine, Mr. F. experienced a long wait in the x-ray department while he was in severe pain. He was not told the cause for the delay, and he worried, "Waiting this long makes you worry that they've forgotten you and you'll end up sitting here all day before someone notices you." Although he made this statement to the author upon her arrival in the department, he had not attempted to ask any x-ray personnel the reason for the delay or to remind them of his presence.

Hospitalized patients, as well as those on dialysis, often exhibit behaviors indicative of powerlessness that can affect their ability to learn. Individuals who feel powerless often demonstrate a marked failure to seek information about their health states. They seem to feel that any action they might take based on such information will not influence what happens to them; therefore, the information seems useless. Although Mr. O. had kept careful records of his weight and blood pressure before starting dialysis, he never asked what they were before or after dialysis runs. The staff contributed to this by failing to volunteer this information to him. At times, hospitalized individuals do not ask questions of health-care professionals, even though they do not understand something about the management of their illness.

In addition to lack of information seeking, the individual who feels powerless often displays a lack of information sharing. When Mrs. M. was reprimanded because she had gained too much weight between dialysis runs and was told to weigh herself at home daily, she did not inform the nurse that she had no scale. Miss L. allowed the medical staff to proceed with the scheduling of pretransplant tests, without telling them that she had serious reservations about having a transplant. When the physician and social worker informed Mr. O. that he was to be transferred to another dialysis center, he was quite unhappy, but he did not discuss this with them or tell them that going to the proposed center would present difficult travel problems for him. When the author asked him why he had not discussed this with the physician, Mr. O. responded, "It wouldn't do any good. If they want me to go there, then I'll have to go."

## Patient/Staff Relationships

Interactions with the staff and routines of the hospital or dialysis unit play a large role in causing powerlessness. One patient expressed frustration and feeling of lack of control over the scheduling of appointments in the outpatient department: "They just tell me when to come in, and since the doctors are only here on certain days, it doesn't matter whether the day is convenient for me." This statement also reflects the fact that the medical-care system has control. The patient's options are limited, since survival depends on compliance with the health-care system demands.

The fact that the health-care personnel have more knowledge than the patient about CRF and its management can contribute to feelings of powerlessness in the patient. Patients feel that they must depend on the personnel to tell them what to do. A dialysis patient with diabetes stated, "I just do what they tell me. I don't even try to adjust my insulin dose the way I used to."

Just before the institution of dialysis, Mr. O. expressed anxiety about the level of competence of the dialysis staff. He stated, "But I guess I'll just have to trust them since I don't know enough to tell if they're competent or not. And I can't request only the good ones anyway."

The individual may express feelings that the staff is in control in a joking manner, such as referring to mistreatment by the staff. Mr. O. verbalized this feeling directly when he said, "I guess I'd better not give him (dialysis technician) a hard time while he has me on this thing (dialysis machine)." Although Mr. O. knew that the technician would not "retaliate," the fact remained that the technician certainly had the power to do so.

This feeling that the staff is in control may make the individual reluctant to express anger. Mr. F. reported, "You have to be nice to them—can't get along without them." After three unsuccessful attempts to insert a needle for dialysis, Mr. O. said angrily, "This is your last chance." Then, "Oh, I guess I can't say that, can I? I *have* to have this." Even when the individual attempts to express anger, the staff may not acknowledge it, thus subtly telling the patient that this expression is not appropriate. When Mr. F., a diabetic patient who had had a transplant, said, "I'm sick and tired of getting stuck for these blood sugars," the nurse laughed and said, "Yeah, we're really mean to you, aren't we?"

Health-care personnel may increase the individual's feelings of powerlessness by comments that accentuate the control they have over the patient. A dietitian teased Mr. F. as she helped him fill out his menu, "You're lucky you have that kidney, or I'd never let you order those tomatoes."

## Dialysis Procedure

Not only does the individual feel controlled by the dialysis and hospital staff, but the individual often feels controlled by the dialysis machine, too. People on dialysis commonly refer to the machine as "the monster" or "that thing." One patient stated, "It's scary to think of being attached to that thing—to be at its mercy." He joked about needing a screwdriver "to take the machine apart if I want to, so I can stay in control." His wife gave him a tiny screwdriver, which he wore on a chain around his neck, and he often brought it out when the alarm sounded on the dialysis machine.

The immobility imposed by dialysis contributes to a loss of control by preventing individuals from meeting some of their own needs for several hours. They must ask to have their food cut up, their beds lowered, or a blanket put over them. Mr. O. joked about the "good service" and chided his wife for not providing such good service at home; however, he expressed frustration when trying to eat or hold a book while on dialysis. "You're so doggone helpless when you're hooked up to that thing!"

Once dialysis is begun, the individual has little power to stop it. Mrs. M. cried before and during dialysis, "I don't want to do this. I want to leave." Individuals sometimes experience uncomfortable symptoms that they cannot control during dialysis, such as leg cramps, weakness, and nausea. But no matter how uncomfortable or inconvenient dialysis is, if an individual wants to live, one does not have the power to say "I don't want to do this." The patient is dependent upon a machine for life. Most patients on dialysis are acutely aware of this dependency. As Mrs. A. stated, "You can't get very far from a dialysis machine or stay for very long. It's like there's a chain tying you to that machine." Mr. O. said resignedly, "I guess I'll just have to get used to this (dialysis). I really have no choice."

The feeling of having no choice about the institution of dialysis is a common one, and individuals often express the feeling that "things are moving too fast." This is particularly true if the individual was too ill to participate in the decision to start dialysis.

## Medical Regimen

Other aspects of the medical regimen, besides dialysis, also may contribute to the individual's feelings of powerlessness. Although following the regimen may provide some feeling of power by helping with symptom control, there is still the knowledge that the regimen is necessary for life. Most individuals seem to feel that they have no choice as to whether or not they will follow the regimen.

Dietary management, in particular, poses many difficulties, and feelings of dissatisfaction are often expressed. Mrs. F. cried, "They say I can live a normal life, but I can't. I won't be able to eat or drink what I want and join in the fun." Mrs. Z. reported, "We've stopped eating out completely, and we really miss it. But it was just too hard to stick to my diet." The desire to eat or drink favorite foods is sometimes overwhelming. Mrs. S. repeatedly exceeded her fluid limitation, in spite of the severe discomfort from fluid overload. She expressed the feeling that she was unable to control her fluid intake. "I try not to drink too much—I swell up so bad—but it's really hard. I'm thirsty all the time."

The dependence on medications also contributes to feelings of powerlessness. Although there may be uncomfortable side effects, the individual must take the medications. Mr. O. stated, "Sometimes I think I'll just stop all of them, but I know I can't do that."

## Family Relationships

In addition to factors directly related to the illness and its treatment, the individual with CRF often experiences changes in family relationships that contribute to feelings of powerlessness. Role reversal commonly occurs, with the spouse and children taking on many of the individual's previous role tasks. At the same time, the patient takes on a more dependent role in the family.

The individual often expresses guilt at being unable to fulfill previous role obligations. As Mrs. O. reported, "I can't pull my share of the weight at home." Mrs. S. lamented, "My husband puts in a long day at work. He shouldn't have to do my work, too." Dependency on one's children seems to produce particularly strong feelings. Mrs. Z. said, "My daughter had to wash my hair when I had the shunt. Isn't that a terrible thing to put that job on a 12-year-old for a whole year? But I had no choice." Regarding her young daughters' helping with housework, Mrs. Z. said, "They're just kids. They shouldn't have to work all the time." Many of these individuals express the fear that they have become, or will become, a "burden" to their families.

In spite of the guilt, however, the individual usually recognizes the need for dependence on others. Mrs. S. said, "You can't complain. After all, you're lucky to have someone to help you." This comment was made after Mrs. S. had expressed frustration that her housework was not being done as well as she would like.

The central nervous system manifestations of CRF produce irritability and mood changes that also can influence family relationships. Mr. O. reported, "I get so depressed and irritable. It bothers me a lot, but I can't control it."

The individual's symptoms and treatment regimen also frequently prevent participation in enjoyable family activities. Camping and hiking with his family had been an important part of Mr. O.'s life, and he became very depressed when he was unable to continue these activities. Mrs. S. cried over her inability to join in previously enjoyed physical activities with her daughters. "I used to skate and swim with my daughters, but now I'm a real dud. All I can do is sit. I told them, 'If I can't keep up, please understand.' '' Mr. O. regretted having missed some of the family activities on vacation because of dialysis. "I was stuck with that machine while they were out sightseeing. Then after I'd finished, they'd already seen everything and didn't want to go back."

The incidence of impotence in men and decreased libido in both men and women with CRF interferes with sexual intimacy and provokes marital strain.

All these examples indicate that the individual with CRF has less control over family relationships and activities than before the illness. Because of the value most individuals

### TABLE 7-2. Factors Causing Powerlessness in CRF.

| Factor Category | Example of Specific Causes |
|---|---|
| Disease process | Uncertainty over relief of symptoms. Fatigue, mental changes. Multiple body systems involved. Decreased sexual functioning. |
| Hospitalization | Basic decisions are made for the patient, that is, when to perform ADLs. Routines imposed on the patient without negotiation—timing of medications and treatments. Loss of control over privacy. |
| Patient-staff relationships | Patient acknowledges staff has more control than patient so fears expressing anger in order to avoid being shunned by the staff. Staff knows more about the patient's pathology. Patients not introduced to staff and other patients who occupy the same room. Verbalizations by staff that they are making the decisions regarding room assignments, fluid restriction, and so forth. Patient not informed about progress, weight, or laboratory values. |
| Dialysis procedure | Venipunctures are painful, unavoidable. Unpleasant side effects after dialysis may prevent functioning (headaches, dizziness). During procedure, patient is immobilized. Dependent on others for all needs during dialysis. |
| Medical regimen | Lack of patient involvement and tailoring the regimen to patient's needs beyond the pathology (scheduling dialysis procedure during work time). |
| Family relationships | Role reversal. Spouse assuming breadwinner and/or household-manager roles. Increased dependence on family for needs. Lack of full participation with family during special events. |
| Employment and financial concerns | May miss work because of symptoms and/or treatment. Feels loss of job security due to illness. Job performance may be decreased or job may be lost. Perceived inability to support family. |

place on family relationships, this is an important factor contributing to an overall sense of powerlessness.

## Employment and Financial Concerns

The individual with CRF may experience changes in work role and resulting financial concerns, which contribute to feelings of powerlessness. Time is often lost from work because of physician's appointments and dialysis. Mr. O. expressed fear that his employer would eventually tire of these absences: "They're agreeable now, but I don't know how much longer they'll put up with me missing so much work." This fear, combined with a feeling that his job performance had decreased, caused much anxiety about his job security. He stated, "I'm losing my creativity. I feel thick-headed. I forget things all the time." Although he was unhappy with his job, he also feared losing it. He lamented, "I'm stuck here. I could never get another job with my kidney disease and my age. I'm lucky to have this one, but sometimes I feel like I'm trapped." One indication of Mr. O.'s feelings of powerlessness is his failure to make an effort to plan for the institution of dialysis with his employer, even though this scheduling was a great source of anxiety to him.

Mr. F. expressed frustration that he was no longer able to work and "support my family the way I'm supposed to." When his wife went to the welfare department to apply for assistance and was treated rudely, Mr. F. expressed extreme anger at his lack of control. "I'm stuck here (hospital) and can't do a damn thing about it! I'd like to go down there and just start punching."

Job loss, or fear of job loss, and extraordinary expenses are significant factors contributing to feelings of powerlessness in individuals with CRF.

The factors causing powerlessness in patients with CRF are summarized in Table 7-2.

Lack of information seeking

Failure to disclose relevant health information

Lack of willingness to make decisions

Expressions of loss of hope

Crying and other expressions of depression

Verbal expressions of loss of control

FIGURE 7-1   Indicators of powerlessness in patients with chronic renal failure.

# Summary

Some general verbal and behavioral indicators of powerlessness have been identified as a result of the author's work with individuals with chronic renal failure. Categories of these indicators of powerlessness are presented in Figure 7-1. The powerlessness seen in CRF is typical of that seen in many other chronic illnesses. An awareness of common indicators of powerlessness enables those who work with the chronically ill to recognize when individuals feel that they are not in control. These indicators also have implications for those working with individuals in acute-care settings because that environment, in and of itself, causes powerlessness.

Developing an awareness of factors that contribute to these feelings of powerlessness can help health-care professionals learn to decrease powerlessness. Many of the factors that cause powerlessness can be eliminated. Others can be offset, to some degree, by specific interventions that tend to promote a feeling of control or power. See Chapter 14 for specific nursing interventions for powerlessness in chronic renal failure.

# REFERENCES

1. Bailey, G. (ed.): *Hemodialysis: Principles and Practice.* Academic Press, New York, 1972, pp. 8-46.
2. Harrington, J. and Brenner, E.: *Patient Care in Renal Failure.* W. B. Saunders, Philadelphia, 1973, pp. 48-55.
3. Wright, R., Sand, P., and Goodhue, L.: *Psychological stress during hemodialysis for chronic renal failure.* Ann. Intern. Med. 64:613, 1966.
4. Cummings, J.: *Hemodialysis: Feelings, facts and fantasies.* Am. J. Nurs. 70:71, January 1970.
5. Wittman, J.: *Anxieties and life adaptations of individuals receiving long-term intermittent hemodialysis.* Unpublished material.
6. DeNour, A. K. and Czaczkes, J. W.: *Personality and adjustment to chronic hemodialysis.* In Levy, N. (ed.): *Living or Dying: Adaptation to Hemodialysis.* Charles C Thomas, Springfield, Ill., 1974, p. 532.
7. Abram, H.: *The psychiatrist, the treatment of chronic renal failure, and the prolongation of life: Part II.* Am. J. Psychiatry 126:162, 1969.
8. Abram, H., Moore, G., and Westervelt, F.: *Suicidal behavior in chronic dialysis patients.* Am. J. Psychiatry 127:237, 1970.
9. Roy, Sister Callista: *Introduction to Nursing: An Adaptation Model.* Prentice-Hall, Englewood Cliffs, N.J., 1976, p. 238.
10. Halper, I.: *Psychiatric observations in a chronic hemodialysis program.* Med. Clin. North Am. 55:177, 1971.
11. Anger, D.: *The psychologic stress of chronic renal failure and long-term hemodialysis.* Nurs. Clin. North Am. 10:449, September 1975.
12. Levy, N.: *Sexual adjustment to maintenance hemodialysis and renal transplantation.* Trans. Am. Soc. Artif. Intern. Organs 18:138, 1973.
13. Abram, H., et al.: *Sexual functionings in patients with chronic renal failure.* J. Nerv. Ment. Dis. 160:223, 1975.
14. Finkelstein, F., Finkelstein, S., and Steele, T.: *Assessment of marital relationships of hemodialysis patients.* Am. J. Med. Sci. 271:21, 1976.
15. Steele, T., Finkelstein, S., and Finkelstein, F.: *Hemodialysis patients and spouses: Marital discord, sexual problems and depression.* J. Nerv. Ment. Dis. 162:225, 1976.
16. Shambaugh, P., et al.: *Hemodialysis in the home: Emotional impact on the spouse.* Trans. Am. Soc. Artif. Intern. Organs 13:41, 1967.

17. Beard, B.: *Fear of death and fear of life.* Arch. Gen. Psychiatry 21:373, 1969.
18. Jackle, Sister Mary: *Life satisfaction and kidney dialysis.* Nurs. Forum 13:360, 1974.
19. Abram, H.: *The psychiatrist, the treatment of chronic renal failure and the prolongation of life.* Am. J. Psychiatry 124:1355, 1968.
20. Reischman, F. and Levy, N.: *Problems in adaptation to maintenance dialysis.* Arch. Intern. Med. 130:864, 1972.
21. Maurin, J. and Schenkel, J.: *A study of the family unit's response to hemodialysis.* J. Psychosom. Res. 20:163, 1976.
22. Anger, op. cit. p. 453.
23. Brand, L. and Komorita, N.: *Adapting to long-term hemodialysis.* Am. J. Nurs. 66:1778, August 1966.
24. Comty, C., Leonard, A., and Shapiro, F.: *Psychosocial problems in dialyzed diabetic patients.* Kidney Int. Suppl. 6(1):150, 1974.

# SELECTED READINGS

Buchanan, D. and Abram, H.: *Psychological adaptation to hemodialysis.* Dialysis and Transplantation 5:36, February-March 1976.
Dean, D.: *Alienation: Its meaning and measurement.* Am. Sociol. Rev. 24:753, 1961.
DeNour, A. and Czaczkes, J.: *The influence of patient's personality on adjustment to chronic dialysis.* J. Nerv. Ment. Dis. 162:323, 1976.
DeNour, A. K., Shaltier, J., and Czaczkes, J. W.: *Emotional reactions of patients on chronic hemodialysis.* Psychosom. Med. 30:521, 1968.
Dimond, M.: *Patients strategies for managing maintenance hemodialysis.* Western Journal of Nursing Research 2:555, Summer 1980.
Greenberg, I., et al.: *Factors of adjustment in chronic hemodialysis patients.* Psychosomatics 15:178, 1975.
Levy, N. and Wynbrandt, G.: *The quality of life on maintenance hemodialysis.* Lancet 1:1328, June 14, 1975.
Lohmann, R., et al.: *Psychopathology and psychotherapy in chronic physically ill patients.* Psychother. Psychosom. 31:267, 1979.
Perlmuter, L. and Monty, R.: *Choice and Perceived Control.* Lawrence Erlbaum Associates, Hillsdale, N.J., 1979.
Shanan, J., DeNour, A., and Garty, I.: *Effects of prolonged stress on coping style in terminal renal failure patients.* J. Human Stress 2:19, 1976.
Ulrich, B.: *Psychological adaptation of ESRD: A review and proposed model.* Nephrology Nurse 2:48, May-June 1980.

# 8

# QUALITATIVE STUDY OF LOCUS OF CONTROL IN PATIENTS WITH PERIPHERAL VASCULAR DISEASE

PATRICIA S. SCHROEDER
JUDITH FITZGERALD MILLER

Individuals with altered health states have been described in previous chapters as experiencing powerlessness. Because circumstances and events appear to be beyond the ill person's control, powerlessness is situationally determined. The chronically ill person's powerlessness may be caused by many factors—including illness-related changes, the health-care environment, and the health team's interactions with the ill individual. In addition to this situationally determined powerlessness, a personality trait—locus of control—influences the chronically ill patient's response to the health problem. Locus of control refers to the individual's perception of whether rewards are dependent on the individual's own behavior or are dependent on forces external to the individual. If outcomes (rewards) are perceived to be contingent on the individual's own behavior, the individual is said to have an internal locus of control. If events are perceived to be contingent upon external forces of fate, chance, or powerful others, the individual has an external locus of control.[1-3] (To avoid cumbersome phrases, such individuals will be referred to as "internals" and "externals" throughout this chapter.)

The purpose of this chapter is to describe behavioral indices of locus of control derived from the qualitative study of eight patients with peripheral vascular disease. Locus of control is an important variable for nurses to understand. Knowing the patients' locus-of-control tendency enables the nurse to anticipate:

—how independent the patient will seek to become.
—how anxiety provoking the situational powerlessness will be for individuals (inter-

nals may have more anxiety in powerlessness situations than externals).
—the importance of mastering control-relevant health information for internals.[4]

It is also important for nurses to understand how coping strategies vary, with internals using approach and direct confrontation strategies and externals using withdrawal, hostility, and aggression.[5] Understanding the patient's locus-of-control tendencies enables the nurse to have a more holistic approach to the patient.

# LITERATURE REVIEW

Locus of control has been measured by using objective tests such as Rotter's Social Attitude Survey or the I-E (Internal-External) Scale,[2] the Health Locus of Control (HLC) Scale,[6] or the Multidimensional Health Locus of Control (MHLC).[7] The advantages of using a quantitative approach to such a concept are obvious. Data are gathered by scales with established validity and reliability, and the score is a clear, definitive indication of the subject's locus-of-control tendency. However, administering written psychologic tests could be cumbersome and impractical for nurses. Traditionally, nurses have not used quantitative measures to validate clinical impressions. This type of validation will become a routine component of practice as more valid and reliable tools to measure select patient phenomena are developed.

Even though quantitative measures are not always feasible, nurses *can* use observational skills to note behavioral indices of locus-of-control tendencies. This chapter presents the initial progress in developing a behavioral observation index for nurses to use in assessing locus-of-control tendencies.

A participant-observer methodology was used to determine the patient's locus of control and individual coping strategies. The eight subjects studied were hospitalized for evaluation and treatment of peripheral vascular disease. The process of participant-observer research is well defined by Byerly as involving:

a sensitive awareness of the behaviors of the persons being observed, similar insight into the investigators' actions and reactions, a careful and complete recording of these events, and retrospective evaluation and analysis of data.[8]

Research findings on various characteristics of internals and externals provided the framework for making behavioral observations. Seeman[9] and Seeman and Evans[10] found that internals readily mastered control-relevant information. Lefcourt[11] concluded from a review of literature on locus of control and cognitive activity that internals are more perceptive to, and ready to learn about, their surroundings. They are more inquisitive, curious, and efficient in processing information than are externals. Internals with high health values sought more information about a threat to health—hypertension—than did externals or the internals with low health values.[12] Fish and Karabenick[13] studied self-esteem and locus of control in college freshmen. Their findings suggest that persons with an internal locus of control exhibit higher self-esteem.

The necessity of congruency between an individual's actual environment and locus of control was discussed by Watson and Baumal.[14] An incongruency is bound to produce anxiety. That is, a person with an external locus of control placed in a nonstructured environment and required to do a task that necessitates more self-direction will experience more anxiety than if the person were placed in an authoritative, structured situation.[14]

Williams, Poon, and Burdette[15] studied the effect of the cardiovascular response on 29 subjects during sensory processing, using forearm blood flow to determine response to sensory intake and sensory rejection. Forearm blood flow increased in externals but remained the same in internals during sensory intake. In association with previous studies done by Williams and coworkers,[16] it was thought that the smaller forearm blood flow could be associated with active vasoconstriction during sensory intake. In accord with other research, Williams and coworkers found that the sensory intake of internals reflected a greater involvement in the task at hand than that of externals and that vascular resistance occurred in internals. The vasomotor response could be considered a means of physiologic coping. Lack of vascular resistance in externals may be significant. A number of questions can be raised, such as, do the personality characteristics of internals serve as a prerequisite for developing vascular disease or other diseases that may have a psychosomatic component? What other psychosocial factors are involved in developing cardiovascular disease?

Lowery and DuCette[17] found that internals with long-term diabetes were less compliant than externals with long-term diabetes. Internality is also related to preventive actions such as wearing seat belts and using preventive dental care.[18] A review of additional literature specific to locus of control is presented in Chapters 3 and 9.

## CLINICAL DATA

Hospitalized patients were provided with professional nursing care by the registered nurse investigator, with careful documentation of the indicators of internal and external locus of control in a clinical journal. The following are profiles of eight subjects and their feelings of control, as well as coping behaviors observed by the investigator. Four subjects were classified as having an internal locus-of-control tendency, and four were considered to have an external locus-of-control tendency. A behavioral assessment tool of locus of control is also presented.

## Internals

### MR. K.

Mr. K. is a 53-year-old white man, an engineer, with an 8-year history of peripheral vascular disease for which he had 10 operations, including lower limb bypass grafts and embolectomies, before having one leg amputated above the knee. He was independent and strong willed and had a well-developed self-care agency. His behaviors and conversations centered on how he could regain complete independence and autonomy, not just when discharged to his home but during his hospitalization. His internal locus of control was also demonstrated by statements he made during interviews:

—"I am responsible for the loss of my leg. I have continued to smoke cigarettes. If I wouldn't have gone back to work so fast after my other surgeries, maybe they could have saved it."
—"A person is only a cripple if he lets himself be one, and I won't."
—"I've been a professional person all of my life, and I know that sometimes professionals can be stupid too, so I won't let my doctors railroad me. I let them know how I feel about what they're doing."
"It's up to me to follow through on the therapy so I can get out of here (hospital)."

Of course, these statements were taken out of context, but Mr. K.'s attitudes and behaviors were compatible with the description of an internal locus of control as noted in the literature.

Mr. K. exhibited coping strategies that one would expect of a person with an internal locus of control. He read a great deal to be current and knowledgeable about his pathology, thereby enhancing his control. He actively participated in self-care and worked to be autonomous. He planned aspects of his care, such as routines to care for his remaining foot, and took special vitamins (including vitamin E) that he perceived as vital in maintaining his health. When he had nothing to do, he would daydream about inventions he could develop for amputees, "It would take someone creative and with my background to think this stuff up." Toward the end of his hospitalization, he began to act out sexually. Playful propositions to nurses and therapists, jokes about sex, and a flirtatious attitude could be interpreted as evidence of his altered body image and masculinity; by utilizing this behavior, he was able to cope with the situation and demonstrate his virility. He expressed that he was still sexually potent in spite of his impaired circulation. It seemed important to him that he reinforce the nurses' understanding of this fact.

## MRS. L.

Mrs. L. is a 50-year-old black woman, a housewife, with a 9-year history of peripheral vascular disease and arteriosclerotic heart disease. Like Mr. K., she has had several lower limb bypass grafts, both aortoiliac and femoral-popliteal. Unlike him, she has not had an amputation. Mrs. L. is strong-willed and takes pride that she was able to walk unassisted in the intensive-care unit after her aortoiliac bypass surgery. Even during exacerbations of her illness, she continued to exhibit a strong self-care agency and internal locus of control. Some of the following statements show further indications:

—"I'm the strong one in my family."
—"You've got to help yourself get better around here. No one can do it but you."
—"God can give me strength and courage to do anything, even to quit smoking."
—"What I do to take care of myself will make the difference; it's not up to the nurses."

Mrs. L. coped by striving for autonomy and utilizing self-care practices. She had a daily routine of walking the halls and sitting in the lounges so that she could meet new friends, and through her encouragement to them, she herself became encouraged. She was very aware of her health regimen, and felt she was more in control if she knew what was going on. Prayer and religion were very important to her and were a source of strength. In regard to her family supports, she stated that she had to support her husband and children whenever she was hospitalized because, "I am the strong one."

## MRS. B.

Mrs. B. is a 46-year-old white woman, a housewife, who has a medical history of two myocardial infarctions within the previous 2 years and began to develop intermittent claudication at the same time. She had several lower limb bypass grafts on both legs, and because the grafts failed, she had a left above-knee amputation after a prolonged hospitalization in attempts to save the leg.

Mrs. B. speaks freely about her pathologies and hospitalizations; although she has a limited vocabulary, she uses all the appropriate medical terminology with obvious understanding. She, too, has a very strong self-care agency and works to do as much for herself as possible. She maintains control of her environment by being up in her wheelchair whenever possible. She is assertive. For example, when the medical team told her that they wanted to attempt another bypass graft, she stated she would not sign the permit until her husband came. She informed them that when her husband arrived, *she* would page the doctors to return and have them provide her and her husband with information needed to make an informed decision.

In coping with her chronic illness, Mrs. B.'s basic strategy was to be knowledgeable about her disease and treatment. This allowed her to relate better to her caretakers and to take a more active role in decision making. She stated that when she felt "blue," she would call her husband to cry or complain, and he would be able to support her enough to allow her to regain control of herself and her surroundings. When she felt stressed, Mrs. B. would increase her smoking. Although alternate methods of tension control were encouraged, Mrs. B. stated that she had decided it was "too late" to quit smoking. She also devised ways of adapting her environment to her chronic illness, such as developing a makeshift waist restraint "in case I fall asleep in my chair" and bringing her belongings into easy reach from her sitting position.

## MRS. H.

Mrs. H. is a 65-year-old white woman who has a 2-year history of peripheral vascular disease. She had many lower limb bypass grafts and arteriograms, which resulted in wrist-drop, foot-drop, acute tubular necrosis, and congestive heart failure. All these conditions have been successfully treated.

On original contact with her, she appeared to have an external locus of control. She had recently been transferred to a general unit from the intensive-care unit after femoral-popliteal bypass surgery that resulted in a cardiac arrest during surgery. While she was receiving intravenous medications, the IV infiltrated, and her left hand became

ecchymotic and very edematous. This additional complication proved to be very traumatic for Mrs. H., and she became withdrawn and did not remember events or visitors
from one day to the next. She was passive to treatment by the health-care team and did
not participate in her own care. Although her short-term and long-term memory was
accurate on various subjects, she stated, "They must have given me too much anes-
thetic because it takes so long after surgery for my mind to clear," and "They make me
take too many pills," even though she took only an oral analgesic approximately every
6 hours for pain.

However, about 1 week after surgery, when it was obvious that she was improving
physically, she began to exhibit indications of an internal locus of control. She asked
questions about her condition and prognosis, and she became more involved in self-
care. When assistance was offered in bathing, she stated, "I have to learn to do this
myself. It bothers me terribly to be dependent on my husband." She also began to take
a very active role in the rehabilitation of her left hand. Before discharge, she questioned
her doctor as to when she could discontinue physical therapy. When he replied "One to
2 weeks," she stated, "One will be enough; I'm doing very well."

Mrs. H. is an excellent example of the hypothesis proposed by Smith.[19] At a time of
life crisis, one is more likely to react with an external locus of control, and as it resolves,
one again becomes more internally oriented.[19] Consideration could also be given to the
fact that during the acute episode, the behaviors manifested resulted from situational
powerlessness. In the long run, her behaviors indicated an internal locus of control. An
interesting problem to consider is do internals display apathy and give up more readily
than externals when placed in powerless positions?

When she was externally oriented, Mrs. H. coped by being passive and dependent.
She also slept a great deal, perhaps indicating a lack of energy and physical debilitation,
or depression.

When she became more internally oriented, she took an active role in her care and
stated that she received satisfaction in her ability to exercise her hand or meet her own
hygienic needs. She received support from her husband but directed his actions when
he offered help.

## Externals

### MRS. E.

Mrs. E. is a 56-year-old white woman who exhibits an external locus of control. She has
diabetes and reportedly did not take her hypoglycemic medications for 4 years because
of the cost. She also reports that because of poor heating in her home, she wore boots
for several months without caring for her feet. On admission, she had a large necrotic
area on the inner aspect of her right foot, probably caused by the boots, and subsequently had a below-knee amputation of the right leg.

Mrs. E. is hesitant to do anything for herself and feels helpless. Although she is
not "submissive" to authority, she relies on persons in authority to make all decisions.
Her physical condition improved greatly since admission, and psychologically she be-

came more pleasant and has learned a small amount about diabetes. When asked her attitude about herself, she replies:

—"I know I'm helpless, and I'll always be helpless."
—"My husband won't wait on me when I get home, so I don't know what I'll do."
—"I lost my leg because my husband didn't repair the furnace."
—"Do you think my wearing boots for those months made my foot bad, or do you think it was the diabetes?"

Mrs. E. exhibits behaviors that, in general, demonstrate a very dependent role.

Initially, Mrs. E. coped with noncompliance through total immobility or dependence. She was disinterested in learning self-care practices and refused to attempt them. She was withdrawn and depressed. Later she became more responsive to teaching but remained far from becoming an information seeker. She socialized minimally but did follow directions. She had no helping relationships with any supportive significant others in her life.

## MRS. R.

Mrs. R. is a 58-year-old white woman who reportedly had psychotic episodes during several hospitalizations. She has had peripheral vascular problems for 4 years that required 4 femoral-popliteal bypass procedures. She now has had a right above-knee amputation and previously had a left transmetatarsal amputation. Mrs. R. also has an external locus of control. She has been a "problem patient" to the staff because they feel she is never satisfied with the care by her therapist and therefore does not seem to them to cooperate with authority figures. She does, however, exhibit evidence of help-lessness and uses religion unrealistically.

—She complained of being tired from taking Librium more often than at home. When encouraged to refuse the extra dose, she stated, "The doctor ordered it, so I have to take it."
—"You have to eat everything they give you or they'll get mad."

Mrs. R. copes through anger and depression. She has an occasional angry outburst but often remains quiet and passive. She is very dependent on a close friend and her family. Religion does provide her with some strength. She participates little in self-care and is not receptive to suggestions of alternative coping and self-care strategies.

## MRS. K.

Mrs. K. is a 48-year-old white woman who has had peripheral vascular disease for 2 years for which she had a femoral-popliteal bypass on the left leg. Her disease had increasingly been limiting her activity, and she was hospitalized to be evaluated for a graft on the right leg. Although she had much pain, she did not elect to have surgery at that time because of the uncertainty of its long-range success.

An evidence of Mrs. K.'s external locus of control was her lack of knowledge of her disease and the treatments. She was unsure why these painful tests were being performed, yet she consented to them. She stated there was nothing she could do to "alter the course of her fate" and prayed that medical science would find a cure for diabetes and her vascular problems. Her conversations were laced with statements such as "You can't win—there's no way you can come out on top with this (disease)." She takes all her medications at home but is unable to identify their names or actions. When discussing her plan of care, she stated, "You have to do what they say."

The coping behaviors Mrs. K. used appear to be based heavily on denial and expressions of guilt. She did not look to ways she could function maximally despite her disease, but instead focused on praying for a cure and expressed much guilt at her inability to fulfill her roles within the home. She used religion in a basically unrealistic way. She avoided confronting the realities of her situation.

## MRS. T.

Mrs. T. is a 61-year-old white woman, a widow, who lives with her daughter and family. She has had peripheral vascular disease for 3 years and had a femoral-popliteal bypass graft on the left leg approximately 1 year ago. She now has been hospitalized for the same procedure on her right leg.

Mrs. T. is a very passive woman who generally agrees with anything that is said, even if it is contradictory. When asked how she felt about impending surgery, she stated, "I don't know, you've got to do what they say." Although her surgery was canceled three times because of laboratory tests not being completed or scheduling difficulties, she never became overtly angry. Postoperatively, she participated little in self-care, even to the day of discharge.

Religion was used by Mrs. T. as a coping strategy. She would pray for relief of pain and strength to handle it, which was quite realistic. Another thing that Mrs. T. did when stressed was to close her eyes and turn her head away as if to block out the undesired stimuli. Her coping reflected nonverbal avoidance. She remained dependent and tolerant of everything because "you have to go along with it."

# BEHAVIORAL INDICATORS OF LOCUS OF CONTROL

In examining these data as a whole, many commonalities specific for internals and externals were noted. An assessment tool has been developed[20] to assist nurses in determining their patients' locus-of-control tendencies. This tool has not been widely tested and is still in its early stages of development. The applicability, accuracy, and usefulness of the tool in all clinical situations cannot be generalized until further study is completed.

Based on the review of research on locus of control, patient behaviors were categorized as indicating an internal or external control tendency. Two nurse educators who had knowledge of locus-of-control research and had conducted locus-of-control studies independently rated the behaviors. Only those behaviors for which there was 100 percent agreement were included on the assessment tool. Items that prompted a discrepancy between the raters were omitted. The assessment tool provides a framework for the organization of observations of behavioral indices of internal and external locus-of-control tendencies. See Table 8-1.

Patients may not exhibit behaviors related to each category noted in Table 8-1, as was true of the patient examples presented in this chapter. Through observations of some of these behaviors, a general tendency toward internal or external control can be discovered.

Caution needs to be used to avoid rigidly categorizing patients as being at one or the other extreme of locus of control. Locus of control is to be viewed as a continuum, with most persons falling somewhere between the extremes. Although quick interpretation of Table 8-1 may lead nurses to believe that externality is negative, this may not be the case in terms of patients' experiences of anxiety, recovery rates, and select patient outcomes after illness episodes. Too little data exist to draw conclusions at this point. Strickland[21] suggests that type A patients with cardiovascular disease may be extremely internally oriented. Increasing internality in the type A person may increase personal striving, stress, and eventually maladaptation.[7]

In a review of literature on locus of control and health, Wallston and Wallston[22] concluded that although internals seemed to engage in more positive health- and sick-role behaviors than externals did, findings are contradictory, and in some instances it is more functional to hold external beliefs. In general, internals were more positive in seeking health information, adhering to prescribed medications, keeping physician appointments, maintaining a diet, and giving up smoking.[22] Lack of consistency in findings may stem from use of Rotter's I-E Scale without validating findings using other locus-of-control measures as well as using convenience samples and not controlling samples' variance in terms of severity and length of illness.[23]

## TABLE 8-1. Behavioral Indicators of Locus of Control

|  | *Internals* | *Externals* |
|---|---|---|
| Role definition and satisfaction | More clearly defined, more satisfying | Less clearly defined, less satisfying |
| Relating to authority | Peer-like interactions | Passive-like interactions |
| Self-esteem | Higher or more stable self-esteem | Lower or less stable self-esteem |
| Responsibility for self-care | Active knowledge-seeking behavior | Do not actively seek information, accept what is given |
| Compliance with health-care regimen | Manipulate regimen | Compliant |
| Confidence in abilities | Self-confident | Lack self-confidence |
| Problem-solving abilities | More successful | Less successful |
| Goal-setting behavior | Realistic in goals set | Unrealistic |
| Level of motivation | Motivation | Tend toward helplessness at times |
| Involvement in decision making | More involvement | Less involvement |

Careful study needs to be conducted to determine the desirability of internality training and the circumstances that warrant strategies to develop patients' internality. Arakelian[23] reviewed literature on locus of control and suggested means of internalization. Three types of internalization strategies include (1) reconstruction of stimuli—helping patients change their perceptions of stimuli (reinterpretation of stimuli); (2) action orientation—helping patients learn problem-solving techniques and eliminate self-defeating behaviors; and (3) counseling—helping patients recognize contingencies between their own behavior and outcomes.

## COPING BEHAVIORS

The case examples in this chapter suggest that the coping strategies used by internals are similar, as are those used by externals. Internals obtained strength from maintaining control over their environment, if only through their knowledge of what was occurring. This knowledge provided internals with the opportunity to make informed choices and accept, reject, or supplement their therapy. Internals also worked to develop self-care abilities. Religion or spouses were frequent sources of support that were generally aimed at returning the patients' strength to handle the situation rather than removing the situation.

Externals more frequently coped through the use of denial or expression of guilt feelings, which was not followed by actions to alter the situation. They were passively accepting and did little to increase their own self-care abilities. Religion was used by some externals but was directed at unrealistic goals such as a "cure" for their chronic disease or a return of an amputated part. In general, the externals' coping strategies did not deal directly with the situation. The use of denial did seem to decrease anxiety for the externals.

Similar findings of coping behaviors of internals and externals were found by Ewig,[24] who used two quantitative locus-of-control measures. Ewig studied coping behaviors of patients who had chronic pain to determine differences in coping between internals and externals. Subjects were classified as internal or external based on both a modified Rotter scale[10] and the original Rotter scale.[2] Ewig's findings support the descriptive research presented in this chapter. Externals used passive coping behaviors (withdrawal, lack of goal setting, lack of self-care involvement, denial, lack of information seeking). Internals used active coping behaviors (initiation of action based on self-care knowledge and skills, goal setting, use of appropriate decision-making strategies, purposeful use of relaxation and/or distraction, pride in self-care strides, and information seeking).[24] A comparison of the coping behaviors of internals and externals is presented in Table 8-2.

## NURSING IMPLICATIONS

Because of the uncertain course of peripheral vascular disease, like any chronic illness, patients are placed in "uncontrollable" situations. How chronically ill patients react to their health problem is very individual. This chapter has reinforced that knowledge about patients' locus of control is important in understanding patients' behavioral response. Knowledge of a patient's locus-of-control tendency can give direction for appro-

TABLE 8-2. Coping Behaviors of Internals and Externals

| Internals | Externals |
|---|---|
| Active in self-care.<br>  Helped others recognize self-<br>    care strides, boasted of ability.<br>  Planned for care needs, made<br>    suggestions to health worker. | Passive dependence.<br>  Sleeping.<br><br>Lack of self-care skills.<br>  Disinterested. |
| Social interaction.<br>  Active interest in others, helped<br>    them solve problems. | Social isolation.<br>  Withdrawn. |
| Set goals.<br>  Modified environment, planned<br>    for safety needs.<br>  Used problem solving. | Focused on unrealistic cures.<br><br>Refused therapies that increase<br>mobility (physical therapy). |
| Information seeking.<br>  Asked specific, relevant<br>    questions.<br>  Read about condition. | Verbal expressions of there is nothing<br>more to be done. |
| Shared perceptions of self as being important.<br>  Described positive role as strong person in<br>    family. | |
| Deliberate use of prayer to provide strength. | |
| Purposeful distraction. | |

priate nursing approaches. For example, in interpersonal relationships, persons with an internal locus of control might best respond to "one-to-one" collaborative planning with the nurse in which maximum involvement of the patient is encouraged. Persons with a more external locus of control might be more responsive to an "authority-to-subordinate" approach, as this is in accord with their perceived view of success in interaction with authority figures. The nurse would need to demonstrate competence and knowledge and share experience so that the patient can surrender planning and involvement and look to the nurse as the authority.

Internals may be more capable of dealing with situations that affect their concepts of themselves. They may be able to preserve a positive self-concept in the face of chronic illness, whereas externals may be in greater need of nursing interventions to maintain a positive self-concept. Externals perceive physical disorders as more disabling than mental disorders, and internals perceive mental disorders as more disabling than physical disorders.[25] Likewise, self-esteem of externals may be more vulnerable to physical health changes than is the self-esteem of internals.

Responsibility for self-care is a major area with divergent approaches based on the patient's locus of control. Internally oriented persons might be eager to receive as much information as possible about their health and plan of care. They could then approach prescribed regimens with confidence and enthusiasm and feel better able to deal with unforeseen situations. Much of the health education could be unstructured or self-directed. Externally oriented persons, however, might be best approached by a structured teaching plan including only the information that is absolutely necessary for safely implementing self-care. Externally oriented persons can be anticipated to be initially unsure of abilities, to need more direction in assuming self-care responsibilities, and to have potentially greater difficulty in problem solving regarding unplanned situations.

The amount of structure and self-direction did influence internals' and externals' success in a weight-control program.[6] Wallston and coworkers found that externals lost more weight in a group-structured, externally controlled program, whereas internals lost more weight in a self-directed, internally oriented program.[6]

Goal-setting behaviors of internally oriented persons are generally more realistic, requiring an honest and supportive approach by the nurse. Throughout the problem-solving process, the patient would benefit optimally from being the focal point of decision making. Because of a higher level of motivation, internal persons have a good chance of achieving realistic goals that tend to be self-determined. Patients with an external tendency can be expected to be responsive to having some decisions made for them. Because of the externals' tendency to set unrealistic goals, they may need more assistance in identifying achievable outcomes and support in believing that the goals are actually attainable.

Locus of control is a fertile area for research and is relevant for nursing. Controversy exists over appropriate means of measuring locus of control and the desirability of internal versus external tendencies. Both qualitative and quantitative studies are needed on locus of control in the chronically ill. Health professionals must continue to develop locus-of-control theory through use of pooled data, validation of observations, and testing of hypotheses. Valuable studies could include how individuals' control tendencies influence compliance, help seeking, anxiety levels, health-maintenance behaviors, perceived vulnerability to diseases, and other sick-role behavior.

Planning and providing care appropriately designed for the individual patient's unique needs and personality are dependent on understanding the patient's control tendency. By developing sensitivity to their own locus-of-control tendencies, nurses will not expect similar control behaviors in their patients. It is possible that an astute practitioner may be routinely assessing patients' locus of control and coping behavior; however, few nurses choose to organize care plans considering the locus-of-control variable, as this variable is not widely familiar to nurses. Omitting locus-of-control data in the assessment may lead to inappropriate nursing approaches that are incongruent with the patient's unique control tendency. The patient's behavior may be one of noncompliance unless effort is made to tailor nursing approaches congruent with the patient's control tendencies. Success in achieving health results may depend, to some extent, on designing strategies tailored to the patient's control tendencies.

# REFERENCES

1. Rotter, J. B.: *Social Learning and Clinical Psychology.* Prentice-Hall, Englewood Cliffs, N.J., 1954.
2. Rotter, J. B.: *Generalized expectancies for internal versus external control of reinforcement.* Psychol. Monogr. 80:1, 1966.

3. Rotter, J. B.: *Some problems and misconceptions related to the construction of internal versus external control of reinforcement.* J. Consult. Clin. Psychol. 21:56, 1975.
4. Kirscht, J.: *Perceptions of control and health belief.* Canadian Journal of Behavioral Science 4:225, 1972.
5. Anderson, C.: *Locus of control, coping behaviors, and performance in a stress setting: A longitudinal study.* J. Appl. Psychol. 62:446, 1977.
6. Wallston, B. S., et al.: *Development and validation of the health locus of control (HLC) scale.* J. Consult. Clin. Psychol. 44:580, 1976.
7. Wallston, K., Wallston, B., and DeVellis, R.: *Development of the multidimensional health locus of control (MHLC) scales.* Health Educ. Monogr. 6:160, 1978.
8. Byerly, E.: *The nurse researcher as participant-observer in a nursing setting.* Nurs. Res. 18:236, May-June 1969.
9. Seeman, M.: *Alienation and social learning in a reformatory.* American Journal of Sociology 69:270, 1963.
10. Seeman, M. and Evans, J.: *Alienation and learning in a hospital setting.* Am. Sociol. Rev. 27:772, 1962.
11. Lefcourt, H.: *Locus of Control: Current Trends in Theory and Research.* Lawrence Erlbaum Associates, Hillsdale, N.J., 1976.
12. Wallston, K. A., Maides, S., and Wallston, B. S.: *Health-related information seeking as a function of health-related locus of control and health value.* Journal of Research and Personality 10:215, 1976.
13. Fish, B. and Karabenick, S. A.: *Relationship between self-esteem and locus of control.* Psychol. Rep. 29:784, 1971.
14. Watson, D. and Baumal, E.: *Effects of locus of control and expectations of future control upon present performance.* J. Pers. Soc. Psychol. 6:212, 1967.
15. Williams, R. B., Poon, L., and Burdette, L.: *Locus of control and vasomotor response to sensory processing.* Psychosom. Med. 39:127, 1977.
16. Williams, R. B., et al.: *Cardiovascular and neurophysiologic correlates of sensory intake and rejection: I. Effect of cognitive tasks.* Psychophysiology 12:427, 1975.
17. Lowery, B. J. and DuCette, J. P.: *Disease-related learning and disease control in diabetics as a function of locus of control.* Nurs. Res. 25:358, September-October 1976.
18. Williams, A. F.: *Personality characteristics associated with preventive dental health practices.* J. Am. Coll. Dent. 39:225, 1972.
19. Smith, R. E.: *Changes in locus of control as a function of life crisis resolution.* J. Abnorm. Psychol. 75:328, 1970.
20. Schroeder, P. S.: *Behavioral indices of internal-external locus of control and a comparison of the coping mechanisms used by each group.* Unpublished material.
21. Strickland, V. R.: *IE and cardiovascular functioning.* In Perlmuter, L. C. and Monty, R. A. (eds.): *Choice and Perceived Control.* Lawrence Erlbaum Associates, Hillsdale, N.J., 1979, pp. 221-231.
22. Wallston, B. and Wallston, K.: *Locus of control and health: A review of the literature.* Health Educ. Monogr. 6:107, 1978.
23. Arakelian, M.: *An assessment and nursing application of the concept of locus of control.* Advances in Nursing Science 3:25, October 1980.
24. Ewig, J. A.: *The relationship between locus of control and pain coping style.* Unpublished material.
25. MacDonald, A. P. and Hall, J.: *Internal-external locus of control and perception of disability.* J. Consult. Clin. Psychol. 36:338, 1971.

# SELECTED READINGS

Wortman, C. B. and Brehm, J. W.: *Responses to uncontrollable outcomes: An integration of reactance theory and the learned helplessness model.* In Berkowitz, L. (ed.): *Advances in Experimental Social Psychology, Vol. 8.* Academic Press, New York, 1975, pp. 279-336.

# 9

# LOCUS OF CONTROL AND IMPLEMENTATION OF HEALTH REGIMENS IN ADULTS WITH INSULIN-DEPENDENT DIABETES

## PAMELA MILLER GOTCH

An estimated 6 million Americans have diabetes mellitus.[1] With improvements in diagnostic techniques and treatment modalities, patients with diabetes are living longer, comprising a substantial proportion of the population utilizing inpatient and outpatient health-care facilities. In spite of the increasing number of patients with diabetes, few nursing studies have been published in reference to this client group. There is little guiding research for the nurse on how people adjust to the diagnosis of diabetes, what coping styles are beneficial, what factors determine the patient's ability to invest in the learning process, or what influences the patient's ability to implement a health regimen that is demanding and complex. This study examines some of these factors.

A cursory examination of medical and nursing literature on diabetes mellitus will lead the reader to appreciate the importance ascribed to the patient's role in the management of the disease.[2-4] Diabetes mellitus is a disease that requires skillful and continuous care. Because supervision by health-care professionals is only occasional, the patient must assume responsibility for the daily implementation of the recommended regimen. Individuals with diabetes have and must exert some personal control over the day-to-day maintenance of their disease if a stable health state is to be achieved.

The importance assigned to patient participation in diabetes management is communicated to the patient by health-care professionals. Such communication may be meaningful to individuals who have always perceived that they exert a great deal of control over their lives. To individuals whose life experiences have led them to believe that they are able to exert little control over life events, patient participation may seem irrelevant. The latter individuals may feel powerless, a term Seeman[5] defined as the expectancy held by the individual that one's own behavior cannot determine the outcomes that one seeks. Seeman postulated that powerlessness exerts a negative effect on seeking and retaining control-relevant information, including health knowledge, since individuals become insensitive to and uninformed about an environment over which they believe they have little control.[6] Further consideration has been given to the concept of personal control by Rotter[7] in his theory of social learning. In Rotter's theory, locus of control has been identified as a variable that describes the degree to which individuals perceive that they are able to control life events.[7]

Williams and associates[8] developed a model describing salient elements relative to control of diabetes, one of which was the degree to which the patient performs the recommended therapy. The degree of personal control individuals feel they have over life events is perhaps related to their ability to implement the health regimen. If individuals perceive that external forces control their lives, they may be unable to implement a health regimen, resulting in noncompliance. Noncompliance may be due to an inability to relate one's own actions to the achievement of diabetic stability and relative good health, as well as an inability to seek and retain control-relevant information.

This study examined the relationship between the individual's perceived locus of control and ability to implement the health regimen associated with insulin-dependent diabetes mellitus. The study tested the null hypothesis that there will be no correlation between the individual's perceived locus of control and the individual's ability to implement the diabetic regimen, as measured by an abbreviated form of Rotter's Internal-External Locus of Control Scale and the Interview Guide for Assessing Implementation of the Diabetic Regimen.

The following terms are discussed below so that their use throughout the chapter is clear:

*Internal locus of control* is the perception that positive and negative life events are a consequence of one's own actions or attributes and thereby are under personal control. Behavior is therefore perceived as affecting one's life and determining one's future.[9-11]

*External locus of control* is the perception that positive and negative life events are unrelated to one's own behavior and thereby are beyond personal control. Life events are perceived as being contingent upon chance, fate, powerful others, or unpredictable elements.[11,12]

*Implementation of a diabetic regimen*—the ability of an individual to carry out a diabetic health regimen—has often been defined in terms of disease control. Frequently used measurements have included blood glucose values, body weights, and the occurrence of hypoglycemic episodes and ketoacidosis.[13,14] Because current diabetic therapy is inexact, disease control and execution of the diabetic regimen cannot be considered synonymous. This study examined the implementation of a diabetic health regimen in terms of the participant's verbalizations and actual skill performance that demonstrated ability to execute health-care actions that are in accordance with the disease requirements. Evaluation of the individual's ability to implement the health regimen included demonstration of general knowledge about diabetes, correct performance of urine testing and insulin administration, meal planning that indicated use of the diabetic exchanges, and the ability to solve problems in given situations.

# LITERATURE REVIEW

## Locus of Control

There has been tremendous interest in and utilization of the concept of locus of control in published and unpublished studies. (See chapters 3 and 8.) The following literature review will include an examination of selected studies employing the concept, with more detailed discussions of the research relevant to health care.

Early studies on locus of control demonstrated the presence of ethnic differences. Blacks and American Indians were significantly more external than whites, which has led to the speculation that external control participates in the development of hopelessness and apathy in the socioeconomically disadvantaged.[15] Various studies examining achievement motivation have utilized I-E measurements. Rotter[16] summarized these findings by stating that internal individuals were more alert to those aspects of their environment that provide for useful information relative to their future behavior and that they were more likely to take steps to improve their environmental condition.

Naditch[17] combined measurements of locus of control and relative discontent to define a population composed of persons who believe they are unable to affect what they subjectively believe to be deficiencies in their lives. He hypothesized and found support for the association of external control, high discontent, and hypertension in his population of black subjects.[17] An unpredicted finding was that internal individuals high on relative discontent had a lower incidence of hypertension.[18] It was postulated that this finding was due to these persons' ability to take advantage of opportunities to express their frustrations through civic action or perhaps was due to a more generalized tendency for these persons to actively cope with their life situations.[18]

The term "crisis" implies that an individual is temporarily overwhelmed by negative influences, with subsequent perceptions of powerlessness. Smith hypothesized that a crisis and its accompanying feelings of powerlessness would be reflected in a more external I-E score. As the crisis resolved, there will be a corresponding decrease in the score. Smith[19] studied two groups of patients in psychologic crises: one group that received crisis intervention and the other group that was beginning psychotherapy. Smith found that the locus of control in the crisis group became significantly more internal 6 weeks after the crisis. No significant changes were noted in I-E scores of the psychotherapy group. In another study of psychiatric patients, Harrow and Ferrante[20] found that depressed patients became significantly more internal as their emotional conditions improved. Harrow and Ferrante interpreted these findings as the result of the patients' increased confidence in their ability to master their life situations.

Several studies have examined locus of control in patients on hemodialysis. Kilpatrick and associates[21] found no support for the hypothesis that the I-E scores of patients on hemodialysis would become more external with increased duration of the disease. They also found no significant relationship between a more internal score and adherence to the medical regimen, although it appeared that the only measurement of compliance was the physician's perceptions of the patients' adjustment.[21] In reexamining their results, the researchers postulated that the scores did not become more external because externality may be associated with noncompliance, the consequences of which would be death, in effect eliminating these patients from their study.[21]

Goldstein and Reznikoff[22] reviewed previous research on suicidal behavior in patients on hemodialysis, which is manifested by noncompliance with the medical regimen. These authors proposed that noncompliance was not a manifestation of suicidal ideation but was a reflection of the patients' external locus of control. When compared with patients with other medical conditions, patients on hemodialysis were significantly more external in their I-E scores.[22] The authors proposed that failure to comply with the regimen may be a result of the patients' inability to see the relationship between their own behavior and the stability of their disease.[22]

Other studies examining locus of control include that of Kirscht,[23] who found internal control was strongly related to the belief that general health was protectable. James and associates[24] found that more internally oriented persons quit smoking after the release of the surgeon general's report in the mid-1960s.[24] Balch and Ross[25] found significant correlations between I-E scores and completion of, and success in, a weight-reduction program in that subjects with an internal locus of control completed the program. Duke and Cohen[26] noted that externally oriented patients were rated significantly lower in cooperation and progress relative to dental health, although the criteria for the ratings were not described.

Nursing research has used the locus-of-control construct. Johnson, Dobbs, and Leventhal[27] found that postsurgical patients with an internal locus of control used more analgesics than did postsurgical patients with an external locus of control. The authors suggested that control over one's environment was associated with the ability to influence others so as to achieve one's own ends. Lowery, Jacobsen, and Keane[28] noted that presurgical patients with an external locus of control were significantly more anxious than presurgical patients with an internal locus of control. The authors proposed that the individual with an external locus of control may be made more anxious by preoperative situations that encourage him to understand, cooperate, and in some ways take control of this life experience. Windwer[29] hypothesized that prospective parents with an internal locus of control would pursue psychoprophylaxis, a method of childbirth that allows active parental participation; however, no support was found for such a prediction.

Utilizing an all-black sample of patients with adult-onset diabetes, one third of whom were newly diagnosed, Lowery and DuCette[30] proposed that the diabetic patient with an internal locus of control would differ from the diabetic patient with an external locus of control in both the extent to which health information was sought and the degree of disease control that was achieved. Data relative to health knowledge, disease control, and locus of control were obtained from each participant. The results of the study supported the prediction that individuals with an internal locus of control are more active information seekers, especially in the early stages of diabetes, although this activity diminshes with time.[30] Interestingly, the researchers found that over time the diabetic patients with an external locus of control showed a significant decrease in the frequency of diabetic health problems, while patients with an internal locus of control showed no such decrease.[30] The authors proposed that there are conditions in which the advantages of the internal locus of control are diminished. Such may occur when individuals with internal locus of control, who have always sought information as a means of control over life situations, discover that such activity is not beneficial in stabilizing their diabetes. A decrease in the effectiveness of their usual behavioral repertoire may lead individuals with internal locus of control to exert less control over health and subsequently incur more diabetic problems than would be expected.[30] This is in contrast to individuals with external locus of control, whose accumulation of facts about diabetes does not have the same significance. Instead, externally oriented persons follow a course of complying with the directions of a powerful other—the physician—and subsequently encounter fewer health problems.[31]

In summary, the literature appears to support Rotter's statement that locus of control influences the ability of individuals to regulate their behavior from relevant cues in their environment. Locus of control appears to influence persons' abilities to seek and retain control-relevant information. Research suggests that locus of control is related to ability to implement a health regimen and to the belief in persons' ability to protect their health.

# Compliance with Therapy

The term compliance is used to describe the patient's adherence to a prescribed course of therapy. It has become clear that noncompliance is a prevalent phenomenon that prevents the realization of potential benefits from therapy and produces inestimable costs in both human and economic terms. At least one third of all participants in most compliance studies do not implement the health regimen as recommended.[32]

Davis,[33] a social scientist, has conducted extensive research on compliance. Studying a rural population of cardiac patients, Davis examined patients' health-care activities relative to advised alterations in work, diet, and personal habits. The population studied most often complied with work regimens or work and dietary regimens. Davis proposed that work compliance reflected individuals' eagerness to regain health so that they may resume their former role responsibilities.[33] Further compliance research determined that there was a significant difference in patient compliance based on communication patterns between patient and physician. Davis found that interactions based on mutual problem solving and the use of tension-releasing mechanisms were positively associated with patient compliance.[34] Negatively associated with compliance were communication patterns based on mutual hostility and lack of adequate feedback from the physician.[35] Relative to the illness itself, Davis found that complex regimens were less likely to be implemented as prescribed.[36]

Caldwell and associates[37] interviewed 42 patients who developed hypertensive emergencies after discontinuation of their antihypertensive medications. Stated reasons for discontinuing the regimen included that the patient felt good, had received inadequate instructions, experienced financial difficulties, lacked family support, had become dissatisfied or discouraged, or had experienced alarming side effects from the medication.[37] Examination of patients who had continued their therapy revealed that these patients had good knowledge of their disease, knew the harmful effects of inadequate treatment, had seen the harmful effects of hypertension in their families, found emotional satisfaction and personal comfort in continuing therapy (including satisfaction with their relationships with clinic staff), and had family support.[38] Finding higher dropout rates in clinics with rotating physicians, the authors proposed that failure to follow a prescribed health regimen was enhanced by lack of continuity in the patient-physician relationship.[39]

Hulka and associates[40] gathered data relative to home medication administration from more than 300 patients with diagnoses of either diabetes mellitus or congestive heart failure. The researchers found that medication errors were associated with complex medication regimens and lack of medication knowledge. No demographic data could be consistently correlated with medication errors.

Nurses have conducted research on self-administration of medications. Neely and Patrick[41] also found that demographic data were not significantly related to medication errors in elderly persons. Serious medication errors were related to the number of prescribed medications, the methods employed to remember to take the medications, and the patients' perceptions of their health as being burdensome. In a study of patients with glaucoma, Vincent[42] found that eye drop administration was correlated with knowledge of the action of the drops and with recognition of the importance of decreasing intraocular pressure. Other nursing research endeavors include that of Bille,[43] who found a higher degree of compliance with such post-hospital recommendations as medications, diet, and exercise in post–myocardial infarction patients who possessed a more positive body image.

Several studies have examined self-management of diabetes mellitus. In a study conducted in the early 1960s, Stone investigated management techniques of patients with diabetes in an attempt to identify factors that contributed to variations in disease control.[44] Even though Stone found that he could not relate control to demographic data, four factors recurrently accompanying poor control were ignorance about the regimen, social and environmental difficulties, emotional problems, and patient refusal to share the goal of good control.[44]

A group of physician and nurse researchers studied diabetic patients at home to determine the relationships among health practices, health knowledge, and diabetic control. The nurse researchers were particularly interested in the way the patients executed the regimens of insulin administration, urine testing, meal planning, and foot care. Examination of home health practices revealed that 80 percent of the patients were rated as unacceptable in insulin administration, 30 percent tested their urine correctly, 25 percent properly spaced their meals, and 50 percent practiced adequate foot care.[45] Although there was no relationship between performance of self-care practices and disease control,[46] patients who knew more about their disease were more successful in implementing the recommended health practices.[47]

Interviews conducted with 65 patients with adult-onset diabetes revealed that the majority of these patients routinely adjusted the dose of their oral hypoglycemic agent without consulting a physician and several participants allowed prescriptions to go unfilled for weeks.[48] It was also noted that urine testing was usually discontinued after the sample supply was exhausted. Home records on diabetic self-care activities were discontinued if the physician did not use the records in planning diabetic management.[48] By establishing a diabetic clinic staffed primarily by a nurse practitioner and a nutritionist, Myers[48] noted a 75 percent compliance rate with clinic protocols, which included dietary and urine-testing records and weekly weight loss of 1 or 2 lb. Analyzing data obtained from 145 interviews with adults with diabetes, Infante[49] demonstrated that factors such as perception of self, cost of care, boredom with the health regimen, anxiety, financial problems, and relationships with significant others had a notable impact on the diabetic patient's ability to comply with the therapeutic regimen.

West[50] examined factors relative to the implementation of dietary prescriptions, a well recognized area of diabetic noncompliance. The investigator noted that inattention to personal preferences, peer group food patterns, and cultural and economic considerations had a negative effect on the implementation of the dietary prescription.[50]

Blackwell[51] encourages health professionals to continue to engage in compliance research so that the individual at risk may be identified and appropriate interventions planned. Factors that are presently accepted as associated with noncompliance include complex health regimens; difficult encounters with the therapeutic source, such as inefficient and inconvenient clinics; problematic patient-therapist interactions, such as dissatisfying communications and inadequate supervision; history of health noncompliance; family instability; and inappropriate health beliefs.[52]

Considering the studies on locus of control and health activities as well as the impact of perceived personal control on learning, nursing research on locus of control and health regimen implementation may add to the growing body of knowledge on patient compliance.

# METHODOLOGY

## The Sample

The participants in this study were patients with newly diagnosed adult insulin-dependent diabetes who were admitted to two private general hospitals in southeastern Wisconsin. Each health-care agency employed a registered nurse in the role of patient educator, whose responsibilities included coordinating a weekly series of five classes on diabetes mellitus. The criteria for participation in the study were:

1. Patient with newly diagnosed diabetes mellitus, at least 21 years of age.
2. Prescribed health regimen that included insulin therapy, a specified-calorie diet, and urine testing.
3. Ability to speak and read English.
4. Personal responsibility of the participant for implementing the health regimen associated with diabetes. Thus excluded were residents of extended-care facilities and those elderly or disabled persons effectively managed by significant others.
5. Willingness to be interviewed in the home 8 weeks after discharge from the hospital. This interval controlled the possibility of an inflated I-E score owing to the crisis phenomenon as reported by Smith.[19]

Twenty adults with newly diagnosed insulin-dependent diabetes were studied to determine the relationship between locus of control and implementation of the diabetic regimen. All participants were white, with an equal number of men and women. The participants ranged in age from 24 to 68 years; 75 percent were 50 years of age or older.

## Development of the Instruments

Two instruments, an abbreviated form of Rotter's Internal-External Locus of Control Scale and the Interview Guide for Assessing Implementation of the Diabetic Regimen, were used in the study. A discussion of the development of the instruments follows.

Included in the 1966 *Psychological Monograph* is a discussion of the development of the Internal-External Locus of Control Scale.[9] Rotter's I-E scale, consisting of 23 forced-choice items and 6 fillers, was designed to test perceived locus of control across a wide range of situations. Included in this monograph are a discussion of the scale's reliability and validity and instructions for the administration and scoring of the scale.[9]

After permission to utilize the I-E scale was obtained from the original researcher, an abbreviated version was developed. Nine locus-of-control items, each having a correlation of at least 0.271 with the total I-E score, were selected. An additional item was selected from the research of Kirscht[53] on perceived personal control and health beliefs. Thus a 10-item forced-choice test was constructed from previously tested locus-of-control items.

The author developed the Interview Guide for Assessing Implementation of the Diabetic Regimen. The interview guide was constructed to assess the participants' knowledge of diabetes; determine their current health practices relative to diabetic requirements; assess their skill in urine testing, insulin administration, and meal planning; and evaluate their problem-solving abilities in given situations.

Before the study was begun, the interview guide was critiqued by a clinical nurse specialist in endocrinology and by two nurse educators who were knowledgeable about diabetes. Revisions were based on the recommendations of these nurse experts. A scoring system was developed in collaboration with the nurse educators. Acceptable responses were defined for each item, and a point system was developed. The scoring system allowed a maximum of 20 points for pathophysiology, 13 points for diet, 11 points for urine testing, 15 points for insulin administration, and 8 points for problem-solving abilities.

## Data Collection

The Interview Guide for Assessing Implementation of the Diabetic Regimen and the Internal-External Locus of Control Scale were completed during a home visit 8 weeks after discharge from the hospital. An assessment kit was used as a component of the interview to evaluate the patient's skills in implementing the diabetic regimen. The kit included:

1. Various commercial diabetic urine-testing products.
2. Artificial urine, composed of fruit juice and commercial fingernail polish remover. The liquid was designed to give a positive glucose and ketone reading.
3. Ampul of sterile water labeled "insulin."
4. Various commercial U-100 insulin syringes.

5. Alcohol wipes.
6. Large foam rubber ball, designed to receive insulin injections.
7. Tape recorder to record the interview.

The Interview Guide for Assessing Implementation of the Diabetic Regimen was used to structure a discussion of the participant's knowledge, current health practices, skills, and problem-solving abilities relative to the health requirements associated with diabetes. It should be noted that skill in urine testing and insulin administration was evaluated by using equipment identical to that which the participant used in daily self-care activities.

# CLINICAL DATA

The data analysis utilized the participant's I-E score as measured by the abbreviated form of Rotter's Internal-External Locus of Control Scale and the participant's diabetic regimen implementation score as measured by the Interview Guide for Assessing Implementation of the Diabetic Regimen. The abbreviated form of Rotter's Internal-External Locus of Control scale was scored in accordance with the author's recommendations as reported in *Psychological Monographs*.[9] The participant was given one point for each response that reflected an external locus of control. Thus, a maximum score of 10 points would indicate that the participant operated from an external locus of control; the minimum score of zero would indicate that the participant operated from an internal locus of control. It was not my intent to categorize participants as possessing either an internal or external locus of control, but rather to note their relative positions on a scale of 0 to 10. The Interview Guide for Assessing Implementation of the Diabetic Regimen was scored in accordance with the point system previously described. Assessment of the participant's knowledge, current health practices, skills, and problem-solving abilities enabled participants to achieve a maximum of 67 points for their ability to implement the health regimen associated with insulin-dependent diabetes.

Table 9-1 presents the locus-of-control scores and diabetic regimen implementation scores for each of the 20 participants.

Since this study sought to examine the degree of relationship between the two variables locus of control and diabetic regimen implementation, a scatter diagram was constructed by plotting the 20 paired measurements. Inspection of the scatter diagram allowed the researcher to visualize the relationship that existed between the two variables.[54] Figure 9-1 illustrates the relationship between locus of control and diabetic regimen implementation in the 20 adults with newly diagnosed insulin-dependent diabetes who participated in the study.

As demonstrated by Figure 9-1, the relationship that existed between the two variables, locus of control and diabetic regimen implementation, was not linear. There appeared to be no systematic tendency for a more external locus of control to be associated with a lower diabetic regimen implementation score.

A Pearson product-moment correlation coefficient was calculated to be $-0.184$. There was a tendency for a more external locus-of-control score to be correlated with a lower diabetic regimen implementation score, but this relationship was so small that it was considered statistically insignificant. Thus, the null hypothesis was accepted.

**TABLE 9-1. Locus of Control and Diabetic Regimen Implementation Scores of Study Participants**

| Participant Number | Locus of Control Score | Diabetic Regimen Implementation Score |
|:---:|:---:|:---:|
| 1 | 2 | 62 |
| 2 | 6 | 55 |
| 3 | 4 | 55 |
| 4 | 6 | 57 |
| 5 | 3 | 45 |
| 6 | 3 | 53 |
| 7 | 1 | 54 |
| 8 | 3 | 41 |
| 9 | 1 | 51 |
| 10 | 5 | 46 |
| 11 | 5 | 46 |
| 12 | 9 | 52 |
| 13 | 2 | 59 |
| 14 | 4 | 59 |
| 15 | 0 | 55 |
| 16 | 2 | 58 |
| 17 | 2 | 56 |
| 18 | 3 | 59 |
| 19 | 6 | 55 |
| 20 | 2 | 59 |

# DISCUSSION OF FINDINGS

The findings of this study (although it consisted of a limited sample of 20) did not lend support to past locus-of-control research that suggested that locus of control is related to one's ability to implement a health regimen and to one's ability to seek and retain control-relevant information. This may be due in part to the difficulty encountered in securing study participants.

To secure a sample of 20 adults with newly diagnosed insulin-dependent diabetes, 39 candidates were approached. Of these candidates, 13 had physician approval for their participation but declined to participate because of family problems, ill health, lack of interest, or insufficient time. An additional six candidates were not contacted by the researcher because the attending physician preferred that the individual not be included in the study. It may be that those individuals who did not participate in the study were in some respects different from those who did participate. Only one participant had a locus-of-control score above six; willingness to participate in a study of this nature may be related to one's locus of control.

# RECOMMENDATIONS FOR FUTURE RESEARCH AND NURSING IMPLICATIONS

This study should be repeated, using a larger sample of participants secured through an outpatient facility. Data could be collected as part of the clinic protocol for all patients

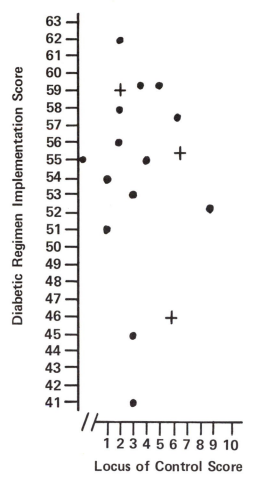

**FIGURE 9-1.** Scatter diagram of locus of control and diabetic regimen implementation scores.

with insulin-dependent diabetes. Baseline data regarding locus of control and diabetic regimen implementation could be secured on all adults with newly diagnosed insulin-dependent diabetes, and a correlation coefficient could be calculated on these data. The individuals could also participate in a longitudinal study that could examine the relationships among locus of control, compliance with clinic follow-up appointments, participation in continuing diabetes patient-education activities, long-term diabetic regimen implementation, and disease control. Research activities that would identify study methodologies that allow systematic examination of the health behaviors of clients in a noninstitutional setting are also needed. Such research endeavors may assist health-care professionals in identifying factors that influence one's ability to implement the recommended therapies associated with chronic illnesses.

Knowledge about control tendencies alone is not sufficient information about individuals to predict compliance. Other data to be considered in planning appropriate nursing approaches to maximize patient implementation of the health regimen are discussed in Chapter 12. As indicated in Chapter 8, the individual's control tendency influences nursing approaches in terms of patient teaching, goal setting, problem solving, and overall interpersonal communication.

# REFERENCES

1. Smith, M.: *Diabetes mellitus: Facts and statistics.* In Guthrie, D. W. and Guthrie, R. A. (eds.): *Nursing Management of Diabetes Mellitus.* C. V. Mosby, St. Louis, 1977, p. 7.
2. Allison, A. E.: *A framework for nursing action in a nurse-conducted diabetic management clinic.* Journal of Nursing Administration 3:54, July-August 1973.
3. Bruhn, J. G.: *Psychosocial influences in diabetes mellitus.* Postgrad. Med. 56:114, 1974.
4. Myers, S. A.: *Diabetes management by the patient and a nurse practitioner.* Nurs. Clin. North Am. 12:420, September 1977.
5. Seeman, M.: *On the meaning of alienation.* Am. Sociol. Rev. 24:784, 1959.
6. Seeman, M.: *Powerlessness and knowledge: A comparative study of alienation and learning.* Sociometry 30:106, 1967.
7. Rotter, J. B.: *Some problems and misconceptions related to the construct of internal versus external control of reinforcement.* J. Consult. Clin. Psychol. 43:57, 1975.
8. Williams, T. F., et al.: *The clinical picture of diabetic control, studied in four settings.* Am. J. Public Health 57:441, 1967.
9. Rotter, J. B.: *Generalized expectancies for internal versus external control of reinforcement.* Psychol. Monogr. 80:1, 1966.
10. Goldstein, A. M. and Reznikoff, M.: *Suicide in chronic hemodialysis patients from an external locus of control framework.* Am. J. Psychiatry 127:1205, 1971.
11. Lefcourt, H. M.: *Belief in personal control: Research and implications.* J. Individ. Psychol. 22:186, 1966.
12. Rotter: *Some problems and misconceptions related to the construct of internal versus external control of reinforcement,* op. cit. p. 1.
13. Williams, et al., op. cit. pp. 450-451.
14. Stone, D. B.: *A study of the incidence and causes of poor control in patients with diabetes mellitus.* Am. J. Med. Sci. 241:436, 1961.
15. MacDonald, A. P.: *Internal-external locus of control: A promising rehabilitation variable.* Journal of Counseling Psychology 18:111, 1971.
16. Rotter: *Generalized expectancies for internal versus external control of reinforcement,* op. cit. p. 25.
17. Naditch, M. P.: *Locus of control, relative discontent and hypertension.* Social Psychiatry 9:113, 1974.
18. Ibid. p. 116.
19. Smith, R. E.: *Changes in locus of control as a function of life crisis resolution.* J. Abnorm. Psychol. 75:331, 1970.
20. Harrow, M. and Ferrante, A.: *Locus of control in psychiatric patients.* J. Consult. Clin. Psychol. 33:587, 1969.
21. Kilpatrick, D. G., Miller, W. C., and Williams, A. V.: *Locus of control and adjustment to long-term hemodialysis.* In *Proceedings of the 80th Annual Convention of the American Psychological Association.* American Psychological Association, New York, 1972, p. 728.
22. Goldstein and Reznikoff, op. cit. p. 1206.
23. Kirscht, J. P.: *Perceptions of control and health beliefs.* Canadian Journal of Behavioral Sciences 41:232, 1972.
24. James, W. H., Woodruff, A. B., and Werner, W.: *Effect of internal and external control upon changes in smoking behavior.* J. Consult. Psychol. 29:185, 1965.
25. Balch, P. and Ross, A. W.: *Predicting success in weight reduction as a function of locus of control: A unidimensional and multidimensional approach.* J. Consult. Clin. Psychol. 43:119, 1975.
26. Duke, M. P. and Cohen, B.: *Locus of control as an indicator of patient compliance.* J. Am. Coll. Dent. 42:177, 1975.

27. Johnson, J. E., Dobbs, J. M., and Leventhal, H.: *Psychosocial factors in the welfare of surgical patients.* Nurs. Res. 19:26, January-February 1970.
28. Lowery, B., Jacobsen, B., and Keane, A.: *Relationship of locus of control to preoperative anxiety.* Psychol. Rep. 37:1120, 1975.
29. Windwer, C.: *Relationship among prospective parents' locus of control, social desirability, and choice of psychoprophylaxis.* Nurs. Res. 26:97, March-April 1977.
30. Lowery, B. and DuCette, J.: *Disease-related learning and disease control in diabetics as a function of locus of control.* Nurs. Res. 25:360, September-October 1976.
31. Ibid. p. 361.
32. Gillum, R. R. and Barsky, A. J.: *Diagnosis and management of patient noncompliance.* J.A.M.A. 228:1563, 1974.
33. Davis, M. S.: *Predicting non-compliant behavior.* J. Health Soc. Behav. 8:270, 1967.
34. Davis, M. S.: *Variations in patients' compliance with doctor's advice: An empirical analysis of patterns of communications.* Am. J. Public Health 58:283, 1968.
35. Ibid. pp. 282-283.
36. Davis, M. S.: *Physiologic, psychological and demographic factors in patient compliance with doctor's orders.* Med. Care 6:121, 1968.
37. Caldwell, J., et al.: *The dropout problem in antihypertensive treatment.* J. Chronic Dis. 22:585, 1970.
38. Ibid. p. 586.
39. Ibid. p. 590.
40. Hulka, B. S., et al.: *Communication, compliance, and concordance between physicians and patients with prescribed medications.* Am. J. Public Health 66:852, 1976.
41. Neely, E. and Patrick, M.: *Problems of aged persons taking medications at home.* Nurs. Res. 17:54, January-February 1968.
42. Vincent, P.: *Factors influencing patient noncompliance: A theoretical approach.* Nurs. Res. 20:512, November-December 1971.
43. Bille, D. A.: *The role of body image in patient compliance and education.* Heart Lung 6:145, 1977.
44. Stone, op. cit. p. 437.
45. Watkins, J. D., et al.: *A study of diabetic patients at home.* Am. J. Public Health 57:453, 1967.
46. Williams, et al., op. cit. p. 445.
47. Watkins, et al., op. cit. p. 454.
48. Myers, op. cit. pp. 416-418.
49. Infante, M.S.: *A study of factors related to levels of compliance of diabetics to a therapeutic regimen.* American Nurses' Foundation: Nursing Research Report 12:427, December 1977.
50. West, K. M.: *Diet therapy of diabetics: An analysis of failure.* Ann. Intern. Med. 79:427, 1973.
51. Blackwell, B.: *Patient compliance.* N. Engl. J. Med. 289:251, 1973.
52. Haynes, R. B.: *A critical review of the "determinants" of patient compliance with therapeutic regimens.* In Sackett, D. L. and Haynes, R. B. (eds.): *Compliance with Therapeutic Regimens.* Johns Hopkins University Press, Baltimore, 1976, p. 39.
53. Kirscht, op. cit. p. 236.
54. Ferguson, G. A.: *Statistical Analysis in Psychology and Education,* ed. 3. McGraw-Hill, New York, 1971, p. 98.

# SELECTED READINGS

Alogna, M.: *Perception of severity of disease and health locus of control in compliant and noncompliant diabetic patients.* Diabetes Care 3:544, 1980.
Beebe, M.: *Diabetes mellitus.* In Anderson, S. V. and Bauwens, E. (eds.): *Chronic Health Problems: Concepts and Applications.* C. V. Mosby, St. Louis, 1981, pp. 210-218.
Blevins, D.: *The Diabetic and Nursing Care.* McGraw-Hill, New York, 1979.
Clark, A.: *The individual who has a metabolic imbalance.* In Leonard, B. and Redland, A. (eds.): *Process in Clinical Nursing.* Prentice-Hall, Englewood Cliffs, N.J., 1981, pp. 384-440.

Davis, W., Hull, A., and Boutaugh, M.: *Factors affecting the educational diagnosis of diabetic patients.* Diabetes Care 4:275, 1981.

Guthrie, D. and Guthrie, R. (eds.): *Nursing Management of Diabetes Mellitus.* C. V. Mosby, St. Louis, 1977.

Hamburg, B., et al.: *Behavioral and Psychosocial Issues in Diabetes: Proceedings of the National Conference.* U.S. Department of Health and Human Services, Washington, D.C., 1979.

Joe, V. C.: *Review of the internal-external control construct as a personality variable.* Psychol. Rep. 28:619, 1971.

Johnson, D. E.: *Powerlessness: A significant determinant in patient behavior?* J. Nurs. Educ. 6:39, April 1967.

Lawrence, P. and Cheely, J.: *Deterioration of diabetic patients' knowledge and management skills as determined during outpatient visits.* Diabetes Care 3:214, 1980.

McCusker, J. and Morrow, G.: The *The relationship of health locus of control to preventive health behaviors and health belief.* Patient Counseling and Health Education 2:146, Summer-Fall 1979.

MacDonald, A. P. and Hall, J.: *Internal-external locus of control and perception of disability.* J. Consult. Clin. Psychol. 36:338, 1971.

Rosenstock, I. M.: *Patients' compliance with health regimens.* J.A.M.A. 234:402, 1975.

Seeman, M. and Evans, J.: *Alienation and learning in a hospital setting.* Am. Sociol. Rev. 27:772, 1962.

Wendland, C.: *Internal-external control expectancies of institutionalized physically disabled.* Rehabilitation Psychology 20:180, 1973.

# 10

# STRESSORS AND BEHAVIORAL RESPONSES OF PATIENTS WITH INFECTIOUS PROCESSES

## BONNIE HILDEBRANDT HOWE

Massive infection within the body creates an incapacitating physiologic response. In order for the human organism to survive, all possible physiologic and psychologic resources must be mobilized. Structural isolation, body-image changes, changes in self-esteem, and deteriorating physiologic status are problems of the patient with a massive infection. These threats contribute to the patient's sense of powerlessness. Mobilization of resources enables the individual to deal with the threat, preserve physical integrity, and avoid prolonged powerlessness. Patients with overwhelming infections use specific coping behaviors that preserve integrity. These behaviors need to be identified. When nurses recognize patients' selected coping mechanisms, they can successfully promote patient adaptation to the stress. The coping behaviors, when recognized as such, are supported and not challenged by nurses.

Stressors and psychologic coping mechanisms of individuals experiencing massive infectious processes are described in this chapter. The following questions are studied: (1) What are the stressors inducing powerlessness in five patients hospitalized with overwhelming infections? (2) What coping behaviors are manifested by patients who are situationally powerless in isolation? (3) What nursing strategies can be employed to assist the patient in adaptation to structural isolation and subsequent feelings of powerlessness?

A participant-observer method was used to study five patients hospitalized with systemic infections. The patients were interviewed weekly during their 10-week hospital stay (except for one patient who died after 5 weeks). All five patients had been placed in wound and skin isolation because of the various organisms cultured from their wounds.

Roy's adaptation model[1] was utilized to compile a comprehensive data base on each patient. Roy's model is based on the following adaptive modes:

1. Basic physiologic needs
   a. Exercise and rest
   b. Nutrition
   c. Elimination
   d. Fluid and electrolytes
   e. Oxygen and circulation
   f. Regulation: Temperature
   g. Regulation: The senses
   h. Regulation: Endocrine system
2. Self-concept
   a. Physical self
   b. Moral-ethical self
   c. Self-consistency
   d. Self-ideal and expectancy
   e. Self-esteem
3. Role function
4. Interdependence[1]

The goal of nursing action, according to the Roy model, is to promote adaptation in all four adaptive modes (physiologic, self-concept, role mastery, and interdependence).[2] In implementing Roy's framework, consideration is given to three types of stimuli: (1) focal—stimuli immediately confronting the individual; (2) contextual—other stimuli present in the immediate environment; and (3) residual—all background stimuli (patients' past experiences, culture, religion, and so forth).[3]

Field notes were used to record observations of patients' responses to stimuli. Everything observed by the researcher's five senses is recorded.[4] Time the author spent with the patients varied from 1 to 2 hours per visit.

## CLINICAL DATA

Stressors experienced by each patient were identified. A list of 46 stressors was compiled, and stressors were ranked from those experienced most frequently to those experienced least frequently (Table 10-1).

The list of stressors (stimuli) was then analyzed using Roy's framework in the form of a care plan; the analysis included nursing diagnoses, patient behaviors and coping mechanisms exhibited, and nursing goals and strategies (Table 10-2).

## Patient Profiles

A brief profile of each of the five patients is included.

Patient #1, Mrs. A., was a 60-year-old divorced white woman who had received a diagnosis of carcinoma of the larynx and pharynx a year earlier. (She had smoked two

## TABLE 10-1. Stressors Experienced by Five Patients with Infections*

1. Decreased physical activity (5)
2. Pain, pronounced on movement (5)
3. Feelings of alienation, isolation (5)
4. Feelings of powerlessness (5)
5. Sense of insecurity (5)
6. Wound and skin isolation (5)
7. Social displacement (family far away) (5)
8. Loss of body part—body-image disturbance (5)
9. Challenged by developmental needs (5)
10. Emotional neglect by staff (5)
11. Lack of self-disclosure (5)
12. Increased metabolism rate due to infection (5)
13. Anxiety (5)
14. Surgery (5)
15. Denial (5)
16. Busy hospital unit (5)
17. Perceived insensitivity of staff to feelings (4)
18. Fear of diagnosis (4)
19. Fear of more surgery (4)
20. Bed rest—immobility (3)
21. Fear of disturbing various tubings (3)
22. Deficient calorie intake (3)
23. Sensory deprivation—no windows and/or TV and/or radio (3)
24. Weakness (3)
25. Decreased GI activity (3)
26. Long history of infections (3)
27. Long history of pain (3)
28. Inability to assume breadwinner role (3)
29. Conflict between dependency needs and need for complete control (3)
30. Low level of knowledge about illness (2)
31. Receipt of messages of anger and frustration from staff (2)
32. Fear of exacerbation of ulcers (2)
33. Unemployed last 2 years (2)
34. Noisy environment (1)
35. Prolonged intubation (tracheostomy) (1)
36. People frequently bumping painful body part (1)
37. Large numbers of people in patient's room at once (1)
38. Financial worry over hospitalization costs and no employment (1)
39. 100% disabled by arthritis (1)
40. Lack of trusting significant other (1)
41. Past coping mechanisms ineffective now (stoicism) (1)
42. Unresolved grief over deceased father (1)
43. Significant other died within last year (1)
44. Guilt over past failures (1)
45. Poor nutrition before illness (1)
46. Restrained with wrist restraints (1)

*The number in parentheses refers to the number of patients experiencing that particular stressor.

**TABLE 10-2. Exemplar Portion of a Care Plan for Patients with Infections**

| Stressors (Stimuli) | Nursing Diagnostic Categories* | Behaviors and Coping Mechanisms |
|---|---|---|
| Self-concept<br>  Physical self<br>  (loss):<br>  1. Body-image<br>     disturbance | 1. Acute grieving<br>2. Delayed grieving<br>3. Alteration in body image<br>4. Alteration in communication<br>5. Social disengagement<br>6. Fear of impending death<br>7. Dehumanization | 1. Denial (not communicating true feelings—not talking about wound, prognosis, tending to talk about hobbies or the past. One patient became very apprehensive when researchers talked about his feelings about surgery; immediately he stood up, washed his hands, and changed the subject.)<br>2. Inappropriate behavior at times (hallucinations)<br>3. Time disorientation<br>4. Anger at staff and researcher at times<br>5. "Ostrich reaction"<br>6. Shut eyes tightly during stressful situations<br>7. End state—passive (eyes closed most of the time, even when the nurse was trying to initiate interaction)<br>8. Loss of body integrity (large, gaping wounds)<br>9. Use of phrases such as, "Boy, I must be shedding like a snake," when rubbing bald head |
| Self-ideal and<br>  expectancy<br>  (powerlessness)<br>  1. Feelings of<br>     isolation (5)<br>  2. Sense of<br>     insecurity (5)<br>  3. Feelings of<br>     powerlessness<br>     (5)<br>  4. Hectic<br>     hospital floor<br>     with<br>     task-oriented<br>     personnel (5)<br>  5. Insensitivity<br>     to patient's<br>     feelings by<br>     staff (4) | 1. Powerlessness | 1. Low knowledge of illness<br>2. Lack of decision making<br>3. "Ostrich reaction"<br>4. Anger—refusing treatments<br>5. Expressions such as, "My adhesions are a losing battle"; "Why can't I talk to the other nurses like you?"; after being asked to express when pain is felt during dressing change, "Oh, so what?" (disgusted)<br>6. Anxiety leading to increased pain<br>7. Restlessness<br>8. "Sleeps a lot"<br>9. When patient asked if ever feels depressed, "Oh, yeah, but nobody knows" |

| Goals | Strategies |
| --- | --- |
| 1. Patient will interact with nurses regarding feelings about illness<br>2. Patient will remain oriented to time and place<br>3. Patient will understand own loss and grief | 1. Encourage patient to make more and more decisions regarding care as soon after the crisis as possible<br>2. Spend time (5-10 min a shift) at bedside to interact and establish a trusting relationship<br>   a. Ask clarifying questions to assist patient to explore feelings (use of self therapeutically)<br>3. Frequent orientation to time and place<br>4. When changing wound dressings, do not show repulsion in facial expression, mannerisms<br>5. Hang personal cards and so forth within sight of patient<br>6. Support significant others in their possible grief process regarding the illness |
| 1. Patient will gain some amount of control over own activities<br>2. Patient will set some expectations for self and future | 1. Use patient's name when interacting with patient (personalize care)<br>2. Assist patient in making as many decisions regarding care as possible (bath, walk, naps, turning, and so forth)<br>3. Be available to talk if patient wants to<br>4. Keep overbed table and call light within reach |

**TABLE 10-2.** *Continued.*

| Stressors (Stimuli) | Nursing Diagnostic Categories* | Behaviors and Coping Mechanisms |
|---|---|---|
| 6. No presence of trusted person (other than researcher) (1) | | 10. Decreased alertness to environment<br>11. Passive, apathetic, withdrawal |
| Self-esteem<br>1. Some emotional neglect by staff leading to lack of true interactions (5)<br>2. Possible maturational crises (5)<br>3. Messages from staff of anger and frustration with the patient (2) | 1. Alteration in body image—self-esteem<br>2. Alteration in self-determination<br>3. Alteration in communication | 1. "Ostrich reaction"<br>2. Anxiety<br>3. Unable to express true wants and feelings, e.g., when asked if ever gets depressed, patient replied, "Oh yeah, but nobody knows"<br>4. Avoidance of situations of self-disclosure<br>5. Decreased motivation and concentration<br>6. Using terms such as "storm troopers" for physicians, "gone to pot" regarding tasting ability, "I'm a cripple" regarding osteoarthritis condition, "all washed out" regarding present state of health<br>7. Complaints of "rough handling" by the physicians<br>8. Dwelling on cleanliness and odor: Upset when bath not given early in morning; told researcher numerous times that he's used to taking a bath or shower every day; when IV (subclavian) came apart, patient said, "It smelled like a horse barn; that bothers me"; "I never perspire much so I don't have a body odor; my skin is like a baby's except when my arthritis pain shoots hard—then I smell like a skunk's nest"; other comments like, "I like the staff here except for a couple people—I bet they'll be glad to see me go" and regarding loss of memory, "I'm old, so it doesn't make any difference anyway." |

*Specific etiologies are not included in the nursing diagnostic statement because all five patients are considered collectively. Etiologies would be patient-specific in individualized care plans.

| Goals | Strategies |
| --- | --- |
| 1. Patient will express feelings about self | 1. Therapeutic use of self to assist the patient in discussing feelings<br>  a. Gently assist the patient in grieving (if applicable)<br>2. To some patients, suggest literature on adult development |

packs of cigarettes a day.) A laryngectomy and cobalt treatments were completed at that time.

Mrs. A.'s present hospitalization resulted in a right radical neck dissection. Three weeks postoperatively, she developed herpes zoster on the left side of her face and a wound infection (Escherichia coli), with ensuing respiratory difficulty. She was placed in isolation and attached to a ventilator via her tracheostomy tube. Her neck wound would not heal in spite of tube feedings and hyperalimentation. Eventually, the wound eroded into the innominate artery anterior to the trachea, causing bleeding and requiring emergency surgery and ligation of the carotid artery.

She slowly began to lose consciousness and during the fifth week was transferred to another floor, since it was felt nothing more could be done for her in this intensive-care unit. She died 2 days later.

Patient #2, Mr. B., was a retired 54-year-old white man who lived with his wife and two of their three sons. He was disabled from rheumatoid arthritis that particularly affected his back. Mr. B. had a history of borderline diabetes.

He was admitted to this medical center from another hospital in his home town approximately 40 miles away, with the diagnosis of coagulopathy. He was bleeding from a drained left subphrenic abscess site. A subtotal gastric resection had been performed 3 years earlier for a bleeding ulcer, but a postoperative anastomotic leak required drainage at that time. Since discharge, frequent small stitch abscesses and extruded sutures had been a problem.

He was admitted to his hometown hospital for an abdominal wall abscess in the left upper quadrant 3 weeks before his transfer. He was discharged after an incision and drainage were performed. Then, 2 weeks later he was readmitted with fever and left pleural effusion and a left subphrenic abscess, and another incision and drainage were performed. Finally 2 days before his transfer to the present facility, he began bleeding around the drain tracts and complained of left abdominal pain.

The coagulopathy was due to a vitamin K deficiency and was treated. A series of antibiotic wound irrigations and a high-protein diet were instituted, and in 3 weeks the wound was healed.

Patient #3, Miss C., was a 25-year-old obese white woman who was single, lived alone, and had been unemployed for 2 years because of recurrent infected lesions on her chest. Her father, with whom she had been very close, died 1 year ago. Her mother had been dead for a number of years. She was especially close to her sister who lived in the state.

She was currently admitted with a large abscess on the right breast. The abscesses began 2 years ago, 2 weeks after she had had a cholecystectomy. She has had numerous abscesses since, for which several surgical incisions and drainages were done over the 2-year period. Two months before this admission she underwent a 20 percent right mastectomy at this hospital, in which the surgeon found focal necrosis and areas of fat necrosis. A simple mastectomy was performed during the second week of this hospitalization.

Patient #4, Miss D., was a 68-year-old white woman who lived with her sister and worked part-time in a central supply department of one of the hospitals in the city. She was a retired registered nurse. A diagnosis of cancer was made 23 years ago, and bilateral lymph node dissection in the groin area was performed. Six years later, another groin dissection was performed, which never healed and currently drains. That same year, staph osteomyelitis in the lumbar region was diagnosed.

Before admission, Mrs. D. experienced fever and an increasing left flank mass. She was anorexic for 3 weeks and lost 25 lb. An exploration of the left flank was done, and 1 liter of exudate was removed from an abscess deep into the iliac crest that extended into the pelvis with extensive necrosis of subcutaneous tissue and fascia. There was loss of abdominal wall musculature over the iliac crest.

Patient #5, Mr. E., was a 50-year-old white man who lived with his wife and one of three daughters.

Two weeks before admission he experienced left testicular and lower back pain after lifting a patient by himself at work. The following day his urine was bloody; cultures were done, which came back negative. Acute epididymitis was diagnosed and antibiotics were ordered.

However, 2 weeks after the initial incident, he exhibited scrotal swelling and clear drainage. The prostate was mildly enlarged. The scrotum was inflamed and indurated over both testicles, especially the right one. A left hemiscrotal orchiectomy and debridement were done to control the infection.

Behavioral responses of these patients were observed and recorded throughout their hospitalization. Stressful stimuli experienced by each patient were used to formulate a generalized nursing-care plan.

# LITERATURE REVIEW AND PATIENT BEHAVIORAL RESPONSES

How an individual copes with the stress of hospitalization, infection, and isolation is unique and varied. Some patients manifested overt anger, while others manifested withdrawn passivity. Roy's adaptation model was used to systematically organize the coping behaviors observed in these patients. The specific and varied behaviors are part of the care plan at the end of this chapter. Common categories of behaviors were noted in all the patients struggling to cope with stress of infection. All the patients studied manifested behaviors from each of the following seven categories:

1. Anxiety:
   —Sense of insecurity.
2. Body-image changes.
3. Decreased pain thresholds.
4. Denial of condition.
5. Depression.
6. Alienation:
   —Feelings of isolation; withdrawal.
   —Feelings of powerlessness, lack of control.
   —Social displacement.
   —Mutual withdrawal; emotional neglect by others.
7. Death or death anxiety.

# Anxiety

Patients experience moderate to intense anxiety when admitted to a hospital, because of the strange environment and the uncertainty over the disease. Selye describes stress as the nonspecific reaction of the body to a stressor as well as a highly specific reaction.[5] A situation is stressful if certain aspects of the physical and emotional environment lead to discomfort for the person in that environment. This discomfort is reflected by psychologic and social responses. Hospitalized patients are stripped of a familiar environment and everything in that environment that contributed to their security—routine activities of daily living, dietary patterns, personal clothing, daily interactions, mobility, and sleep patterns. Stress arises from a situation based largely on the way the person perceives it. This perception depends on factors such as genetic equipment, basic individual needs, early conditioning influencing life experiences, and cultural pressures.[6]

Selye divided the stress syndrome into three stages: alarm, resistance, and exhaustion. Alarm involves the physiologic and psychologic preparation to meet the perceived stress (threat). The body adapts or copes to maintain homeostasis. This adaptation is assisted by acclimatization, which is resistance. Acclimatization prepares the body to meet stress by exposing it to a series of minor, though related, stresses. If this coping process fails, exhaustion ensues, which may rapidly become fatal. Exposure to greater or repeated stresses, with inadequate rests between them, produces exhaustion.[7] Death follows exhaustion, and one of the five patients in the sample (Mrs. A.) died after the physiologic and psychologic stress created an irreversible exhausted state. Selye's emphasis is on the internal state of the organism and its consequences rather than on the situation that produces it.

Lazarus, on the other hand, speaks of stress as an extreme instance of disturbed equilibrium. He defines stressors as the conditions that bring about the stress states. Sources of stress can occur in two types of situations: one that produces deprivation of biologic needs, or makes extreme physical demands upon the individual, and one that involves threats to the self-esteem of the person.[8] These stressors produce a sense of insecurity. It is the uncertainty, the unpredictability of disease, as well as the health-care environment, that accounts for patient's anxiety.

Some behaviors indicative of distress or anxiety, as identified by Minckley,[9] include restlessness; meaningless, rapid speech; crying or angry behavior; and withdrawal. Physiologic signs and symptoms could include nausea, vomiting, headache, unstable vital signs, diffuse pains in joints and muscles, exhaustion, hypersensitivity to noise and lights, breathlessness, and sweating of palms and soles. All five patients studied exhibited these behaviors during the course of their hospitalization.

Other examples of anxiety behaviors in this sample of patients included a look of panic in their eyes at times, shutting eyes during specific anxiety-producing circumstances, anger, denial (not wanting to talk about feelings regarding the disease), false cheerfulness, increased muscular tension, inappropriate verbalization at times, holding the researcher's hand tightly, fatigue, fine tremor of hands, describing feelings of confusion as "being way out there," turning off the conversation when the topic got too personal, time disorientation, memory loss, and hallucinations.

# Body Image

Body-image changes result from the physical deterioration of the body and can lead to identity disturbances. Kuha studied identity disturbances in patients with tuberculosis and stated:

> It is of course natural for the onset of a chronic illness forming a threat to the patient's existence, and for the consequent institutionalization, to lead secondarily to an increase in his psychic symptoms as well. It has been described that low spirits and depression—mainly in the form of intense feelings of helplessness and hopelessness, associated with a paralysis of the psychological defense mechanisms or ego functions—have already been observed in patients prior to the onset of psychosomatic illness.[10]

This disturbance in identity precipitates a level of anxiety in each patient that is exhibited by increased muscular tension and sometimes false cheerfulness. Many of the patients in the present study felt extremely tired; when given a chance to hold someone's hand, such as mine, these patients held it very tightly.

Some specific examples of behaviors and coping mechanisms related to body-image changes in this sample included statements and behaviors such as the following:

—"I'm old, so it doesn't make any difference anyway."
—"Boy, I must be shedding like a snake," when rubbing his bald head.
—References to self such as "gone to pot," "gone to the dogs."
—When noted lack of taste sensations, said, "I'm incapable of even performing that basic function."
—Describes present health state as being "all washed out."
—One patient looked at her exposed, gaping wound, gasped, covered her eyes, and turned away. She stated, "I figured it would look that awful." During later dressing changes she was asked to communicate any pain the procedure caused her. She stated, "What's the use?" or "So what?"

Some patients manifested apologetic comments such as the following: "I'm sorry you have to work with my smelly wound." "I'm used to taking a bath every day and not perspiring in bed." "When my IV (subclavian) came apart, it smelled like a horse barn, and that bothers me." "I like the staff here except for a couple people . . . I bet they'll be glad to see me go." These cues are indicative of perceived body-image changes and a concern of appearing repulsive to others.

# Pain Threshold

Decreased pain thresholds seemed to correspond to increasing anxiety. Patients asked for pain medications to be given "on the dot" when they were due. In a discussion on the psychology of illness, Smith said, "The greater the anxiety in the patient's responses to his illness, the more crippling the pain; not only because of the manifest physical reaction, but also because of its unconscious determinants."[11] It was also noted that the youngest patient (25 years old) tended to have the lowest pain reaction threshold. Volicer studied stress levels of patients during hospitalization and found that younger people rated the stress value of events higher in magnitude than did older people.[12] One patient also felt paranoid that the nurses were purposefully stalling in giving her the prescribed pain medication when it was due.

# Denial

Denial has been studied extensively and has been found to be the most common method of handling anxiety.[13-18] Denial is a normal human defense mechanism against frightening or threatening symptoms of illness despite repeated explanation by the physician. It exists until the diagnosis is accepted. Patients may use denial by thinking, "I know it wasn't as bad as they say."[15]

Denial was exhibited by all the patients in this study by their inability to communicate their true feelings about their illnesses. Until they looked at their infected wound, some patients denied having a wound at all. One patient had used denial for years after her diagnosis of cancer of the throat. She continued smoking 2 packs of cigarettes a day. This same patient never was able to talk openly about cancer or express her feelings about herself and the illness. She died in the hospital without having disclosed her feelings.

# Depression

Roy's description of depression is pertinent to the patients observed in this study:

> When the adult person experiences a loss of a valued object, he struggles to deal with the loss of support-feedback. He also has to deal with the response pattern of not showing anger. Such a response pattern makes it difficult to be aware of and deal with the feelings of sadness and anger that the loss provokes. Thus the person turns the anger and sadness inward and feels less of worth to himself.[19]

Depression is the most profoundly disturbing emotional problem because of its immobilizing characteristics.[15,20]

The patients in this study experienced depression and expressed sadness, inattention to grooming and activities of daily living, decreased interest in activity, slowing of response, irritability, and inability to concentrate. The patients expressed feeling "blue" and "hopeless" and had symptoms of sleep disturbance, anorexia, crying spells, constipation, fatigue, and listlessness. Depression was the longest-lasting emotional state, persisting until the patient was ambulatory on the general hospital unit.

Depression is defined by Schmale as "the ego's shocking awareness of its helplessness in regard to its aspirations." "The effects of helplessness and hopelessness which seem to prevail at the time of disease onset were used as evidence for giving up the 'fight or flight,' in an external objective direction (helplessness), and/or giving up the self-directed, internally oriented fight or flight (hopelessness)."[21] The exact influence of such psychic giving up on resistance, immunity, organ dysfunction, healing, and abnormal cell growth needs to be studied.

# Alienation

Alienation is pronounced in patients with infections. Patients are physically removed from others when they are placed in protective isolation. They also feel unclean and repugnant. Friends and health-care workers avoid contact with the patient. Patients feel powerless in this environment. They are no longer able to become angry. Their affects become "flat," and they are unable to make decisions. They are no longer motivated to engage in diversional activities and, for that matter, are unable to concentrate. They sleep a good deal of the time and are totally dependent on the staff for care. Alienated behavior was especially prominent in one patient. When nurses entered her room, Mrs. A. would have her eyes closed or would close them suddenly. Sometimes she would not open her eyes for the entire time of the nurses' presence in her room. Many times she did not want to talk; her comment to the staff would be, "Let me sleep."

The nursing staff may contribute to this vicious downward spiraling of the patient's psychic defenses by also withdrawing. As Smith states, "In some cases the nursing staff withdraws from the seriously ill patient or from the patient whose death is imminent. The withdrawal of emotional investment in such a patient is a defensive maneuver on the part of the nurse, who must manage her feelings of failure and her own emotional reaction to the meaning of illness and death. It is not easy to see the nursing function as one of helping the patient to accept his illness."[11] Unfortunately, mutual withdrawal constitutes an unhelpful way of dealing with helpless and hopeless feelings. In looking at helplessness in animals, Seligman noted, "An animal who expects that responding is futile becomes passive because passivity costs less. . . ."[22] This concept can be applied to both the patient and the staff.

# Death

According to Mandler, helplessness in its extreme state is hopelessness. When helplessness builds up over a variety of situations and continues unchecked for a time, a general feeling of not having control in any situation ensues.[23] All of life may seem hopeless. The patient with a long-term infection experiences day after day of sensory deprivation, personal exposure of wounds, and lack of control. The feeling of helplessness is prevalent. A sense of hopelessness—a giving-up syndrome—needs to be avoided to prevent death.

I suggest that a patient in the lifesaving environment of a hospital is vulnerable to death from hopelessness. The idea of death from a feeling of loss of control is not a new one. Cannon studied the phenomenon of voodoo death and identified that psychologic factors influenced the death. Cannon reported that extreme fear results in excessive sympathicoadrenal stimulation, which precipitates death.[24] Pattison studied 12 chronically ill patients with emphysema and measured physiologic, psychologic, and sociologic parameters through the use of various scales. Neither the physiologic nor the psychologic measures were predictive of clinical outcome, but the sociologic measures were predictive. In other words, the clinical outcome of the patient's illness was in part reflected by the individual's ability to use social resources, most specifically, significant others. Those individuals who had someone and something to live for lived longer. The data showed that severely ill persons tend to "flatten out" emotionally. This is interpreted as denial, repression, suppression, and rationalization. Severely ill patients cannot maintain their investment and involvement with others and, in a sense, withdraw into themselves. "In essence, if one experiences critical object loss, then there is no will to live, there is no hope to regain loving relationships, and therefore one gives up the attempt to live."[25]

It is believed that Mrs. A. died sooner than her physiologic state dictated because of her feelings of total powerlessness. The entire life situation caused her to give up the will to live.

The dying patient, according to Robinson, needs to be treated with respect. She says, "Care should include allowing a patient to talk of these things (realization of death) with doctors, nurses, and others. On the other hand, a patient should be allowed *not* to talk of such things if he preferred and never relinquish hope or the denial of fear."[26]

Mrs. A. never was able to truly express her feelings about her impending death. Mrs. A.'s wishes for silence were respected, but it was communicated to her that if she did want to talk, her primary nurse care giver wanted to listen.

The pattern of behaviors observed as anxiety, body-image changes, decreased pain thresholds, denial, depression, alienation, and death resulted from specific stressors (see Table 10-1). A nursing-care plan based on the Roy adaptation model to assist the patient experiencing an infectious process is included in Table 10-2.

## NURSING IMPLICATIONS

The identified stressors are the foci for nursing intervention. In implemenation of the Roy adaptation model, stressors or stimuli would be assessed in terms of four adapative modes: (1) physiologic (exercise and rest, nutrition, fluids and electrolytes, oxygen and circulation, temperature, the senses, and endocrine regulation); (2) self-concept (physical self, moral-ethical self, self-consistency, self-ideal and self-expectancy, and self-esteem); (3) role function; and (4) interdependence.[27] Nursing strategies for physical self, self-ideal and self-expectancy, and self-esteem components within the adaptive mode of self-concept are presented in an exemplar portion of a care plan in Table 10-2.

## SUMMARY

Patients' behaviors in response to massive infection included withdrawing, becoming uncommunicative, not participating in simple decisions, being passive during painful intrusive procedures, sleeping, requesting pain medications, and dwelling on cleanliness. The Roy adaptation model was used to organize the data and generate nursing strategies. Stressors specific to the five patients were identified by the participant-observer approach. Exemplar nursing goals and strategies were proposed to minimize patient maladaptive behavior within the self-concept mode.

As noted in the beginning of this chapter, patient adaptation behaviors and responses to infection can be grouped into seven types of manifestations: (1) anxiety, (2) body-image changes, (3) decreased pain thresholds, (4) denial, (5) depression, (6) alienation, and (7) death.

The person experiencing a massive infectious process enters the health-care facility (hospital) in a vulnerable, debilitated state. The stressors of the hospital environment are many and varied, and they are perceived differently by individuals. The resulting stress experienced by the patient is exhibited by behaviors of *anxiety.*

As the stressors of illness and the environment ravage the patient's body and mind, the person experiences changes in self-perception. The altered *body image* is always accompanied by a feeling of self-degradation, and self-esteem plummets. Along with the increasing anxiety levels and negative body image experienced, one's *threshold to tolerate pain* decreases. There is an irony that develops as therapeutic regimens are employed by health-care personnel to help the patient regain health. Many times, in order to promote health, patients are made to endure many painful, dehumanizing procedures during the entire hospital stay (pain in order to achieve no pain and health).

It is not surprising that because of the negative stressors already experienced, the person adapts to this predicament by totally denying the severity of the condition. *Denial* can be a lifesaving coping mechanism when the threat of exhaustion (mental and physical) appears imminent. *Depression* also is inevitable when someone experiences continual loss—loss of body integrity, loss of self-esteem, loss of dignity, loss of interaction with others, and loss of control. As Seligman so convincingly shows, there is a direct relationship between depression and "learned helplessness" behaviors.[28] The *alienation* syndrome results from social displacement, feelings of isolation, loss of physical control, powerlessness, and a mutual withdrawal of patient and staff. Eventually, hopelessness becomes a reality; if hopelessness is not reversed, *death* ensues, as in one of the patients studied.

Nurses can make a difference in this progression of adaptation in patients experiencing complete powerlessness. The use of a nursing model empowers the nurse to systematically help patients overcome powerlessness. Roy's adaptation model gives the nurse a thorough guide for making assessments, arriving at nursing diagnoses, and devising strategies. *Physiologic needs* of the patient comprise the first mode in which the nurse must develop strategies to support the patient's physiologic coping. These needs include exercise and rest, nutrition, elimination, fluid and electrolyte balance, oxygen and circulation, and regulation of temperature, senses, and endocrine system.

The second and probably the most important adaptive mode is the patient's *self-concept.* This mode is comprised of five submodes: body image, moral-ethical self, self-consistency, self-ideal and self-expectancy, and self-esteem. The first submode is physical self. The patient needs assistance in coping with the negative body image that has developed. A trusting, genuine relationship must be developed between nurse and patient in which the patient can feel comfortable in venting some of the pent-up feelings regarding body image. This means spending unhurried time with the patient. A prime concern of the nurse must always be a sensitivity to the feelings of the patient, that is, being careful not to show repulsion when changing wound dressings or not to make comments to other staff members at the patient's bedside. Personal articles, cards, and pictures help remind patients that they are loved and missed and are worthy of these expressions of esteem. Significant others need to be supported in their adaptation to the patient's condition so that their strength can be maximized in assisting the patient to achieve health. The moral-ethical submode needs to be dealt with in a nonjudgmental manner. The patient may be experiencing severe guilt feelings regarding past noncompliant behavior and needs a trusting relationship with the nurse to talk about these emotions. The self-consistency submode is dealt with by trying to reduce the patient's resulting anxiety. The nurse must understand a patient's outbursts of emotion at possibly inappropriate times. The nurse needs to realize that these outbursts are necessary for the patient to progress in a positive adaptive process. Staff members should not become frustrated or take outbursts as personal attacks, but rather should act as a sounding board for the frustrated patient. It is important that the patient be able to express feelings.

When self-ideal and self-expectancy are thwarted, feelings of powerlessness can result. Measures are taken to help the patient regain and maintain as much control over the situation as possible. The patient must be included in decision making such as deciding when to bathe or nap, as well as being asked for input into the medical-care regimen, that is, diagnostic tests and medication schedule. The patient's territory (room) must facilitate as much comfort and privacy as possible.

The self-esteem submode is the fifth and last within the self-concept mode. Again, through humanistic, holistic caring, the nurse shows patients that they are worthwhile persons who deserve care, love, and health.

Role function is the third mode to be assessed. The nurse must identify the primary, secondary, and tertiary roles of patients and then determine whether patients are experiencing role distance, conflict, or failure. In all cases, the sick role disrupts all other roles, and the nurse needs to foster positive role behavior. Again, the nurse tries to foster as much control for the patient as possible.

The fourth and last mode is that of interdependence. Potential difficulties (diagnoses) can be dysfunctional dependence or independence. The nurse helps patients decide rationally what activities and decisions they can make in light of their conditions. This is done in a manner that respects each person's integrity and dignity. As already described, the rapport between the patient and nurse is such that mutual respect is established. The patient must perceive that health-care personnel care about the patient.

Nursing can make the difference between a hopeless, withdrawn, dying person and someone who is sick and vulnerable but who also knows that he or she is worthy of trying to achieve a healthy equilibrium. Nurses provide the patient with support in coping so that successful adaptation occurs.

# REFERENCES

1. Roy, Sister Callista: *Introduction to Nursing: An Adaptation Model.* Prentice-Hall, Englewood Cliffs, N.J., 1976, pp. 379-385.
2. Riehl, J. and Roy, Sister Callista: *Conceptual Models for Nursing Practice,* ed. 2. Appleton-Century-Crofts, New York, 1980, p. 179.
3. Roy, Sister Callista and Roberts, S.: *Theory Construction in Nursing: An Adaptation Model.* Prentice-Hall, Englewood Cliffs, N.J., 1981, pp. 44-45.

4. Bogdan, R. and Taylor, S. J.: *Introduction to Qualitative Research Methods.* John Wiley & Sons, New York, 1975, pp. 6, 32, 36, 42, 60-62.
5. Selye, H.: *Stress.* Psychology Today 3(4):24, 1969.
6. Wolff, H. G.: *Life stress and bodily disease.* In Weider, A. (ed.): *Contributions Toward Medical Psychology, Vol. 1.* Ronald Press, New York, 1953.
7. Selye, H.: *The Stress of Life.* McGraw-Hill, New York, 1956.
8. Lazarus, R.: *Adjustment and Personality.* McGraw-Hill, New York, 1961, p. 309.
9. Minckley, B.: *Emotional aspects of intensive care.* In Meltzer, L., Abdellah, F. G., and Kitchell, J. R. (eds.): *Concepts and Practices of Intensive Care for Nurse Specialists.* Charles Press Publishers, Bowie, Md., 1976, p. 383.
10. Kuha, S.: *Identity disturbances in patients with pulmonary tuberculosis.* Acta Psychiatr. Scand. 49:557, 1973.
11. Smith, S.: *The psychology of illness.* Nurs. Forum 3:46, 1964.
12. Volicer, B.: *Perceived stress levels of events associated with the experience of hospitalizations: Developing and testing of a measurement tool.* Nurs. Res. 22:493, November 1973.
13. Geiger, W. J.: *Behavioral perspectives in coronary care.* J. Fam. Pract. 2:245, 1975.
14. Jones, B.: *The patient and his responses.* Am. J. Nurs. 67:2313, 1967.
15. Hackett, T. P., Cassem, N. G., and Wishire, H. A.: *The coronary care unit: An appraisal of its psychological hazards.* N. Engl. J. Med. 277:1366, 1968.
16. Foster, S. and Andreoli, K. G.: *Behavior following acute myocardial infarction.* Am. J. Nurs. 70:2344, 1970.
17. Druss, R. and Kornfeld, D. S.: *The survivors of cardiac arrest.* J.A.M.A. 201:291, 1967.
18. Cleveland, S. E. and Johnson, D. L.: *Personality patterns in young males with coronary disease.* Psychosom. Med. 24:600, 1962.
19. Roy, op. cit. p. 229.
20. Sobel, D. S.: *Personalization in the coronary care unit.* Am. J. Nurs. 69:1439, 1969.
21. Schmale, A. H.: *Relationship of separation and depression to disease.* Psychosom. Med. 20:260, 1958.
22. Seligman, M.: *Helplessness: On Depression, Development, and Death.* W. H. Freeman, San Francisco, 1975, p. 50.
23. Mandler, G.: *Helplessness: Theory and research in anxiety.* In Spielberger, C. (ed.): *Anxiety: Current Trends in Theory and Research.* Academic Press, New York, 1972, p. 371.
24. Cannon, W. B.: *Voodoo death.* American Anthropologist 44:1969, 1942.
25. Pattison, E. M.: *Psychosocial predictors of death prognosis.* Omega 5:147, 1974.
26. Robinson, W.: *The dying patient and his relatives.* Nurs. Times 69:651, May 17, 1973.
27. Roy, Sister Callista: *Introduction to Nursing: An Adaptation Model.* Prentice-Hall, Englewood Cliffs, N.J., 1976.
28. Seligman, M.: *Helplessness: On Depression, Development, and Death.* W. H. Freeman, San Francisco, 1975.

## SELECTED READINGS

Cassem, N. G., et al.: *Reactions of coronary patients to the coronary care nurse.* Am. J. Nurs. 70:319, 1970.
Dellipiani, A. W., et al.: *Anxiety after a heart attack.* Br. Heart J. 38:752, 1976.
Glass, D. C., Singer, J. E., and Friedman, L. N.: *Psychic cost of adaptation to an environmental stressor.* J. Pers. Soc. Psychol. 12:200, 1969.
Lefcourt, H.: *The function of the illusions of control and freedom.* Am. Psychol. 28:421, 1973.
Mowrer, O. H. and Viek, P.: *An experimental analogue of fear from a sense of helplessness.* Harvard Educational Review 15:200, 1945.
Miller, W. P., Seligman, M. E. P., and Kurlander, H. M.: *Learned helplessness, depression and anxiety.* J. Nerv. Ment. Dis. 161:347, 1975.
Overmeir, J. B. and Seligman, M. E. P.: *Effects of inescapable shock upon subsequent escape and avoidance responding.* J. Comp. Physiol. Psychol. 63:28, 1967.

Seligman, M. and Maier, S.: *Failure to escape traumatic shock.* J. Exp. Psychol. 74:19, 1967.

Staub, E., Tursky, B., and Schwartz, G.: *Self-control and predictability: Their effects on reactions to aversive stimuli.* J. Pers. Soc. Psychol. 18:157, 1971.

Stotland, E. and Blumenthal, A.: *The reduction of anxiety as a result of the expectation of making a choice.* Can. J. Psychol. 18:139, 1964.

Thornton, J. and Jacobs, P.: *Learned helplessness in human subjects.* J. Exp. Psychol. 87:367, 1971.

Visotsky, H. M., et al.: *Coping behavior under extreme stress.* Arch. Gen. Psychiatry 5:430, 1961.

# 11

# ENERGY DEFICITS IN THE CHRONICALLY ILL: THE PATIENT WITH ARTHRITIS

## JUDITH FITZGERALD MILLER

Energy is the capacity to do work. Within the complexity of the human system, work takes place on a variety of planes. In a biologic sense, energy is a requirement for cell metabolism. In a psychologic sense, energy is needed for mobilizing psychologic defense mechanisms. Cognitively, energy is needed for learning, generating ideas, solving problems, and striving for goal attainment. Social energy includes being able to interact with others as members of family and community systems. Social energy is needed for interacting with persons for whom the individual has a cathexis as well as with persons for whom there is no attachment.

## ENERGY AS A POWER RESOURCE

Energy is viewed as a power resource because of the vastly important role it plays biologically, psychologically, cognitively, and socially. Energy provides power in the following ways: It is a resource for mobility,[1] a factor in promoting well-being and a feeling of physical reserve, a means of providing confidence in task accomplishment, and a means of responding to unexpected stress. An energy deficit contributes to powerlessness. When the capacity to do work is lacking, powerlessness exists. The term entropy is used to describe disorganization resulting from energy loss.[2] When a state of entropy exists, the organism is powerless. Energy deficits are a common problem in chronically ill patients.

In nursing care of chronically ill patients, helping the patient become aware of energy resources and manage energy deficits is an empowerment strategy. Specific aspects of energy as a power resource will be examined more closely.

# Energy Is a Basic Mobility Resource

Fagerhaugh[1] describes energy, time, and money as basic mobility resources. Individuals draw on basic mobility resources for physical mobility and sociability. The individual's needs for physical mobility and sociability are easily met during various states of health, if adequate financial resources are present. However, basic mobility resources are decreased and continue to dwindle in persons with chronic health problems. Persons who have low energy resources but sufficient money resources can purchase the basic mobility resources of another. Mobility assistants can be hired[1] to help with various living tasks—cleaning, cooking, transportation, and so forth.

Typically, the chronically ill person suffers from a deficit of the basic mobility resource energy. Furthermore, when the ill person also lacks sufficient financial resources, the only remaining basic mobility resource is time. Having all the time available that is needed, the patient will spend it to accomplish the mobility task. For example, the patient with emphysema may require the entire morning to get dressed and perform normal morning hygiene activities. The same patient may also spend twice as much time performing routine errands such as walking to the store, since the patient may have to stop to "catch a breath" at puffing stations along the way. Figuring out which route has the least resistance (terrain without walking uphill) and allowing sufficient time to avoid the routes with difficult terrain are ways of using time as a basic mobility resource.[1]

# Energy Promotes Well-being

A sense of self-satisfaction and well-being is felt when energy is present. The individual can control interactions with the environment and can engage in meaningful activities. Meaningful activities and interactions provide positive feedback about self and give a sense of joy.

# Energy Enables Task Accomplishment and Ability to Respond to Needs

Energy is a basic necessity for task accomplishment. Whether the tasks be providing self-care, learning new skills, working on the job, performing other roles, or responding to unexpected stress, energy gives the individual confidence in ability to complete the task successfully. Because of the extensive energy requirements in individuals with chronic illness, energy deficits may be a problem. Analysis of the energy state is important.

# ENERGY ANALYSIS FORMAT

## Energy Sources and Transformation

Ryden[3] presents a comprehensive format to examine energy. Three constructs proposed in Ryden's energy utilization model are (1) energy sources, (2) energy transformation, and (3) energy expenditure or storage. Energy sources include nutrients, oxygen, and water; other sources are rest and motivation. Energy transformation refers to the body's physiologic processing and distribution of energy sources.[3] In chronically ill persons, energy is affected by pathophysiologic changes that may interfere with digestion, circulation, respiration, endocrine balance, and cellular metabolism. The third construct is energy expenditure. According to Ryden, energy expenditure takes place on three levels: compensation, mobility, and growth. At the compensation level, energy is used for restoration of physical and psychosocial equilibrium. At the mobility level, energy is spent in work, hobbies, and dealing with the external environment. At the growth level, energy is spent in learning. Figure 11-1 contains Knoebel's interpretation[4] of Ryden's model.[3]

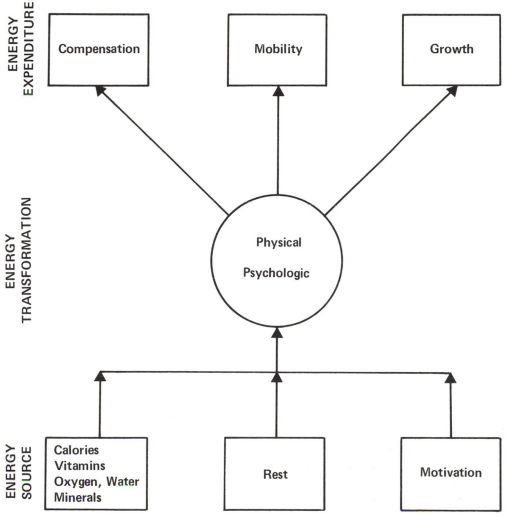

FIGURE 11-1.   Knoebel interpretation of Ryden energy source-utilization model.

# Energy Requirements in Chronically Ill Persons

In order to understand the energy deficits in chronically ill persons, a more specific analysis of energy requirements is needed. Energy requirements will be discussed in terms of restoration of physical integrity, role expansion and coping with the effects of illness, daily activities that cannot be omitted, activities that provide social stimulation, recreation, exercise, and learning. In this light, energy requirements include specific energy needs above and beyond that energy needed for basal metabolism. The model presented in Figure 11-2 forms the basis for discussion throughout this chapter.

Restoration of physical integrity refers to wound healing (soft tissue and bones), recovering from inflammatory processes, achieving a metabolic balance (as between nutrients, insulin level, and exercise), generating new cells after cell destruction from medical therapy (chemotherapy and radiation therapy), and participating in physical therapy regimens to restore muscle strength. Pathophysiologic demands and therapy demands create a compromised energy state in chronically ill persons.

Role expansion and coping with the effects of illness require energy. Illness demands the individual learn new self-care practices, monitor self-response to therapy, and become sensitive to cues that need action to avert a crisis. Role expansion includes learning the goals, behaviors, and sentiments of the new role. For chronically ill patients, the new role is self-care agent. A self-care agent is the individual (or designate) who carries out self-care practices to meet requisites presented to the individual. Such requisites arise from therapies, developmental needs, and universal needs.[5] The role of self-care agent includes varied activities, for example, calculating diet according to prescribed calories and fat restriction, administering prescribed medications, or irrigating a wound.

The new role expectations of self-care agent are beyond the continuing roles and role expectations. Those continuing roles may include mother, housewife, participant in children's school events, member of the symphony women's league, and part-time teacher of an adult art education course. The role expansion increases energy demands, adding new time pressures, problem solving, and anxieties because of role insufficiency. Role insufficiency is any difficulty in learning and/or performing new role behavior.

Coping with the tasks of a chronic illness requires energy. Because coping has been discussed in detail in Chapter 2, only brief examples of energy depletion and coping are presented here. The examples selected are those that do not require extreme physical exertion such as jogging. Coping strategies such as self-disclosure, examining feelings, developing insights to the feelings, and relating feelings to behaviors are challenging and drain energy. Other preferred verbal modes of expression used as coping mechanisms—such as laughing, crying, and singing—may be especially taxing to a person with a chronic condition such as severe pulmonary emphysema. The coping tasks of chronic illness identified in Chapter 2 and the psychosocial challenges of illness discussed later in this chapter require energy.

Energy is required for daily activities that satisfy basic needs. These activities cannot be omitted and can be considered synonymous with daily activities that satisfy some of the universal self-care requisites proposed by Orem.[5] The universal self-care requisites include air, water, food, elimination, activity and rest, solitude and social interaction, and

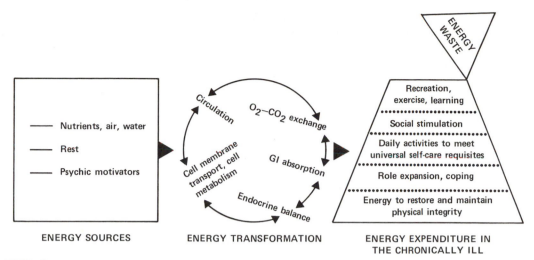

FIGURE 11-2. Energy analysis model for chronically ill persons.

protection from harm. Maintaining personal hygiene and getting dressed are other examples of activities of daily living.

Activities that may not be required daily but are essential to preventing loneliness, low self-esteem, or distorted self-concept are those which provide for social interaction. Social activities, although they require energy, provide an opportunity for human interaction. The result of this communication is, indirectly, feedback about self. The person may feel, "I was successful in relating to another; she seemed to enjoy my company; I was able to be of assistance to another; and I received positive feedback about how I am doing."

Recreation, exercise, and learning are essential for enjoying life. Adequate energy sources are needed for all three activities to take place.

While energy expenditure in the above categories is required, energy is depleted or wasted in many ways in chronically ill persons.

## Energy Wasters

Preventing energy depletion by eliminating energy waste is a responsibility of nursing. Energy is wasted through physical means, lack of environmental management, and unchanneled psychologic reactions and feelings (Table 11-1). Nursing interventions can be directed toward alleviating physical discomforts that waste energy. These physical discomforts may include inadequate pain management, anorexia, fever, infection, diarrhea, and interrupted sleep. Forced immobility, which occurs when patients are in traction or casts or on bed rest, causes diminished muscle strength and muscle atrophy. Lack of environmental management by poor planning—for example, by making unnecessary trips up and down stairs—or by lack of priority setting in undertaking the day's activities can be alleviated by the nurse. Nurses can help patients gain insight into their behavior and recognize specific ways their environment can be managed to eliminate

**TABLE 11-1.  Energy Depletion from Waste**

| Physical | Lack of Environmental Management | Psychologic |
|---|---|---|
| Pain—inadequate pain-management resources | Uncoordinated efforts directed at a variety of tasks to be accomplished | Uncontrolled anxiety |
| Anorexia | Lack of planning before engaging in physical activities | Unexpressed anger, hostility |
| Fever | No priorities identified so as to eliminate frustration when least | Unresolved grief |
| Infection | important tasks are not accomplished | |
| Diarrhea | Procrastination; working at avoiding getting started | |
| Interrupted sleep | Giving up quickly, necessitating repetitious starting over in task-accomplishment efforts | |
| Forced immobility—traction, casts, bed rest | | |

energy waste. Psychologic energy wasters may include uncontrolled anxiety, unexpressed anger, and unresolved grief. Identifying the patient's energy wasters is an important component of the energy-analysis format (see Fig. 11-1). It is nursing's responsibility to assess energy sources, transformation, and expenditure. Specific nursing diagnoses describing energy deficits can be identified.

# Nursing Diagnoses and Patient-Identified Dilemmas

Specific nursing diagnostic statements relating to energy can be made as a result of the energy analysis. Exemplar nursing diagnoses are included in the following:

— Guilt due to an inability to fulfill expected roles according to personally established criteria.
— Anxiety due to lack of knowledge regarding the meaning of energy depletion.
— Unpredictable daily work-rest pattern due to changing energy availability.
— Inability to recognize depleted energy states due to lack of internal awareness.
— Helplessness due to a perceived lack of control over energy expenditure.
— Frustration related to inability to complete desired tasks within a specified time.

Although it is easy to empathize with patients who may have to eliminate certain activities because of energy deficits, the real impact of energy dilemmas can be felt and expressed only by the patients themselves. Consider the following abbreviated descriptions of dilemmas that occur in patients with rheumatoid arthritis:

A 56-year-old woman described what difficulty she felt because she could not even plan ahead during a day. A friend called her at 9:00 A.M. and suggested that they meet for lunch. Because the patient was feeling stiff with increased pain and fatigue at that particular time, she refused lunch, only to be symptom-free by noon. The patient described the uncertainty of how she would feel (how much energy she would have), being unable to plan ahead, feeling somewhat embarrassed over having misjudged her status, and being unable to begin to explain the uncertainty dilemma to her healthy friend. She regretted needlessly missing an opportunity to alleviate her loneliness (she lived in a rural area, her husband was at work all day, and there were no neighbors who dropped by). She was hesitant to initiate social plans with others because of her uncertainty in being able to carry out the plans.

A middle-aged woman who had majored in music and enjoyed playing classical music on the piano was forced to give up style and grace of playing the piece properly because of arthritic changes (lack of strength and dexterity, and increased pain) in her hands. For someone who had taught music and proper interpretation of musical works, this posed a difficult problem. She would have to refrain from playing for months at a time during exacerbations in order to protect her joints and provide them with rest. Absence of this important part of her life caused real grief.

Another woman expressed role insufficiency because of the weakness and fatigue caused by the arthritis. She stated, "Now that I finally have grandchildren, I am unable to enjoy them. With my arthritis, I'm afraid I will drop the baby. I looked forward to running in the back yard with them; by the time they're old enough to run, I'll be lucky if I'm able to get myself to the table to eat." She expressed feeling deprived of a role that belonged to her and looked forward to a future filled with disability and dependence.

John was a middle-aged factory worker with newly diagnosed rheumatoid arthritis. For a number of years, John and his fellow workers played cards during breaks and lunch hour, keeping a running tally of wins, losses, and so forth. Now, instead of playing cards, John uses the time to rest and relax in a lounge chair within view of the card playing. John feels his buddies resent his behavior and view it as an abnormal withdrawal. He feels it is impossible to convince the other men of his necessity to rest so he can complete his 8-hour shift. The fellow workers have commented to him, "You're making too much of this arthritis thing. You don't look any different than you ever did." John feels socially isolated at work as a result of his careful use of time to restore energy.

A grade-school teacher in her 30s discovered that standing outside for playground duty in the morning and at noon precipitated pain and unnecessarily depleted energy. She felt guilty in trying to be excused from this duty even though she would exchange this activity with lunch room monitoring. She felt it was a reflection of her inadequacy as a teacher.

The feelings of being a burden are readily described by Mrs. T. Since her rheumatoid disease has progressively worsened, she has been unable to keep up her own apartment. "Now I have to live with my son, daughter-in-law, and their family. They don't like it any more than I do. I feel so in the way, so always present—someone extra who is monitoring their fights and their times of intimacy."

The defining characteristics of energy-deficit diagnoses identified by Pinekenstein[6] in her study of patients with cancer has relevance for analysis of energy states in general. Two categories of defining characteristics of the nursing diagnosis "energy deficiencies" were patient verbalizations and nonverbal responses. Patients' verbalizations of actual or perceived changes in energy level included references to past energy, "I used to be able to work all day, make supper, and attend an evening class. Now it's difficult to set the table." Patients' references to present energy level may include, "I'm weak, just don't have any strength." Patients may verbalize hopelessness by stating, "I'm just the same, as weak as ever, despite the physical therapy. It's no use."

The nonverbal responses to energy changes include decreased social involvement (irritability, use of frequent rest periods, decreased socialization with family and friends), weight loss and muscle wasting, decreased activity tolerance, excessive use of routine patterns, and use of others' basic mobility resources.

Analysis of energy in patients with rheumatoid arthritis serves as a prototype for energy analysis in chronically ill persons. The unique problems of patients with arthritis are discussed.

# ENERGY DEPLETION IN PATIENTS WITH RHEUMATOID ARTHRITIS

Arthritis afflicts more than 31.6 million Americans; of these, 6.5 million have rheumatoid arthritis.[7] Rheumatoid arthritis is a systemic autoimmune disease that affects joints and connective tissue. The effects of the disease can be widespread and completely debilitating. The outstanding patient challenges are to maintain comfort, preserve joint mobility and function, protect joints during exacerbations, complete prescribed exercise routines to maintain muscle strength and joint function, adhere to medicine regimens, pace activities to conserve energy, and obtain emotional and systemic rest.[8] Because of these challenges, the patient with arthritis is described as a prototype for understanding energy deficits in chronically ill patients. Energy depletion in patients with arthritis results from physiologic and psychologic processes.

## Physiologic Energy Depletion

Physiologically, energy depletion is due to inflammation, metabolic changes, and pain. The connective tissue and joints become inflamed. The resultant swelling, stiffness, and muscle spasm cause pain that depletes energy. Metabolic changes occur, such as synovial membrane hypertrophy, articular cartilage destruction, and invasion of pannus into the bone. The resultant swelling, stiffness, and muscle spasm cause pain that depletes energy. Other systemic effects of the disease include muscle atrophy, myositis, fever, anorexia, and malaise. The inflammatory process can be widespread, as in arteritis, iritis, pneumonitis, and carditis.[9] Anemia contributes to poor energy reserve in patients with arthritis and results from the blockage of iron release from the reticuloendothelial cells to the erythropoietic cells.[10]

Because pain is chronic, the patient with arthritis cannot anticipate an end; relief would be a pleasant outcome, as in the healing of a surgical incision or the birth of a baby. However, as Swartz[11] puts it, "Arthritis is so damned daily."

# Energy Is Affected by Psychologic State

The psychologic and social processes and characteristics that accompany chronic illness deplete energy. Psychologic characteristics of individuals with chronic illness and those specifically prevalent in patients with arthritis may include anger, contained hostility,[12] depression, hypochondriasis, hysteria,[13] and mourning.[14] Energy is wasted in anxiety. Patients have anxiety over uncertainty of energy availability from day to day.[15] Anxiety is also present in terms of pain control. Patients ask themselves, ''Where will it hit next? How bad will it be? What residual weakness and deformity will I suffer?''

Myerowitz[16] categorized the research on psychosocial variables in rheumatoid arthritis into three groups of studies:

1. Studies that focused on characteristics present in subjects before disease onset (rheumatoid arthritis personality studies).
2. Studies that examined relationships of life experiences and psychologic states just before disease onset.
3. Studies that suggest psychologic responses during the course of the illness.

It is beyond the scope of this chapter to replicate a review of the literature on psychosocial variables and arthritis. The reader is directed to major literature-review works of King,[17] Moos,[18] and Hoffman.[19] However, findings of studies in Myerowitz' first category have been refuted. Zeitlin[14] states that there is no convincing evidence that a premorbid ''rheumatoid personality'' exists.

The studies on psychologic experience and related disease onset have been critiqued because of the retrospective recall of the subjects and investigator bias.[14] Two groups of patients have been identified by Rimon.[20] One group of patients with arthritis has acute disease onset, rapid symptom progression, and lack of hereditary predisposition. These patients have had a significant conflicting situation in their lives. The other type of patient has an insidious onset, delayed symptom progression, and no identifiable psychologic conflict at the disease onset or at times of exacerbation.

Research on psychologic findings throughout the course of the disease is not unique to the patient with arthritis but is applicable to all patients coping with chronic health problems.[13] It is understandable that behaviors of anger, frustration, anxiety, and depression would result from the symptoms and disability of the disease. There are some unique differences in responses between patients with arthritis and patients with other health problems. Patients with rheumatoid arthritis anticipate the course of their disease to get worse, whereas patients with peptic ulcers do not believe this is the future course for their illness.[21]

# Disabling Themes in Arthritis

The diagnosis of rheumatoid arthritis is accompanied by disabling themes in that the patient fears becoming crippled, being perceived as being old and nonproductive, and not being understood by loved ones (being unable to obtain empathy from significant others). Mayville[22] proposed reasons why some patients with newly diagnosed rheumatoid arthritis display disabled behaviors after the diagnosis but displayed no changes in gait, posture, pace of movement, and joint dexterity before the diagnosis. She states their behaviors are due to previous knowledge of arthritis and associations with others who have the disease, patient efforts to reduce joint movement to control pain, low energy levels and joint stiffness, self-concept change of perceiving self as being old and disabled, and acting out a need for empathy as a signal to others to try to understand their plight. Some of the identified responses may be a positive means of coping and a way of decreasing joint aggravation. Other behavior reflecting a distorted self-image may need nursing intervention.

# NORMALIZING

Patient endeavors to normalize (described as a coping task in Chapter 2) expend energy. Wiener[15] described the components of this behavior, which she identified in a study of 21 subjects with rheumatoid arthritis. Normalizing refers to behaviors an individual uses to continue what the individual perceives to be a normal life. The categories of normalizing identified by Wiener were covering up, keeping up, justifying inaction, pacing, eliciting help, and balancing the options.

Covering up allows patients with arthritis to view themselves as they would prefer to be viewed by others. It includes keeping the signs and symptoms of the disease (assistive devices, slowed gait, painful expressions) out of view of others.

Keeping up refers to carrying on with the same schedule one kept before the diagnosis, resulting in exhaustion, excessive time for rest to restore energy, and, in some cases, exacerbation of symptoms and fever. Wiener[15] identifies a paradox in patients who cover up and keep up. These patients long for understanding and sensitivity. They verbalize, "Nobody really knows how bad it is," yet state, "If I acted the way I feel, nobody would want to be around me." The patients use energy in wishing for caring empathy while using energy to guard against turning off family and friends.

Justifying inaction includes providing rationale to others for not being able to engage in activities or meet their expectations. Justifying inaction may be necessary in cases of pain, stiffness, and uncertainty that accompanies the illness. However, justifying inaction becomes especially problematic after a history of covering up and keeping up. Imagine the dilemma of the woman who in the morning refused an afternoon bridge club engagement and then is seen shopping later in the afternoon. With the uncertainty of severity of symptoms, with increased morning stiffness on this particular day—"one of her bad days"—the patient's worry about being able to cover up and keep up during the social event caused her to refuse the social activity. Yet when symptoms subsided and she faced real demands of household management, she proceeded to do her grocery shopping.

Pacing is the balancing of activities of "keeping up" with rest. This is the desired normalizing strategy and one with which nurses can help patients. Pacing is an energy conservation behavior. Patients can be helped to analyze their daily activities, to provide for complete rest of all joints at some point throughout the day, and to obtain 8 to 10 hours of sleep a night.

Balancing the options available to the patient requires energy. Balancing the options includes deciding "whether to keep up and suffer the increased pain and fatigue;

whether to cover up and risk inability to justify inaction when needed; whether to elicit help and risk loss of normalizing. . . ."[23]

# CLINICAL DATA AND NURSING INTERVENTIONS FOR ENERGY CONSERVATION AND RESTORATION

The modified Ryden model[3] provides a framework for nursing intervention for patients with energy deficits. Energy sources can be restored, problems in transformation can be referred for medical therapy, and energy expenditure can be managed. A patient example will be used to demonstrate nursing care. Refer to Figure 11-2.

Mrs. S. is a 54-year-old Mexican-American woman with an 18-year history of rheumatoid arthritis. Her ankles, knees, hands, wrists, and shoulders are the most seriously involved joints. Mrs. S. weighs 205 lb and is 5 ft 4 in tall. Her most recent hospitalization was for rest, weight reduction, and the fitting of hand-wrist splints for nighttime use. Currently, she is receiving health care in an ambulatory arthritis center. Mrs. S. resides with her Mexican-American husband, two or more teenage grandchildren, and nieces and nephews. The exact makeup of the household occupants had been changing from week to week. Neither Mr. S. nor Mrs. S. was employed outside of the home; however, Mrs. S. cared for three infant and toddler grandchildren (all in diapers) while their parents worked. This work was physically taxing and frustrating; for example, Mrs. S. could not readily manipulate the diaper pins.

## Analysis of Energy Sources

### NUTRIENTS

Mrs. S.'s energy sources were inadequate. Despite her obesity, she was malnourished. Her intake of milk, fruit, vegetables, and lean protein was lacking. Dietary counseling with her cultural needs in mind enhanced her understanding but did not change her overeating pattern.

### REST

Mrs. S. was not able to obtain any rest during the day in her current home situation; at night her sleep was interrupted by what Mrs. S. describes as "the same old pains and worry." In completing a sleep history, data regarding time of retiring, bedtime rituals, sleep environment, and the patient's perception of sleep disturbance are obtained. Mrs. S. described her worries as interfering with her sleep.

Mrs. S.'s psychic state served as an energy depleter and not an energy source. She was filled with anxiety over the care of her many grandchildren and anticipating how to inform her children she could no longer keep up the pace the children's care demanded. She resented her husband's seeming lack of understanding of her pain, fatigue, and slow mobility. She resented her husband's lack of productivity and his lack of help with the children. Mrs. S. was worried about their financial status. (They already had their gas turned off on one previous occasion.)

Mrs. S.'s psychologic state accounts for her difficulties with energy sources in all three categories (nutrients, rest, and psychic energizers). To help with underlying anxieties about finances, Mrs. S. was referred to a social worker. The nurse acted as a liaison and accompanied Mrs. S. for the first social-work interview. Mobilizing social-services resources was an initial step in alleviating the financial worries.

Mrs. S.'s concept of self as having been a source of strength within the family (maintained the family network) was enhanced by enabling her to discuss her perceptions of her role and providing honest praise for a job well done.

Helping Mrs. S. with role transition of giving up the role of care provider for the babies (her final decision after much difficult deliberation) was important in helping Mrs. S. rest and alleviate her guilt over the children's care. Mrs. S. needed help with eliminating role strain by having her review the alternatives and make a decision. She determined that giving up the role of care provider would help her obtain needed rest during the day and would alleviate her guilt over not being able to adequately manage the children. Her role transition was helped by having her rehearse how she would inform her daughters and by giving her a mental picture of what her day would be like without this responsibility.[24]

Family counseling was begun. This therapy helped increase Mr. S.'s participation in household tasks and increased his empathy for his wife. The teenaged grandchildren, who had been truant, are less of a behavior problem because their parents and grandparents became more sensitive to the teenagers' needs and demonstrated interest in them and their school activities.

Now that Mrs. S. is less anxious, data obtained in the sleep history can be used to plan strategies to promote sleep. She needed help in reestablishing a bedtime routine. Her pain management at bedtime needed improvement. She was taught not to omit the prescribed sulindac (Clinoril) and aspirin in the evening. Mrs. S. assumed these contributed to her wakefulness. She was taught progressive relaxation through autosuggestion,[25] which promoted rest and well-being and conserved energy.

Since pain-control strategies conserve energy, other means of helping Mrs. S. were to identify and attempt to eliminate the pain promoters that were part of her routine. For example, she was encouraged to avoid extended exposure to cold weather, such as standing outside waiting for public transportation. She was taught principles of joint protection and avoiding joint strain during routines, that is, to avoid struggling to open screw top jars and to seek assistance from Mr. S. to open difficult covers. The necessity of complying with wearing the night splints for joint alignment was reinforced.

As the psychosocial energy expenditure was controlled, Mrs. S. was more motivated to improve her nutritional energy source and to lose weight, thereby further alleviating joint strain caused by excessive weight.

# Energy Transformation

Although there was no real energy transformation problem with Mrs. S., the excessive intake of calories needs to be controlled. There was no other pathologic problem requiring medical intervention.

# Energy Expenditure

## ENERGY TO RESTORE AND MAINTAIN PHYSICAL INTEGRITY

Although Mrs. S. was extremely anxious, she was noncompliant with the night splints, diet, and follow-up clinic visits. Now that her psychologic stresses were less, she completed her prescribed exercise routine twice daily and followed through with other therapeutic requirements. Less energy was wasted when she was compliant.

## ROLE EXPANSION AND COPING

Mrs. S.'s role expansion (learning self-care practices) has been accompanied by role contraction—giving up the child care and related pressures. She was also receiving more attention from her husband, which was a psychic energizer for Mrs. S. Her means of coping was through prayer. Although she no longer attended Mass daily, her active prayer life contributed to her energy source. The positive effect of prayer was emphasized.

## DAILY ACTIVITIES TO MEET UNIVERSAL SELF-CARE REQUIREMENTS

Mrs. S. was taught to use her present energy efficiently by planning for what she would be doing and where she would be, and collecting what she needed in one trip. For example, she was encouraged to complete her personal hygiene and loosening-up exercises in the warm shower in the morning before descending the stairs to make breakfast. (The bedrooms and bathtub are on the second floor.) She was instructed to plan ahead and bring downstairs in the morning what she would need for the rest of the day. When she was working in the kitchen, she was taught ways of supporting her joints and reminded to sit down while working whenever possible. Good body mechanics for proper joint alignment were reviewed.

## SOCIAL STIMULATION

Many of Mrs. S.'s neighborhood friends were members of the Mexican-American culture. These women provide a support group for one another through weekly meetings at each other's houses. Mrs. S. was encouraged to tell them of her uncertainty of being with them for every "get-together." The social and morale benefits of this group of friends were reviewed with Mrs. S., and it was determined that the energy expenditure was well worth her involvement with the group. From the group members, she received feedback about being a worthwhile person. She was also able to express her concerns to people of her own culture and felt truly understood by them. When Mrs. S. is in an energy-depleted state, expenditure in this category could be restricted or eliminated.

## RECREATION, EXERCISE, AND LEARNING

Mrs. S. used little—if any—energy for recreation, exercise, and learning. Her sole means of recreation was watching television. Her exercise was necessarily confined to her prescribed routine of range-of-motion exercises to maintain joint mobility. Developing new enjoyable outlets would assist her psychologic well-being. Examples of new outlets may include singing in the church choir, participating in the weekly Bible study class, and corresponding with residents in her native Mexican village.

## ENERGY WASTE

Mrs. S. wasted energy through anxiety and immobilized problem solving. Ways to handle anxiety (practicing relaxation exercises, verbalizing feelings to nurse, taking problems one at a time) were discussed. Mrs. S. was helped to feel self-confident and to have increased self-esteem so that she could resume the role of family decision maker with ease. During periods of disease exacerbations, the increased pain and occasional fever wasted energy. Eliminating routine exercises and increasing rest and analgesics during exacerbations helped conserve energy.

Although not needed for Mrs. S., other nursing strategies can be used to conserve energy for patients with arthritis.

# GENERAL NURSING INTERVENTIONS FOR ENERGY CONSERVATION AND RESTORATION

A comprehensive nursing approach to conserving and restoring energy includes restoring energy sources, helping the patient evaluate energy expenditure, increasing energy reserve, and eliminating energy waste.

The energy sources of nutrients (food, vitamins, minerals, and water) have been discussed in relation to Mrs. S. Patients need to be advised of the necessity to make diet adjustments because of deficiencies or excesses of certain foods. Maintaining intact, healthy autoimmune systems to prevent infections and therefore prevent energy waste depends in part on adequate nutrition. The energy sources of sleep-rest have also been described in relation to Mrs. S. Through use of a sleep history, promoting relaxation at bedtime and helping the patient establish a bedtime routine are helpful nursing activities.

The role of psychic energizers in restoration of energy states needs further emphasis. Energy is obtained through psychic renewal. Psychic renewal takes place through meditation (prayerful or other), routine progressive relaxation, creative imagery, and autogenic suggestion.

Physiologic changes during meditation that indicate a calming effect are decreased respiratory and heart rates, decreased oxygen consumption, lowered or stabilized blood pressure, and decreased skin conductivity.[26] Autogenic training is a self-induced meditation-relaxation procedure.[27] Briefly, the procedure includes six stages. During the first stage, the individual focuses "passive attention"[26] on each limb, while repeating,

"My right arm feels heavy," and progressing throughout the body—all limbs, torso, neck, jaw, forehead. In the next stage, the same progression of limbs is used to review warmth: "My right arm feels warm." In the third stage, the individual is to emphasize, "My heartbeat is calm and regular." Focusing on depth and ease of respiration takes place in the fourth stage, while the individual repeats the phrase, "It breathes me." During the fifth stage, the individual focuses on warmth in the upper abdomen (solar plexus), stating, "My solar plexus is warm." Instructions for the last stage are to repeat, "My forehead is cool." Pelletier states that after practice ranging from 2 months to 1 year, the entire series of six stages can be completed in 2 to 4 minutes.

Progressive relaxation in which the person is taught to focus on the extremes of muscle tenseness and complete relaxation of the same muscle group is another relaxation method.[28]

Mental imagery is a device for promoting calmness and well-being. By creating tranquil images in the mind, mind-body pathways extend this feeling from a mental state to an actual physical state. For example, the patient with arthritis may visualize lying on a warm sunny beach at the ocean. The patient pictures the warm sun and sand easing out the joint stiffness and imagines the ocean waves washing in and out, washing away the pain. The patient feels the body to be very light, agile, and floating. The outcome should be deep relaxation and renewed energy. The autosuggestion may have improved the comfort state as well.

Facilitating psychic energizers includes helping patients with motivation. Their eagerness to accomplish something, to establish goals, and to anticipate desired outcomes is a psychic energizer.

Any discussion on restoration of energy would be incomplete without referring to the work of Krieger.[29-31] Krieger's premise is that energy from one human being (healer) can be transferred through touch to another (healee). Energy from the healer helps "repattern the patient's energy level to a state that is comparable to that of the healer."[29] Although countless cases of improved health after therapeutic touch have been documented,[31] the only quantifiable variable that increases significantly at the 0.01 level of significance after treatment with therapeutic touch is hemoglobin.[31] The group receiving therapeutic touch had significantly higher hemoglobin than the control no-touch group. Perhaps what was once a maneuver to comfort, share an experience, and reassure that dependence is allowed through touch can now be viewed as a powerful transfer and repatterning of energy from someone who is healthy to someone who is ill. The healing act of touch is not understood scientifically, and no attempt will be made to speculate about what actually happens. For a description of the technique, readers are referred to *The Therapeutic Touch.*[31]

## Enabling the Patient to Evaluate Energy Expenditure

Helping patients plan more precisely for energy utilization in various activities is now possible through use of METs. MET refers to metabolic equivalents, the amount of oxygen used per minute per kilogram of body weight. One MET equals 3.5 ml oxygen per kilogram of body weight per minute. Table 11-2 contains a list of activities and their approximate energy expenditure in METs.

**TABLE 11-2. Approximate Energy Expenditure in METs (Activities of 70-kg Individual)***

| Category of Activity | Light (1-3 METs) | | Moderate (3.5-6 METs) | | Heavy (7+ METs) | |
|---|---|---|---|---|---|---|
| Personal care activities | Rest | 1 | Showering | 3.5 | Ambulation with | |
| | Sitting | 1 | Using bedpan | 4.0 | braces or | |
| | Standing (relaxed) | 1 | Walking downstairs | 4.5 | crutches | 6.5 |
| | | | Conditioning | | Walking upstairs | |
| | Eating | 1 | exercises | 4.5 | with 17-lb load | 7.5 |
| | Conversation | 1 | Walking 3.5 mph | 5.5 | | |
| | Dressing-undressing | 2 | | | | |
| | Wash hands, face; shaving | 2 | | | | |
| | Propelling wheelchair | 2 | | | | |
| | Shaving | 2.8 | | | | |
| | Bedside commode | 3 | | | | |
| | Walking 2.5 mph | 3 | | | | |
| Recreational activities | Walking level, slowly 1 mph | 1.2 | Walking level 3 mph | 3.5 | Tennis | 6.0 |
| | Painting, sitting | 1.5 | Bowling | 3.5 | Trotting horse | 6.5 |
| | Playing piano | 2.0 | Cycling 5.5 mph | 3.5 | Spading | 7.0 |
| | Driving | 2.0 | Badminton | 3.5 | Jogging level | |
| | Canoeing 2.5 mph | 2.5 | Canoeing, sailing | 3.5 | 5 mph | 7.5 |
| | Horseback riding slow | 2.5 | Golfing | 4.0 | Skiing | 8.0 |
| | Volleyball | 2.5 | Swimming | 4.0 | Squash | 8.5 |
| | | | Dancing | 4.5 | Basketball | 8.5 |
| | | | Gardening | 4.5 | Tennis | 8.5 |
| | | | | | Cycling 13 mph | 9.0 |
| | | | | | Gymnastics | 10.0 |
| | | | | | Football competition | 10.0 |
| Housework activities | Hand sewing | 1.0 | Ironing, standing | 3.5 | Mowing lawn by hand | 6.5 |
| | Sweeping floor | 1.5 | Scrubbing floors | 3.5 | Shoveling | 7.0 |
| | Machine sewing | 1.5 | Hanging wash | 3.5 | Ascending stairs | |
| | Polishing furniture | 2.0 | Cleaning windows | 3.5 | with 17-lb load | 7.5 |
| | Peeling potatoes | 2.5 | Beating carpets | 4.0 | Planting | 7.5 |
| | Washing small clothes | 2.5 | Plowing with tractor | 4.5 | Construction physical worker | 6.5 |
| | Kneading dough | 2.5 | Lifting, carrying 20-44 lb | 4.5 | Pick and shovel work | 8.0 |
| | Cleaning windows | 3.0 | Carpentry | 5.5 | Splitting wood by hand | 10.0 |
| | Making beds | 3.0 | Using pneumatic tools | 6.0 | | |
| | Desk work | 1.2 | | | | |
| | Typing (electric) | 1.2 | | | | |
| | Radio-TV repair | 1.2 | | | | |
| | Draftsman | 1.8 | | | | |

*Adapted from Clark;[32] Krusen, Kottke, and Ellwood;[33] and Karvonen and Barry.[34]

Although MET assignment has been used as a specific energy prescription for patients with cardiac disease, specific energy expenditure analysis using METs is helpful for all patients striving to understand energy use and plan for bursts of energy expenditure. Planning includes providing for extra rest and avoiding excessive MET expenditure in a 24-hour period. The anxious patient uses more METs per activity than the individual who is not anxious.

## Increasing Energy Reserve

Energy reserve is increased through physical conditioning. A regular exercise program strengthens muscles (increases muscle fiber size, endurance, and flexibility); burns calories; improves lung aerobic capacity; and affects fat metabolism by increasing high-density lipoproteins (HDL), which is helpful in ridding cholesterol from the blood vessels. Exercise decreases harmful very low-density lipoproteins (VLDL). Exercise increases strength of cardiac contraction and decreases blood pressure and heart rate. In addition, exercise promotes a feeling of well-being. For some, physical exercise not only builds up energy reserve but also decreases an energy waster—anxiety.

Eliminating energy waste as summarized in Table 11-1 in the areas of physical waste, or environmental management, and psychologic waste is a nursing responsibility. For patients with arthritis, pain is a typical energy waster. Eliminating pain promoters, such as joint strain, damp environment, inadequate rest, and ineffective analgesic schedules, eliminates energy waste from pain.

Establishing avenues for self-expression and ventilation of hostility may help alleviate psychologic energy wasters—anxiety, anger, and unresolved grief or guilt. Eliminating disabling themes (person's self-perception of being old, crippled, and dependent) will also eliminate some psychic energy waste.

## SUMMARY

Energy is a power resource. A deficit in energy is often present in individuals with chronic health problems. Analysis of energy states can be guided by using the modified Ryden model,[3] in which energy sources, transformation, and expenditure are determined. Nursing diagnoses are identified, and strategies to alleviate the diagnoses are carried out. Alleviation of energy deficits results in alleviation of a degree of powerlessness. In this chapter, the patient with arthritis was described as a specific patient prototype in applying the energy analysis model summarized in Figure 11-2.

## REFERENCES

1. Fagerhaugh, S.: *Getting around with emphysema.* In Strauss, A. (ed.): *Chronic Illness and the Quality of Life.* C. V. Mosby, St. Louis, 1975, pp. 99-107.
2. Putt, A.: *General Systems Theory Applied to Nursing.* Little, Brown & Co., Boston, 1978.
3. Ryden, M.: *Energy: A crucial consideration in the nursing process.* Nurs. Forum 16:71, 1977.
4. Knoebel, P.: *An analysis of energy utilization through the implementation of the Ryden model.* Unpublished material.

5. Orem, D.: *Nursing: Concepts of Practice*, ed. 2. McGraw-Hill, New York, 1980.
6. Pinekenstein, B.: *Energy, alterations in: Deficiencies, identification and comparison of defining characteristics in five hospitalized clients.* Master's essay, Marquette University, 1979.
7. *Arthritis: The Basic Facts.* Arthritis Foundation, Atlanta, Ga., 1981, p. 2.
8. Kaye, R. and Pemberton, R.: *Treatment of rheumatoid arthritis.* Arch. Intern. Med. 136:1023, 1976.
9. Groer, M. and Shekleton, M.: *Basic Pathophysiology: A Conceptual Approach.* C. V. Mosby, St. Louis, 1979.
10. Tobe, R.: *Anemia.* In Leitch, C. and Tinker, R. (eds.): *Primary Care.* F. A. Davis, Philadelphia, 1978, pp. 91-94.
11. Swartz, F.: *The rehabilitation process—as viewed from the inside.* Rehabil. Lit. 31:203, July 1970.
12. Cobb, S.: *Contained hostility in rheumatoid arthritis.* Arthritis and Rheumatism 2:419, 1959.
13. Spergel, P., Ehrlich, G., and Glass, D.: *The rheumatoid arthritic personality: A psychodiagnostic myth.* Psychosomatics 19:79, 1978.
14. Zeitlin, D.: *Psychological issues in the management of rheumatoid arthritis.* Psychosomatics 18:7, 1977.
15. Wiener, C.: *The burden of rheumatoid arthritis: Tolerating the uncertainty.* Soc. Sci. Med. 9:97, 1975.
16. Myerowitz, S.: *The continuing investigation of psychosocial variables: Rheumatoid arthritis.* In Hill, A. G. (ed.): *Modern Trends in Rheumatology,* ed. 2. Appleton-Century-Crofts, New York, 1966, pp. 92-105.
17. King, S. H.: *Psychosocial factors associated with rheumatoid arthritis.* J. Chronic Dis. 2:287, 1955.
18. Moos, R. H.: *Personality factors associated with rheumatoid arthritis: A review.* J. Chronic Dis. 17:41, 1964.
19. Hoffman, A.: *Psychological factors associated with rheumatoid arthritis: Review of the literature.* Nurs. Res. 23:218, 1974.
20. Rimon, R.: *Social and psychosomatic aspects of rheumatoid arthritis, study of 100 female patients.* Acta Rheumatica Scandinavia Supplement 1:13, 1969.
21. Williams, R. L. and Krasnoff, A. G.: *Body image and physiological patterns in patients with peptic ulcers and rheumatoid arthritis.* Psychosom. Med. 26:708, 1964.
22. Mayville, K.: *The significance of crippling response to rheumatoid arthritis.* Master's essay, Marquette University, 1979.
23. Weiner, op. cit. p. 102.
24. Meleis, A. I. and Swendsen, L.: *Role supplementation: An empirical test of a nursing intervention.* Nurs. Res. 27:11, January-February 1978.
25. Benson, H.: *The Relaxation Response.* William Morrow & Co., New York, 1975.
26. Pelletier, K.: *Mind as Healer, Mind as Slayer.* Dell Publishing, New York, 1977.
27. Luthe, W. (ed.): *Autogenic Therapy.* Grune & Stratton, New York, 1969.
28. Jacobson, E.: *Progressive Relaxation,* ed. 2. Chicago Press, Chicago, 1938.
29. Krieger, D., Pepper, E., and Ancoli, S.: *Therapeutic touch: Searching for evidence of physiological change.* Am. J. Nurs. 79:660, April 1979.
30. Krieger, D.: *Healing by the laying-on of hands as a facilitator of bioenergetic change.* In Kennedy, M. and Pfeifer, G. (eds.): *Current Practice in Nursing Care of the Adult.* C. V. Mosby, St. Louis, 1979, pp. 209-217.
31. Krieger, D.: *The Therapeutic Touch.* Prentice-Hall, Englewood Cliffs, N.J., 1979.
32. Clark, N. F.: *Disturbances in the blood pumping mechanism.* In Jones, D., Dunbar, C. F., and Jirovac, M. M. (eds.): *Medical-Surgical Nursing: A Conceptual Approach.* McGraw-Hill, New York, 1978, pp. 813-839.
33. Krusen, F. H., Kottke, F. J., and Ellwood, P. M.: *Handbook of Physical Medicine and Rehabilitation.* W. B. Saunders, Philadelphia, 1971.
34. Karvonen, M. J. and Barry, A. J.: *Physical Activity and the Heart: Proceedings of a Symposium, Helsinki, Finland.* Charles C Thomas, Springfield, Ill., 1967.

# SELECTED READINGS

American College of Sports Medicine: *Guidelines for Graded Exercise Testing and Exercise Prescription.* Lea & Febiger, Philadelphia, 1976.

Fries, J.: *Arthritis: A Comprehensive Guide.* Addison-Wesley, Reading, Mass., 1979.

McCaffery, M.: *Nursing Management of the Patient with Pain,* ed. 2. J. B. Lippincott, Philadelphia, 1979.

O'Dell, A.: *Pain associated with arthritis and other rheumatic disorders.* In Jacox, A. (ed.): *Pain: A Source Book for Nurses and Other Health Professionals.* Little, Brown & Co., Boston, 1977, pp. 349-372.

# 12

# AN ANALYSIS
# OF COMPLIANCE BEHAVIOR:
# A RESPONSE
# TO POWERLESSNESS

## DIANE HELLENBRAND

All chronically ill individuals are confronted with the coping task of compliance with regimens. Compliance may include adhering to medications and treatment routines, altering life-style, and subjecting oneself to continuous surveillance by medical teams. Compliance is vital in maintaining health. Gillum and Barsky[1] summarized compliance research and found that one third of all studies report a noncompliance rate of 50 percent or greater. Most of these studies used only questionnaires to determine the degree of patient compliance. Reported compliance, as measured by questionnaires alone, has been shown to be inflated by approximately 30 percent. Numerous studies have been undertaken to identify demographic, sociobehavioral, and illness variables that enhance or hinder compliance. The data are contradictory in many instances, primarily because of different methodologies, measuring techniques, and sampling procedures.[2] This inconsistency among approaches causes difficulty in validly comparing various findings with factors causing noncompliance. Health-care professionals must understand the extent and causes of noncompliance so they can positively influence variables that will enhance adherence to therapy. Since nurses have more individualized contact with patients than do any other health-care professionals, nurses have greater opportunity to assess and promote compliance with therapeutic regimens.

The purposes of this chapter are to describe, compare, and analyze variables affecting the degree of compliance exhibited by two black individuals with diabetes mellitus and to determine the relationship of compliance/noncompliance to powerlessness. The identified cultural factors, attitudes, and values of the American black race toward health-related compliance will be presented. Literature will be reviewed according to sociobehavioral, illness, and demographic variables. Two cases will be reported according to sociobehavioral and illness variables, with particular emphasis on individual perceptions and attitudes. Powerlessness is included as a perception influencing compliance. Therapeutic nursing actions that enhance compliance are also presented. Strategies to increase compliance also enhance patient's perceived control. Emphasis is given to the assumption that "the patient is an active participant in dealing with his illness and will take what he regards as appropriate steps within his own life framework."[3] The "life framework" of an individual must be defined in order to completely understand the determinants of compliant/noncompliant behavior and to implement effective therapies based on individual needs and concerns. Parsons notes, "To implement medical techniques effectively is partly a socio-cultural problem."[4] Nursing is instrumental in helping to meet health-care needs with social, cultural, and environmental determinants.

## LITERATURE REVIEW

## Variables Influencing Noncompliance in Blacks

Culture, attitudes, and values of the American black toward health-related compliance are difficult to find in the literature. Not one study has been found that related cultural traits to compliant/noncompliant behaviors. Two general black cultural traits identified by Taylor are (1) high value on personal projection and responsiveness and (2) a great emphasis on categorizing diseases into "natural" and "unnatural" processes.[5] Blacks are characterized by large extended families with strong, extensive kinship bonds referred to as "black togetherness."[6] Nobles further states individual projection and responsiveness are defined and supported by the extended family and are "deeply rooted in African heritage and philosophical orientation." This emphasis on strong social bonds among blacks seems to imply that the degree of compliance could certainly be influenced by blacks' perceived identity in a white-dominant society.

Based on these data, one could assume that the more binding the social ties and identity with black "togetherness," the less likely the black individual would adhere to a therapeutic regimen designed solely for the individual without considering the family, environment, and overall life-style. However, Parsons[7] notes that in the American (white?) value system, the primary focus of evaluation is individual achievement. This probable inconsistency between white-based individual achievement and black-based group "togetherness" can serve as an influential variable in how well blacks comply with individually designed regimens.

Another black cultural trait cited was the significance of "natural" or "unnatural" processes. Bloch[8] reports that black folk medicine is based on several beliefs, one of which consists of classifying illnesses into "natural" and "unnatural" categories. This categorization dictates the type of care and practitioner sought. A "natural" illness is viewed as resulting from strong forces of nature (i.e., cold air, impure food, water, air). "Unnatural" illnesses are seen as evil influences that are not treatable by health-care providers because "the Devil cannot be fought with drugs." Bloch goes on to note that "the fact that an illness has not been cured alerts the believers that it is of 'unnatural' origin."[9]

Since diabetes mellitus is a chronic, incurable illness, it could be viewed as having an "unnatural" origin that cannot be mastered or controlled. On the other hand, the American value system emphasizes activism in which the society is oriented to mastery over its environment by establishing goals and striving for ideals.[7] This value is carried over to illness in that the individual is encouraged to gain mastery and control over the illness. It seems that activism is an important influence in the designing of therapeutic regimens to "control" diabetes mellitus and serves as an evaluative tool in analyzing patient compliance. The usual approach of expecting patients with diabetes to be active participants in their care may not be appropriate for blacks, especially if the black patient perceives diabetes as an "unnatural" illness.

It is recognized that diversity exists within the black culture in terms of intraethnic groups and so forth. Only one generalized view of blacks is presented here.

# Sociobehavioral and Illness Variables Affecting Compliance

## THE HEALTH-BELIEF MODEL

Compliance means a patient's complete and consistent adherence to the prescribed therapeutic regimen. Davis reports, "Compliance depends on many social and psychological factors, particularly salient norms and values which are incongruent with doctors' advice."[10] Some of these norms and values will be examined through a health-belief model as defined by Becker.[11] Becker's model is based on social stratification data, perceived objectivity, patient expectations, work values, and interpersonal relationships between the patient and physician. Norms and values cannot be considered the only determinants of compliant behavior; illness variables must also be examined.

The health-belief model, as proposed by Becker,[11] helps explain behavior according to the perceived value of an outcome (control of diabetes) and the individual's expectation that a given action (adherence to a therapeutic regimen) will result in that outcome. This model has three main components:

1. Readiness and motivation to take action to comply with the therapeutic regimen.
2. An evaluation of the benefits of the actions and the barriers to action. For patients with diabetes, the benefits could be control of diabetes. Barriers to the proposed action include family and/or social problems, finances, attitudes, and so forth.
3. A cue (internal or external) to action must be present to trigger advocated action. The cue may be pain, life-threatening situation, or other powerful stimulus. The patient must perceive that compliance will reduce the threat.[11]

Although not explicated by Becker,[11] powerlessness must be considered a component of the health-belief model. Perceived powerlessness may be a stimulus for compliance or noncompliance. If patients feel their actions will not alter the outcome, powerlessness may cause noncompliance. Conversely, powerlessness stimulates compliance if the individual is feeling powerless because of severe symptoms. When symptoms interfere with desired roles, activities, comfort, and a positive self-concept, powerlessness prevails. The patient may see that complying with the prescribed regimen will minimize immobilizing symptoms, thereby alleviating powerlessness. The Becker model is a guide to identifying factors that enhance or hinder compliant behavior and also is a tool to predict compliance. Research pertinent to select components of the health-belief model is included.

Haynes[12] reports that compliance is hardest to achieve when personal habits (i.e., smoking, drinking) must be broken and is least difficult when compliance involves acquiring new habits (i.e., taking medications). The model states that preexisting behaviors or habits that must be completely changed to comply with a proposed regimen serve as an important hindrance to compliance. Persons are also more likely to adhere to advice that involves the least amount of difficulty in effecting a change.[13] This knowledge helps to predict that compliance decreases with increasingly complicated and difficult regimens.

Ramirez[14] studied 116 Chicano adults to assess the effect a Chicano or Anglo communicator had in influencing the return of a completed questionnaire. He found that compliance was associated with the degree of social stratification (status, expertise, and authority) of the communicator as perceived by Chicano subjects. The Chicano subjects were significantly more compliant with the Anglo communicator's requests than with those of the Chicano communicator because the Chicanos perceived the Anglo individual as having expertise and being an authority. Vincent[15] goes on to note, "The patient must believe that the orders come from a legitimate authority," in order for compliance to occur.

Banks[16] studied 40 black undergraduates who received positive or negative reinforcement upon completion of a task from either a black or white evaluator. He concluded that "the behavioral and self-evaluative reactions of blacks to social reinforcements depend upon the degree to which the source of those reinforcements is perceived as objective." When the practitioner's reinforcements are contingent upon the behaviors and are instrumental to the outcomes of the patient, the practitioner is viewed as being objective. If the health-care practitioner's proposed regimen for an individual has a primary focus on benefiting that individual, then it is likely to contribute to a positive behavioral reaction (compliance).

Practitioners often perceive the success of therapies in controlling or curing disease as a measure of their own expertise, skill, and ego concern, rather than as an achievement of the patient. Failure to comply, resulting in failure of the therapy, was viewed as being caused by the patients' "uncooperative personality," according to 67 percent of senior physicians surveyed.[1] "Noncompliant behavior was further explained by increased difficulty of communication, and attempts by doctors and patients to control each other."[17] Banks and colleagues[16] explain that the major characteristic that seems to distinguish a practitioner who is objectively interested from one who is not is the "degree of manipulativeness" the practitioner uses. If the patient perceives the regimen is imposed without patient input and is manipulative, primarily focusing on the practitioner's self-interest and prestige, then the patient is likely to be noncompliant. The regimen is more likely to be perceived as patient centered when the patient has participated in formulating some aspects of the regimen. Thibaut and coworkers[18] found that encouraging participation entails raising expectations about the quality and acceptance of outcomes. The individual who is involved in planning the regimen is more committed to comply and accept outcomes. Raising patient expectations can result in decreased compliance if the expectations are greater than a perceived possible outcome. A relative balance between expected and actual outcomes must exist for optimal compliance to occur.

The patient-physician relationship is an important determinant affecting compliance. Marston[2] revealed that some of the significant factors supporting compliance were patient satisfaction with the care received, patient choice of a particular physician, and previous patient-physician interactions. Patients with satisfactory physician relationships had significantly better disease control than did those with unsatisfactory relationships.[2] An important variable in promoting compliance is the patient's perception of the physician's concern and competence. Haynes[12] reports a positive correlation between physician supervision and compliance when the supervision consists of a concerned physician who is interested in the patient and regularly inquires about the patient's health, progress, and compliance. Komaroff[19] notes that patients are likely to be compliant "when the physician strongly believes in the worth of treatment, and when the physician regularly and explicitly inquires about compliance." Becker[11] reported that noncompliance was positively correlated with the physician's failure to communicate to the patient the purpose of treatment or the need for follow-up appointments.

## ILLNESS VARIABLES

Illness variables such as perceived susceptibility, severity, duration, illness attitude, regimen complexity, and knowledge of illness and treatment promote or hinder compliance. It is important to remember that the patient's perception of these variables, rather than objective reality, is the major determinant in compliance.

### Severity

Perceived susceptibility, severity, and the likelihood of disease recurrence were positively correlated with degree of compliance.[11] Marston[2] reported, "Compliance was 70% when mothers estimated their children to be moderately or severely ill as opposed to thinking their children were mildly ill (30% compliance)." On the other hand, Hulka and coworkers[20] reported that actual disease severity in diabetic patients studied did not correlate with compliance.

### Illness Duration

Haynes[12] and Marston[2] reported that compliance decreases over time. This can be partly attributed to adjustment to the disease, with correspondingly less attention given to it. No reported research was found on gradual *versus* sudden onset of illness and compliance, as well as the visibility of the illness and compliant behavior.

### Illness-Health Attitude

Davis and Eichhorn[13] report that a positive health attitude *versus* a negative health attitude tends to increase compliance. When perceived desirability of health outweighs the perceived benefits of illness, compliance is more likely to occur. However, with many chronic diseases, including diabetes, a complete return to health is unattainable, and the individual must live and cope with varying degrees of ill health.

## Complexity of Self-Care

The complexity of the therapeutic regimen is negatively correlated with the degree of compliance. In most of these studies, number of different medications per individual was the sole criterion for regimen complexity.[13,20] When considering the complexity of the regimen, often the individual will comply with the regimen in varying degrees or will comply with one part but not with other parts. For example, most patients with diabetes who require insulin and diet restrictions will commonly adhere to the insulin requirement but tend not to comply fully with the diet restriction. These adjustments reflect the individual's striving for control over an imposed regimen.

## Patient Knowledge and Control

Patient knowledge of illness and its treatment did not seem to increase compliance, although compliance increased in correlation with a belief in personal susceptibility to serious problems.[2] Lowery and DuCette[21] studied diabetic patients with internal and external locus of control. The internals, who perceived a relationship between their actions and outcomes, desired a great deal of information about their illness and treatment in order to control the disease, but they exhibited less long-term compliance than the external patients. The externals, who perceived no relationship between their actions and outcomes, did not actively seek information and were not interested in self-control of their disease, but they had a higher rate of compliance since they relied on the authority of the practitioner. However, a lack of patient knowledge about the disease and its treatment does adversely affect compliance. Rosenstock[3] explains that patients must know why they are being treated, how long the treatment will last, and the results of treatment in order for compliance to take place.

## Demographic Variables

There is widespread consensus in the literature that demographic variables (age, sex, socioeconomic status, education, religion, race, and marital status) have minimal or no measurable effects on compliance. A few papers report that low socioeconomic status is related to noncompliance, but this is not consistently supported.[2,15,20] Haynes[12] found that long waiting periods before and during appointments leads to decreased compliance in keeping appointments. Since people with low socioeconomic status are likely to use public health services where waiting periods are long and the benefits of a consistent and continuous patient-physician relationship are lacking, it seems appropriate to assume that socioeconomic status does indirectly affect compliant behavior. No specific research reports support this conclusion. Table 12-1 contains a summary of repeatedly tested variables that significantly influence compliance.

None of the studies reported have emphasized the effect of family and/or significant others on compliance. Although this is a difficult variable to measure, it certainly plays

TABLE 12-1.   Factors Increasing Noncompliance

| Category | Factors Associated with Noncompliance |
|---|---|
| Regimen | Complexity<br>Degree of behavioral change<br>Duration (indefinite or lifelong) |
| Therapeutic source | Inefficient and inconvenient clinics |
| Patient-physician interaction | Inadequate supervision<br>Patient dissatisfaction<br>No explanation of illness given<br>Physician disagreeing with patient<br>Formality or rejection of patient |
| Patient | Inappropriate health beliefs<br>Expectations not met<br>Previous or present noncompliance with<br>   other regimens<br>Family instability |

an important role, since human beings are social beings and derive many of their perceptions and attitudes from the culture, society, social groups, and organizations with which they identify. Vincent[15] proposed that one measure that needed research data was "the importance of the influence of family members in encouraging or discouraging compliance." She found that greater compliance existed among men who had "support" from their wives than among those who did not. Davis and Eichhorn[13] found that 52 percent of their subjects reported they were highly influenced by relatives and friends and that 48 percent were slightly influenced.

Vincent[15] reports that not all patients believe they ought to cooperate with a physician's advice. Yet why do some patients comply fully and others in only varying degrees? In the preceding pages, influencing variables have been reported and have been devoid of individual characteristics and situations. In the last analysis, compliance problems are behavior problems, and these problems can be analyzed best by looking at individual characteristics and situations. To determine the relative importance of these variables, two cases are presented. These two middle-aged black individuals of low socioeconomic status have adult-onset diabetes mellitus that requires insulin and diet control for optimal management. However, overall diabetic control is much more complex than just adhering to a diet and taking insulin. The cases presented will include a brief patient profile and sociobehavioral and illness variables related to the degree of compliance. Data will be categorized according to Becker's health-belief model and will include patient's perceived disease severity, duration of illness, regimen complexity, attitude toward illness, knowledge about the health problem, meaning of the illness, and degree of perceived powerlessness. Demographic variables will not be considered in detail since both individuals have similar demographic data and the literature reviewed did not consistently relate these data to compliant behavior. There are distinct differences in the degree to which each patient complies with the individual regimen.

# CLINICAL DATA

# Mr. G.

### PROFILE

Mr. G. is a 49-year-old black man who has had diabetes mellitus for the past 20 years and has required insulin for control since disease onset. He had been married for about 25 years but was divorced 5 years ago. He has four children, all of whom are alive and well, although one son in his 20s received a diagnosis of diabetes a few years ago. Mr. G.'s family, on both his maternal and paternal sides, has a history of diabetes. Mr. G. has a somewhat uncertain disease pattern. He originally required very small amounts of insulin along with the restricted diet. Then 2 years ago, he developed resistance to beef insulin and began to experience prolonged hyperglycemic episodes that did not respond to increased insulin therapy. During this time, he developed noticeably impaired vision, especially in his right eye, and frequent, moderately severe bilateral foot pain. This condition has persisted for the past 2 years. Good blood sugar control has been accomplished for the past 2 months using pork insulin. Mr. G. lives in a dreary, sparsely furnished apartment above a tavern with a male roommate who is "very easy to get along with." Mr. G. has a girlfriend, who still visits once in a while, with whom he had had a sexual relationship, but he has been impotent for the past 2 years (influenced by diabetes mellitus). He maintains an active social relationship with a number of close friends. When he is confined to the apartment because of ill health (he also has hypertension, which precipitated congestive heart failure on several occasions), his friends perform necessary tasks such as doing laundry and grocery shopping. Within the past 3 years, four close relatives died as a direct result of diabetes " 'cause they wouldn't do what the doctor told them to." Mr. G. reports "having just made up my mind" in adjusting to the prescribed diabetic regimen after seeing "one friend go blind and almost dying myself." When asked, "What's the hardest part of having diabetes?," he answered, "The poor vision and the pain in my feet." Mr. G. had operated a tavern for 18 years until 2 years ago when, "I had to quit 'cause the pain in my feet got too bad." He admits to having drunk alcohol "when I knew better" but denies alcohol consumption in recent years. Mr. G. has complied completely with taking all medications, testing his urine for sugar, and adhering to the 1800-calorie diabetic diet for the past 2 years. In fact, he was so concerned about not eating more than what was on the diet that he was actually eating less than prescribed. The doctors have told Mr. G. that his vision would improve, his pain would decrease, and his sexual ability could possibly return once he was back under consistent control. Mr. G. had a similar, shorter diabetic crisis approximately 5 years ago in which he experienced a great reduction in the pain after diabetic control was regained.

### SOCIOBEHAVIORAL FACTORS

The dominant sociobehavioral factors that appear to influence Mr. G.'s compliance to his diabetic regimen consist of his health expectations, respect for physician's expertise, relationship with the physician, social and family networks, and intense desire to control disease symptoms. Compliance is equated with control of adverse symptoms.

Mr. G.'s expectations of the therapy centered on relief from the symptoms (pain, impaired vision, impotency) that are directly related to hyperglycemia. The desired outcomes of the prescribed therapeutic regimen are congruent with Mr. G.'s major need and expectation.

The expertise and authority of the physicians appear to be highly regarded by Mr. G. Their efforts "saved me those two times when I couldn't even tell them what was wrong." Also, the physicians' previously prescribed regimen was effective in relieving his symptoms, which gives added credibility to Mr. G.'s present expectations and faith to continue complying even though it took 2 years to regain control.

Mr. G. also has a very supportive long-term relationship with his physicians. He has continually seen the same two physicians for the past 2 years, and he telephoned them about three or four times per week about his diabetic reactions, which usually required an insulin adjustment. In his interactions with the physicians, Mr. G. was always very cooperative, attentive, and receptive to their impressions and suggestions (the "ideal patient"). Mr. G. feels that his health concerns are the physicians' primary interest, which enhances his faith in the physicians' therapeutic abilities. Mr. G. seems to perceive that the entire concept of his adult responsibility revolves around his participating and cooperating with the prescribed regimen. He feels his behavior in following their recommendations will achieve desired control.

The support and help from friends prevents social isolation and helps motivate him to keep "fighting" for improved health. Mr. G.'s girlfriend still lends her support even though the relationship has changed since his impotency. The overall relationship with family and friends supports a "togetherness" approach to adjusting to Mr. G.'s diabetes since he has told his friends about his disease and lets them know how they can assist him (i.e., not offering him beer during card playing).

## ILLNESS VARIABLES

The illness variables influencing Mr. G.'s compliance include symptom severity, duration of diagnosis, attitude toward illness, complexity of health regimen, knowledge of the health problem, and the meaning of the illness.

The severity of Mr. G.'s symptoms greatly limits his physical and social activities. He is unable to walk more than one block at a time, has noticeable difficulty seeing cars when crossing the street, sometimes is unable to climb two flights of stairs to his second-floor apartment and thus stays in his apartment the entire day, and has leg pain that wakes him occasionally at night and limits visiting friends and attending card parties during the day. In Mr. G.'s case, the severity of the symptoms does enhance compliance because of the perceived importance that Mr. G. attributes to these physical and social activities. The severity of the symptoms probably prompted him to take action and make a commitment. The severe diabetic symptoms interfered with his role as friend, father, worker, and lover. Therefore, the need to manage these symptoms in order to live as an interdependent person became crucial. Mr. G. chose to comply with the therapeutic regimen to reduce or eliminate the symptoms. Compliance is equated with control—control of symptoms and deteriorating health. Compliance in this case means Mr. G. will be able to engage in important roles by preserving functional abilities.

Even though literature indicates compliance decreases over time, this has not occurred in Mr. G.'s case. Even though he experienced severe symptoms for almost 2 years without relief, he continued to adhere closely to all aspects of the diabetic regimen (as determined by weight, urine-testing record, and observation). Because severe symptoms interfered with his life-style, Mr. G. valued compliance as a means to obtain symptom relief.

Mr. G.'s attitude toward diabetes can be explained by his statement, "Some of my friends tell me that they would sooner have cancer than diabetes, but not me. I can *live* with diabetes but cancer would kill me." This quote implies that Mr. G. recognizes that diabetes can be controlled and he can continue to live if he complies with the diabetic regimen. His illness attitude consists of accepting that he has diabetes, that he has a role in helping to control the adverse effects of uncontrolled diabetes, and that he could be worse off (i.e., have cancer).

Mr. G.'s overall health regimen is rather complex. He is instructed to take three pills once a day (a cardiotonic glycoside and antihypertensives) and two injections of mixed insulin (two types) each day. He is also asked to test his urine for glucose four times a day and to record the results for physician's use in determining his body's insulin requirements. Mr. G. is to adhere to an 1800-calorie diabetic diet. An additional requirement during Mr. G.'s almost 2-year insulin-resistant episode was to attend the clinic nearly every week, which required two bus transfers. This degree of regimen complexity would tend to hinder overall compliance since it requires a substantial time to complete and serves to disrupt life activities (i.e., social). However, the complexity of Mr. G.'s regimen did not hinder his compliance and may even have enhanced it. Since Mr. G. had experienced severe symptoms while he was insulin resistant, he could have perceived that a difficult regimen would be necessary to resolve this problem. According to Mr. G.'s perception, the difficult regimen was credible and likely to work.

Mr. G.'s knowledge of diabetes and its treatment consists of a general and accurate knowledge of diabetic pathophysiology and the need for and action of insulin. Mr. G. did *not* understand the action or the names of his heart and blood pressure medicines. However, this medication seemed to be taken regularly and consistently, as determined by his report and by blood pressure measurements. Therefore, it did seem that detailed knowledge about his disease and treatment was *not* an essential variable in promoting his compliance with the regimen.

Whether diabetes is viewed as a "natural" process by Mr. G. is very difficult to determine. Diabetes was present on both sides of his family and in his former wife's family. Mr. G. had had prolonged exposure to this disease and its treatment, which could serve to enhance his acceptance. However, Mr. G. also reported several immediate family members who died because they would not adhere closely to the treatment and did not accept the disease and its restrictions. Mr. G. has not referred to diabetes as an "evil influence" or "punishment from God," statements that would tend to support diabetes as an "unnatural" process according to Bloch.[8] Since Mr. G. has exhibited a strong commitment in trying to control and manage his diabetes, it seems that he believes his diabetes can be controlled (natural process). This belief supports compliance since in the "natural" process there is an outcome that can be realized.

Mr. G.'s high level of compliance is summarized according to Becker's health-belief model:

1. Mr. G.'s motivation and readiness to take action seem to have been fostered primarily by the severity of his symptoms and their impact on limiting his life-style (long walks, visiting family and friends, working, sexual intercourse, and so forth).
2. The perceived benefits of action consisted of relief from these symptoms, which would result in a return to usual life-style activities. This return to usual life-style activities would reestablish harmony and consistency among Mr. G.'s actions, attitudes, and values. The barriers to act appear to be minimal since compliance did not require a drastic change in any of Mr. G.'s behaviors (i.e., he was not fond of sweets and could easily adhere to the dietary restrictions, and he had been taking insulin and testing urine for the past 20 years while carrying out work and family responsibilities). Regarding his financial situation after leaving work, Mr. G. received disability funds that met his living needs "without any problems." There are no identifiable barriers to hinder compliance.
3. The probability that compliance would reduce threats of impotence and restricted mobility from leg pain was Mr. G.'s perception. He stated, "I just made up my mind to control it."

# Mrs. L.

## PROFILE

Mrs. L. is a 54-year-old obese black woman who has had diabetes for the past 7 years but did not require insulin until 2 months ago. Before taking insulin, Mrs. L. was taking three pills once a day to lower her blood sugar. Mrs. L. has seven children, all of whom are alive and well; none have diabetes. Mrs. L.'s husband died a few years ago. She lives in her own home with two of her unmarried children and two grandchildren. There is no history of diabetes on either side of Mrs. L.'s family. Mrs. L. has been encouraged by the physicians over the past 7 years to lose weight and has lost 10 lb. Mrs. L. remains obese (5 ft 4 in, 207 lb) and has been instructed that her diabetes could probably be controlled with diet alone once her weight was reduced to a normal range. Mrs. L. has not experienced any diabetic crises but does have occasional symptoms of hyperglycemia (frequent urination and thrist). None of these symptoms noticeably restricts her life-style. Mrs. L. was a girl scout counselor until about 5 years ago. She was a chief cook at a local hospital until about 1 year ago when she was hurt in an accident. Since then, she cares for her two grandchildren on weekdays and exerts a minimal amount of activity. She is known for preparing large, delicious meals for her family, especially on weekends when her other children and grandchildren gather at her house. Her role as mother seems to revolve around preparing large and good meals for her family. Also, mealtime serves as the focal point from which social activities develop. Mrs. L. participates in neighborhood activities and has several close friends. She plans to participate actively in the girl scout program this summer, mainly by teaching outdoor cooking. Her diabetic regimen consists of a daily dose of insulin, adherence to a 1000-calorie diet, and urine testing four times a day. The proposed outcome for following this regimen is weight loss, which would probably result in discontinuing or at least reducing insulin use, preventing hyperglycemic side effects (i.e., eye changes, neuropathy), and reducing the urine testing to once a day. Mrs. L. has no other significant health problems requiring compliance. Mrs. L. has been unable to lose any weight in the past 2 months although she states she is "following the diet religiously and the diet is not frustrating at all." Compliance with the diet is very questionable. She is complying with taking the insulin since her blood sugar is now within an acceptable range and her records of urine tests have been normal.

## SOCIOBEHAVIORAL FACTORS

The major sociobehavioral factors analyzed include health expectation, physician objectivity, social and family networks, and relationships with physicians.

Mrs. L.'s expectations regarding following the diabetic regimen consist of keeping her diabetes within an "acceptable range." This has been achieved by just taking the insulin since her blood sugar has returned to an acceptable range and her hyperglycemic symptoms have subsided. Mrs. L. has stated, "I should really lose some weight," but this action does not seem to be a priority since it is worded in the future tense and is probably not her own desire but rather a verbalization of the physician's orders. Her mothering identity and the task of providing good meals for her family are extremely important to her and probably serve as the major deterrent to adherence to dietary restrictions. To prevent hyperglycemic side effects over time is not a strong stimulus to comply, since she does not realize or perceive what hyperglycemic side effects can entail. Also, persons from lower socioeconomic backgrounds tend to be oriented to the present rather than the future and do not see a real need to try to prevent something that, in their estimation, probably would not happen anyway. Mrs. L.'s perceptions about her diabetes have not been influenced by a family history that would enhance her awareness of and experience with varying degrees of diabetic severity. Since Mrs. L.'s orientation seems to revolve around an "acceptable control," which is now achieved by administering insulin, there is no real need to comply with the rest of the regimen.

Parts of the prescribed regimen are in conflict with Mrs. L.'s values and interfere with her life-style. Mrs. L. has social and family acceptance of her obesity and even an expectation that this is a characteristic of a "good" mother. Therefore, a prescribed regimen requiring weight reduction is not consistent with Mrs. L.'s identity, values, and life-style. There is incongruence between physician values and those of Mrs. L. This incongruence enhances noncompliance. Adherence to the diet restrictions requires modifying previous, long-established behavior, which is difficult to achieve and must be strongly stimulated for positive results to occur. Mrs. L.'s expectation of acceptable control is achieved by taking insulin, which involves the least difficulty and with which she complies fully. She probably recognizes the authority and expertise of the physicians, but this does not serve as a strong positive influence to promote full compliance.

The social and family relationships are strong and play a prominent role in Mrs. L.'s values and concerns. There is a cohesiveness among the family members, and the family situation appears stable; therefore, family instability is not a factor in promoting Mrs. L.'s noncompliant behavior. However, the strong family ties and emphasis on Mrs. L.'s role as mother and homemaker probably indirectly reinforce her dietary non-compliance.

Mrs. L.'s relationship with her physicians is friendly and cooperative. She did refuse to start insulin for 6 months because, "I didn't want to take the needle." She states that she adheres to the diet precisely and does not understand why there is not a corresponding weight loss. She denies having any difficulty adhering to the regimen completely. It appears that Mrs. L. is not accepting her disease at this point. She is not able to realize that full compliance with the therapeutic regimen will necessitate changes in life-style. Mrs. L. was not an active participant in deciding her dietary regimen; therefore, the physician was not aware of her values and attitudes about food. This lack of awareness would contribute to noncompliant behavior. Mrs. L.'s noncompliance is used to maintain control in other aspects of her life, that is, family solidarity and the image she portrays in the family as a matriarch with special skills—cooking. Noncompliance alleviates the powerlessness she feels when family doubt her ability to play desired roles and her obese image is changing.

## ILLNESS VARIABLES

The illness variables influencing compliance are perceived susceptibility and symptom severity, attitude toward the illness, complexity of the regimen, knowledge about the problem, and the meaning of the illness.

Mrs. L. was not susceptible to diabetes according to her family history. The duration of her disease has been relatively short (7 years) and rather mild (required pills without acute symptoms). Even before she started taking insulin, her symptoms did not impair her activities or life-style.

When asked, "What's the worst thing about having diabetes?," Mrs. L. replied, "The diet restrictions and taking insulin." Note that her response actually refers to the diabetic treatment rather than the disease. Her expressed attitude toward the illness is not as negative as her expressed attitude toward the treatment. When Mrs. L. was confronted by her 16-year-old daughter who feared that her mother would die young because she had diabetes, Mrs. L. reassured her by saying that "isn't going to happen to me 'cause my diabetes isn't bad at all."

The complexity of Mrs. L.'s regimen is minimal in that she takes one kind of insulin once a day, and is to adhere to 1000-calorie diet and test her urine four times a day. This lack of complexity should serve to enhance overall compliance.

Mrs. L.'s knowledge of her illness and its treatment is very good. She understands both the pathophysiology of diabetes and the prescribed therapy.

Whether Mrs. L. views her disease as a "natural" or "unnatural" process is difficult to evaluate. Since she does not refer to diabetes as a consequence of an evil force or the result of a sin, it seems that she views diabetes as a "natural" process that can be managed and controlled. Also, she expects that her blood sugars will be maintained within an acceptable range, which connotes a belief in disease control.

Mrs. L.'s degree of compliance is summarized according to the health-belief model:

1. Mrs. L. is not significantly motivated to take action. Her diabetes is mild and does not exhibit symptoms that interfere with life-style or role performance. For Mrs. L., to take action and comply with diet regimen require a major change in her habits and eating behavior.
2. In evaluating the regimen's potential benefits versus the barriers to the action, it appears that the barriers outweigh the perceived benefits. The proposed benefits of full compliance involve loss of weight, which may not be desired; prevention of diabetic complications, which may never occur regardless of actions; and control of blood sugar, which has been achieved with insulin. The barriers to act consist largely of family and Mrs. L.'s values regarding motherhood and the homemaker role and the significance of mealtime socialization. From this evaluation, the proposed benefits are weak factors for enhancing full compliance, and the barriers consist of well-established values and congruent behaviors that are difficult to modify even when the benefits are strong forces.
3. Mrs. L. does not perceive any threat from the illness. Compliance, subsequent weight loss, and altered body image and image as a mother are threatening. A cue (powerful stimulus) to act seems to be lacking. There is no strong stimulus available that would serve to promote improved compliance. Mrs. L. manifests powerlessness and an external locus of control, which contribute to noncompliance. She stated, "What's going to happen is going to happen, no matter what I do."

In summary, the factors contributing to compliance/noncompliance with therapeutic regimens are indeed complex and very closely interrelated. By presenting and analyzing the sociobehavioral and illness variables of individual patients, it was impossible to evaluate which variables appear to dominate in compliant/noncompliant behaviors. Compliance was more likely to occur when the proposed treatment outcome was congruent with the individual's desired outcomes, attitudes, and values. The number and importance of the barriers to compliance contributed to noncompliant behavior. Individual characteristics such as personality, perceived control, coping mechanisms, and perceived role tasks also influence the degree of compliance. Health-care providers must focus on the individual, family, and environment in order to fully assess compliance/noncompliance and then to implement therapeutic interventions to improve health-related behaviors.

# NURSING IMPLICATIONS

Nurses play a major role in helping to implement therapeutic regimens and enhancing compliance with these regimens. The Williams model, Process of Diabetes Control,[22] suggests that day-to-day control depends on the patient receiving support, considering specific psychologic factors, and patient teaching to increase patient awareness. Active patient participation and a real sense of patient control for optimal disease management are needed.

Nurses provide support through developing meaningful interpersonal relationships. Patient-expressed needs and concerns are the primary nurse-patient focus. After needs that are the immediate focus of the patient are met, changes due to the prescribed regimen can be implemented. The patient's psychologic factors (motivation, coping styles, personality, perceived control) provide one focus for nursing intervention. One diabetic patient had a poor self-concept; actions were directed to improve her concept of self before compliance could begin. The patient needs to feel worthwhile to exert effort to comply.

Nurses not only teach patients about health, illness, and treatment; they also help patients learn why their participation in the therapy is so important. Patients can learn mechanisms for being in control. Even though the literature did not find a consistent positive correlation between knowledge and compliance, it was reported that a lack of knowledge about the illness was correlated with noncompliance. Since nursing incorporated all aspects of the patient's world with its holistic approach (considering the significant others, environment, psychosocial components, and so forth), nurses are able to teach effectively in the context of the patient's unique life framework. This strategy is developed in more detail in Chapter 13. The supporting, guiding, and teaching aspects of nursing help patients mobilize, enhance, and/or develop resources to resolve dissonance and promote consonance. The prescribing of a therapeutic regimen, if different from a patient's daily patterns of living, will contribute to dissonance, which leads to patient decision making whether or not to comply.[10] Nurses can influence socioeconomic concerns, such as a patient's fear of being unable to afford insulin, by cooperating with social-service agencies to obtain needed resources. When nurses provide continuity in the health team, ongoing helping relationships, and patient teaching to help patients learn control mechanisms, patient consonance and enhanced compliance should result. The literature consistently reports that supervision and follow-up care enhance compliance.

Nursing interventions are directed toward the whole person and emphasize the person's need for involvement in planning and tailoring regimens. Patients develop anxiety in a helper-patient relationship characterized by formality, high structure, and an unquestioning attitude by both helper and patient. When patient anxiety exists, compliance is less likely. Therapeutic regimens that are planned by physicians "in the patient's best interest" without considering the patient's social stresses will be incomplete and probably will not be followed. Detailed assessment of social stress is needed to plan for helping to overcome barriers to compliance. The home setting fosters an unstructured patient-controlled environment, so nurses caring for patients at home may need to emphasize nursing care directed at increasing compliance.

Knowledge obtained through holistic nursing assessment needs to be shared with physicians so that medical recommendations that consider the barriers to compliance can be appropriately prescribed. The feedback patients receive from nurses and physicians influences behavior. Zifferblatt[23] reports that if the consequences of actions are perceived as beneficial, these actions will have a high probability of occurrence since they provoke positive reinforcement. The nurse's role is to help patients realize the benefits, become aware of an improved health state, and receive praise for whatever degree of compliance is detected.

The actual effect of these described nursing interventions in promoting compliance has not yet been studied or reported. The overall emphasis on increasing compliance is to promote patient-perceived control.

## SUMMARY

Patients' compliance or noncompliance is influenced by the factors explicated in Becker's health-belief model.[11] In addition, the concept of powerlessness needs to be considered in that compliance results when patients perceive their actions will influence (control) positive outcomes, that is, eliminate powerlessness caused by troublesome symptoms and/or complications. In this instance, patients perceive they have power to improve the health state, and that power is enhanced through compliance when the end result is increased capability for role fulfillment such as resuming work, increasing socialization, or increasing mobility. Patients' deliberate noncompliance may be geared to achieving control over other aspects of their lives. When there is dissonance between values or self-perception and the imposed regimen, noncompliance may serve to decrease the dissonance. For example, Mrs. L. valued meals for family socialization, prepared a large amount of food, consumed excess calories, and encouraged her family to do likewise. She perceived this was necessary to maintain family solidarity. Her self-perception and her family's perception of her were that weighing less than 200 lb would be unhealthy, making her susceptible to pathogens.

Helping patients perceive a sense of control to alleviate powerlessness should have an impact on improving compliance. The degree of conjoint (patient-nurse or patient-physician) planning to tailor regimens to individual circumstances influences compliance. Mutual determination of compliance strategies is a way of helping the patient develop a perceived sense of control.

## REFERENCES

1. Gillum, R. F. and Barsky, A. J.: *Diagnosis and management of patient noncompliance.* J.A.M.A. 228:1563, 1974.
2. Marston, M. V.: *Compliance with medical regimens: A review of the literature.* Nurs. Res. 20:312, July-August 1970.
3. Rosenstock, I.: *Patients' compliance with health regimens.* J.A.M.A. 234:402, 1975.
4. Parsons, T.: *Definitions of health and illness in the light of American values and social structure.* In Jaco, E. G. (eds.): *Patients, Physicians, and Illness.* The Free Press, New York, 1972, p. 110.
5. Taylor, C.: *Soul talk: A key to black cultural attitudes.* In Luckraft, D. (ed.): *Black Awareness: Implications for Black Patient Care.* American Journal of Nursing, New York, 1976, pp. 1-5.
6. Nobles, W. W. and Nobles, G. M.: *African roots in black families: The social-psychological dynamics of black family life and the implications for nursing care.* In Luckraft, D. (ed.): *Black Awareness: Implications for Black Patient Care.* American Journal of Nursing, New York, 1976, pp. 6-11.
7. Parsons, op. cit. pp. 107-127.
8. Bloch, B.: *Nursing intervention in black patient care.* In Luckraft, D. (ed.): *Black Awareness: Implications for Black Patient Care.* American Journal of Nursing, New York, 1976, pp. 27-35.
9. Ibid. p. 30.
10. Davis, M. S.: *Predicting non-compliant behavior.* J. Health Soc. Behav. 8:265, 1967.

11. Becker, M. H.: *Sociobehavioral determinants of compliance.* In Sackett, D. L. and Haynes, R. B. (eds.): *Compliance with Therapeutic Regimens.* Johns Hopkins University Press, Baltimore, 1976, pp. 40-50.
12. Haynes, R. B.: *A critical review of the determinants of patient compliance with therapeutic regimens.* In Sackett, D. L. and Haynes, R. B. (eds.): *Compliance with Therapeutic Regimens.* Johns Hopkins University Press, Baltimore, 1976, pp. 26-39.
13. Davis, M. S. and Eichhorn, R. L.: *Compliance with medical regimens: A panel study.* J. Health Hum. Behav. 4:240, 1963.
14. Ramirez, A.: *Social influence and ethnicity of the communicator.* J. Soc. Psychol. 102:209, 1977.
15. Vincent, P.: *Factors influencing patient non-compliance: A theoretical approach.* Nurs. Res. 20:509, November-December 1971.
16. Banks, W. C., et al.: *Perceived objectivity and the effects of evaluative reinforcement upon compliance and self-evaluation in blacks.* Journal of Experimental Social Psychology 13:452, 1977.
17. Davis, M. S.: *Variations in patients' compliance with doctors' advice: An empirical analysis of patterns of communication.* Am. J. Public Health 68:274, 1968.
18. Thibaut, J., et al.: *Compliance with rules: Some social determinants.* J. Pers. Soc. Psychol. 30:792, 1974.
19. Komaroff, A. L.: *Practitioner and the compliant patient.* Am. J. Public Health 66:833, 1976.
20. Hulka, B. S., et al.: *Communication, compliance, and concordance between physicians and patients with prescribed medications.* Am. J. Public Health 66:847, 1976.
21. Lowery, B. and DuCette, J.: *Disease-related learning and disease control in diabetics as a function of locus of control.* Nurs. Res. 25:358, September-October 1976.
22. Williams, T. F., et al: *The clinical picture of diabetic control, studied in four settings.* Am. J. Public Health 57:441, 1967.
23. Zifferblatt, S. M.: *Increasing patient compliance through the applied analysis of behavior.* Prev. Med. 4:173, 1975.

# SELECTED READINGS

Barofsky, I.: *Medication Compliance.* Charles B. Slack, Thorofare, N.J., 1977.
Bille, D.: *The role of body image in patient compliance and education.* Heart Lung 6:143, 1977.
Blackwell, B.: *Counselling and compliance.* Patient Counselling and Health Education 1:45, Fall 1978.
Becker, M. and Green, W.: *A family approach to compliance with medical treatment.* Int. J. Health Educ. 18:173, 1975.
Becker, M., Drechman, R., and Kirscht, J.: *A new approach to explaining sick role behavior in low income populations.* Am. J. Public Health 64:205, 1974.
Brand, R., Smith, R., and Brand, P.: *Effect of economic barriers to medical care on patients' noncompliance.* Public Health Rep. 92:72, 1977.
Conway, M. E.: *Are attitudes toward work related to readiness to seek medical care?* Nurs. Res. 22:123, March-April 1973.
Coogan, J. E.: *Motivating the unmotivated patient.* Nursing74 4:31, February 1974.
Dracup, K. and Meleis, A.: *Compliance: An interactionist approach.* Nurs. Res. 31:31, January-February 1982.
DiCicco, L. and Apple, D.: *Health needs and opinions of older adults.* In Apple, D. (ed.): *Sociological Studies of Health and Sickness.* McGraw-Hill, New York, 1960, pp. 26-39.
Given, C., Given, B., and Simoni, L.: *The association of knowledge and perception of medications with compliance and health states among hypertension patients: A prospective study.* Res. Nurs. Health 1:76, 1978.
Green, L.: *Should health education abandon attitude change strategies: Perspectives from recent research.* Health Educ. Monogr. 30:25, 1970.
Guthrie, D. and Guthrie, R.: *Nursing Management of Diabetes Mellitus.* C. V. Mosby, St. Louis, 1977.

Haynes, R. B., Taylor, W., and Sackett, D.: *Compliance in Health Care.* Johns Hopkins University Press, Baltimore, 1979.

Kasl, S.: *The health belief model and behavior related to chronic illness.* Health Educ. Monogr. 2:433, Winter 1974.

Kirscht, J.: *The health belief model and illness behavior.* Health Educ. Monogr. 2:387, Winter 1974.

LaFargue, J. P.: *Role of prejudice in rejection of health care.* Nurs. Res. 21:53, January-February 1972.

Levy, R. L. and Carter, R. D.: *Compliance with practitioner instigations.* Social Work 21:188, 1976.

Loustau, A.: *Using the health belief model to predict patient compliance.* Health Values: Achieving High Level Wellness 3:241, 1979.

Lowe, M.: *Effectiveness of teaching as measured by compliance with recommendations.* Nurs. Res. 19:59, January-February 1970.

Lyman, S.: *The Black American in Sociological Thought.* G. P. Putnam Sons, New York, 1972.

Lytton, H. and Zwirner, W.: *Compliance and its controlling stimuli observed in a natural setting.* Developmental Psychology 11:769, 1975.

Marston, M. V.: *The use of knowledge.* In Hardy, M. and Conway, M. (eds.): *Role Theory: Perspectives for Health Professionals.* Appleton-Century-Crofts, New York, 1978.

Miller, L., Goldstein, J., and Nicolaison, G.: *Evaluation of patients' knowledge of diabetes self care.* Diabetes Care 1:275, 1978.

Peay, M. Y.: *Effects of social power and preexisting attitudes on public and private responses to an induced attitude.* Human Relations 29:1115, 1976.

Rodin, J. and Slochower, J.: *Fat chance for a favor: Obese-normal differences in compliance and incidental learning.* J. Pers. Soc. Psychol. 29:557, 1974.

Scherwitz, L. and Leventhal, H.: *Strategies for increasing patient compliance.* Health Values: Achieving High Level Wellness 2:301, 1978.

Steckel, S.: *Contracting with patient-selected reinforcers.* Am. J. Nurs. 80:1596, September 1980.

Talkington, D.: *Maximizing patient compliance by shaping attitudes of self-directed health care.* J. Fam. Pract. 6:591, 1978.

Tagliacozzo, D. L.: *The patient's view of the patient's role.* In Jaco, E. G.: *Patients, Physicians, and Illness.* The Free Press, New York, 1972, pp. 172-185.

Watkins, J., et al.: *A study of diabetic patients at home.* Am. J. Public Health 57:452, 1967.

**PART 4**

# ALLEVIATING POWERLESSNESS

Complete alleviation of symptoms and cure are not appropriate goals for the chronically ill. The focus on alleviating a prevailing perception—powerlessness—and enhancing quality of life is an appropriate nursing goal. Chronically ill persons have deficits in one or several power resources of the power model (Chapter 1). The more power resources that can be restored, the more quality of life will be enhanced and powerlessness will be alleviated.

Discussion of alleviation of powerlessness in Part 4 takes place from two perspectives: (1) generalized categories of nursing strategies as an exemplar plan for nursing intervention and (2) development of specific components of the power resource model. Generalized strategies for alleviating powerlessness are presented in Chapters 13 and 14. Stapleton presents a prototype of empowerment strategies that could be used for any chronically ill patient. Pfister-Minogue addresses specific power resources of knowledge and motivation. Two power components that are influential in alleviating powerlessness are self-esteem (Chapter 15) and hope (Chapter 16). Detailed analyses of these concepts and specific means of enhancing self-esteem and inspiring hope are included. Developing the power resources of physical strength, psychologic stamina (support network of significant others), positive self-concept (emphasis on self-esteem), energy, knowledge, motivation, and hope alleviates powerlessness.

# 13

# ENABLING STRATEGIES

## KATHY PFISTER-MINOGUE

One of the major roles of nursing is to help persons move toward optimum wellness. For chronically ill persons, this includes assisting them to manage alterations in their health. As has been emphasized throughout this book, a sense of powerlessness, or loss of control, often accompanies the demands made by chronic illness. Initially, nurses manage new demands resulting from these altered health states for patients; ultimately, nurses have a role in helping patients manage these demands for themselves. The interventions nurses use to facilitate self-care and increase patient control are referred to as "enabling strategies." It is necessary to develop and use enabling strategies to effect the patient's sense of control. The purpose of this chapter is to discuss three enabling strategies: patient education, individualization of patient education, and behavior modification. The three enabling strategies are directed at developing specific components of the power resource model (see Fig. 1-1, Chapter 1). Patient motivation and knowledge are patient power resources that are developed through use of enabling strategies such as those described in this chapter. The enabling strategies are implemented through use of a nursing framework.

The use of a nursing framework offers an organized approach to patients who require nursing care. It is a prerequisite to the enabling strategies because it provides a means to view the total, or holistic, health situation of the patient. The nursing framework requires the nurse to be more systematic and predictive in care. The framework is a tool to guide practice. Although individual nurses may choose various frameworks for this purpose, a self-care framework is applied here.

# SELF-CARE FRAMEWORK

"Self-care refers to actions based on culturally or scientifically derived practices freely performed by individuals (or their agents), directed to themselves or to conditions or objects in their environment in the interests of their own life, health, or well-being."[1] According to Orem, the important components of the self-care framework are self-care agency, therapeutic self-care demands, self-care deficits, and nursing agency. Self-care agency is the power of the person to engage in the estimative and productive operations essential for self-care. It comprises all of the person's resources and abilities. Therapeutic self-care demands refer to the work that has to be done by or for an individual to achieve better health. Therapeutic self-care demands have three distinct components: (1) universal self-care requisites, (2) developmental self-care requisites, and (3) health deviation self-care requisites. Universal self-care requisites are common human needs for air, food, water, elimination, activity and rest, solitude and social interaction, safety, and normalcy. Developmental self-care requisites refer to needs related to developmental processes (tasks). Health deviation self-care requisites are needs resulting from an altered health state and/or a prescribed regimen.[2] Self-care demands can also be related to achieving a higher level of wellness and well-being. Self-care deficits arise when the self-care demands exceed a person's self-care agency. The use of nursing agency is important in relation to these deficits. Nursing agency is a set of qualities, knowledge, and skills that the nurse has acquired through specialized study. Nursing agency is used to alter the self-care demands or to supplement or increase a patient's self-care agency in dealing with self-care deficits.

Both patient and nurse are holistic, interactive beings. As shown in Figure 13-1, humans have psychologic, physiologic, social, and spiritual components. All these aspects of humans contribute to self-care agency. The nurse also has these components. In addition, the nurse's personal knowledge base and professional knowledge base contribute to the nursing agency.

The patient is located on a health-illness continuum. If the patient is unable to meet self-care requisites through utilizing the self-care agency, self-care deficits result. When these deficits exist, nursing is needed. Nursing agency is put into operation to resolve self-care deficits.

The nurse uses nursing agency in problem solving or in applying the nursing process, which consists of four steps. *Step 1* is the initial and continuing determination of why a person should receive nursing care. It involves assessment of the person's self-care agency and self-care demands, and the determination of the self-care deficits. *Step 2* is designing a system of nursing to achieve the patient's health goals through therapeutic self-care. *Step 3* is the actual meeting of the patient's requirements for nursing as the nurse uses assisting actions (may act for, provide for, guide, support, decide for or with, teach the patient, and so forth).[1] *Step 4*, evaluation, is the measurement of movement toward health.

Consider an example of the demands resulting from health deviation requisites confronting a person with a newly diagnosed myocardial infarction. These demands may include the need to rest, have the heart monitored for arrhythmias, cope psychologically with this altered health state, take medications, and adhere to special diet. These de-

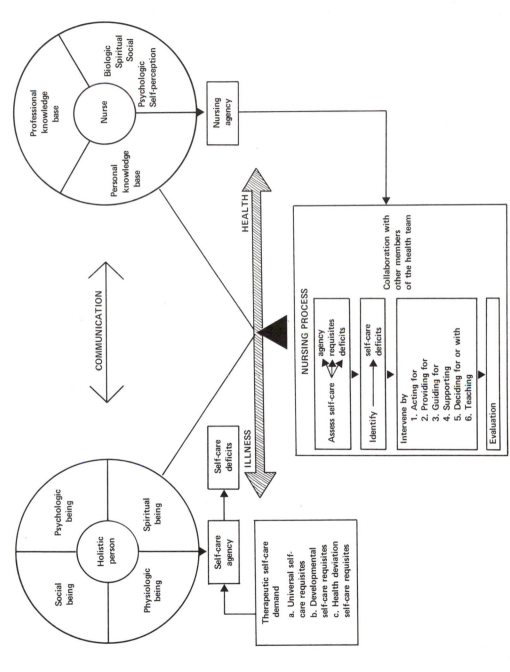

**FIGURE 13-1.  Self-care nursing model.**

mands continue throughout the long-term rehabilitation phase of the illness. New demands—such as the need to alter risk factors appropriate to the patient, to integrate the myocardial infarction into a positive concept of self, and to master roles important to the patient—prevail during the recovery phase of the illness. Nurses must assess this person's self-care agency in managing these long-term demands. During more dependent phases of an illness, nurses supplement the self-care agency by "doing for" the patient. As patients improve physically, they are taught how to care for themselves. Patient education is one of the most widely used enabling strategies. The patient is taught what has happened to the heart and the need to modify activity, diet, and medications; the patient's self-care agency is enhanced, as is the ability to master health needs.

## POWER RESOURCES—KNOWLEDGE AND MOTIVATION

## Knowledge

Patient knowledge is a power resource and an enabling factor in managing chronic illness. Patient education is a powerful tool for enhancing the patient's self-care agency. Recently, health-care professionals have been more cognizant of the patient's need for information. Many pamphlets and audiovisual aids are available to provide information to a patient about a given health situation. Insurance companies are beginning to pay for health education because they realize that if individuals can learn to care for themselves, costly hospital and medical bills will be avoided.

In many settings, however, patient education has been defined only as the provision of information. Although this has assisted many in achieving healthier lives, knowledge alone is often insufficient in assuring that the expected behavior change will continue throughout the life of the chronically ill person. Even though patients have been instructed in what to do, they often do not follow through with the desired behaviors. As noted in Chapter 12, rates of patient noncompliance are as high as 50 percent to 70 percent. So if learning is defined as change in behavior, then our teaching is not consistently accomplishing this.

Even though patients have a knowledge of medications, diets, and exercise programs, they do not follow these prescriptions. What else is lacking in the self-care agencies of these individuals? Various reasons for seeming lack of motivation can be proposed. Patients may be too consumed by the need to cope with their feelings about their diagnoses to have the energy to learn and adopt new practices. They may have a general knowledge of what is appropriate but may not know how to fit it into their own life-styles. It may be just too difficult for persons to alter patterns of behavior that have been established over long periods in spite of the fact that these may no longer be good for their health.

If we assume that all behavior is causally determined, the question of why the patient chooses to comply or not to comply needs to be examined. Motivation theory is important to compliance and thus is a part of the nurse's knowledge base in using the enabling strategies.

# Motivation

Attempts to explain human beings' behavior probably date back to the beginnings of humankind. Many approaches have been used. In the 17th century, the predominant view emphasized humans' free will and ability to exercise rationality.[3] The ability to reason thus allowed humans to control their behavior. Humans were thus morally responsible for their behavior.

With the development of the physical sciences in the 17th and 18th centuries, more mechanistic views of motivation arose. Descartes believed animals acted on the basis of external and internal forces.[3] He felt humans' behavior was caused by a combination of these forces, plus human beings' rationality. Others felt humans were motivated by the pursuit of pleasure and avoidance of pain. This was extended to include learning of behavior on the basis of pleasurable versus adversive outcomes.

After observing animal behavior, Darwin felt that behavior was controlled by the struggle to obtain necessities of life such as food and space.[4] The idea of survival of the fittest grew out of this concept. Darwin believed that instincts largely determined behavior. Freud also felt instinctual urges controlled behavior.[5]

As a commitment to a scientific method of investigation grew in the 20th century, many animal studies were done. Reward versus punishment, reinforcement, adverse stimuli, deprivation of biologically significant stimuli, and stimuli and responses in general were studied in animals. Skinner, Thorndike, Watson, Hull, and Spence are important behavioral theorists.[6] Watson reacted against instinctual causes of behavior and believed behavior was controlled by various stimulus-response situations and was flexible and modifiable.[7] Hull added to this the concept of reduction in biologic drive as a positive reinforcer for behavior. Thus again the biologic needs of humans were the focus. If a behavior had been reinforced over time, Hull felt that this contributed to its maintenance. He referred to this as habit strength.[5] Other theorists proposed that stimuli do not elicit responses; they only strengthen the tendency to respond. Some motive or need is at the basis of the response.

At the same time, other theorists were trying to describe behavior on the bases of neurology, hormones, genetic information, and other physiologic data. Many of the studies related to these theories were done on animals. Recently, more complex species of animals that are closer to humans have been studied. Behaviorists have also been doing more testing in humans in the last century.[3]

Behavior is most likely caused by the interrelationship of nerves, hormones, stimulus conditions, behavioral events, the human being's rational ability, and many other yet-unidentified influencing factors. There is no one answer.

Since these studies have not been well controlled, have focused on isolated units of behavior, and have mostly been done on animals, it is difficult to glean from these data much that is helpful to patient education. Stimulus-response theories of motivation underlie the enabling strategy of behavior modification that will be discussed later in this chapter.

Maslow developed a humanistic theory of motivation. Maslow views the human as an integrated whole; thus, he proposes that one cannot conduct experiments looking at an isolated entity. He feels, therefore, that one cannot accept the tightly controlled experimental approach as the only method of developing science. Maslow proposes that the human being is always in a wanting state. Once a state of satisfaction is reached in one area, another desire wanting to be satisfied appears. He has classified a list of drives to assist in analyzing behavior, acknowledging that these are dynamic and there are many exceptions. He hypothesizes that basic needs are similar from culture to culture but are met in different ways. He emphasizes that goals and barriers to goals may be different for each individual.[8]

It will be recalled that there is a hierarchy of needs in Maslow's theory of human motivation. The hierarchy of needs is composed of physiologic needs, safety needs, belongingness or love needs, esteem needs, and the need for self-actualization. Maslow feels it is quite true that humans live by bread alone when there is no bread; that is, humans, deprived of food, will seek to meet this need first. If hunger is satisfied, humans will go on to meet other higher-order needs. He acknowledges exceptions to these hypotheses at all levels. For example, under certain circumstances, a human has chosen to fast or take one's own life to accomplish the pursuits of higher-level needs.[8]

Maslow's observations may have some implications for patient education. For example, a patient who is in pain or physically threatened may not be able to focus on learning the kind of diet and exercise plan the patient should follow.

Rogers' humanistic theory of motivation is based on a fundamental construct, the "actualizing tendency." This means persons have an inherent tendency to develop all their capacities in ways that maintain or enhance the individual. Two additional sources of motivation are the need for positive regard from others and the need for self-regard.[9]

Perhaps some of the most useful work on motivation in light of our goal—that is, to enhance the self-care agencies of individuals—is the study of why patients choose to behave or not to behave in a way that complies with health-care advice. This is an important question in terms of utilizing education to enhance self-care agencies. The literature regarding compliance has attempted to answer this question.

## Motivation and Compliance

Correlations have been identified between characteristics of patients and their regimens and decreased or increased compliance. Although these do not provide an adequately proven set of recommendations for teaching, they do suggest components of a conceptual framework that may facilitate teaching. Factors that influence compliance are grouped under the following headings to facilitate discussion: demographic factors, sociopsychologic factors, interaction or provider-patient relationship factors, and other factors.

Demographic factors such as age, sex, education, and socioeconomic status have been studied. No correlations were found between age, sex, and motivation to seek help or comply.[10,11] Increased education and socioeconomic status were associated with increased preventive and symptomatic physician visits in some studies, but other studies found no relationship.[10,12-14]

Several sociopsychologic factors have been related to compliance. Input from family, peers, and reference groups is important. Advice from such people is often regarded as highly as advice from health-care providers.[15-17] Side effects of medications were related to decreased compliance. Perceived benefits of following advice and perceived costs are important. Higher perceived benefits resulted in increased compliance. Higher perceived barriers resulted in decreased compliance.[14,18] Detailed information about what drugs would "do for you specifically" has been related to increased compliance.[17] As complexity and feasibility or practicality increase, compliance decreases.[10,11,19] The more the health advice changes one's life-style, the less a person will comply.[20] This is especially true if compliance requires changes in work habits.[13,21] Very high levels of perceived severity of the health problem decrease compliance, whereas moderate levels increase compliance.[22]

Becker and Maiman discuss many of the above variables in terms of a "value-expectancy model." They view compliant behavior as being predicted from the value or outcome that behavior has to an individual and the individual's expectation that a given action will result in that outcome, weighed against the total costs, burdens, and side effects resulting from actions to comply.[23]

The development of this model grew out of the Public Health Service's interest in disease prevention in the 1950s. There was widespread failure of people to accept preventive health measures and screening tests. The concern was particularly for the prevention of tuberculosis, poliomyelitis, dental disease, and rheumatic fever. Thus, the theory was based on studies involving preventive health behavior rather than on studies focusing on the patient with chronic illness. Selected important elements such as the sick role, the influence of family and significant others, and the health provider–patient relationship are not addressed in this model.

Becker and Maiman analyzed the work of five colleagues who have proposed models to describe action in situations involving risk taking or decision making under uncertainty (which they feel is what happens in preventive health). The models of Tollman, Rotter, Edwards, Atkinson, and Feather were compared with Becker and Maiman's health-belief model. All were similar in emphasizing that prediction of behavior depends on two variables: (1) the value placed by the individual on a particular goal, and (2) the individual's estimate of the likelihood that a given action will result in achievement of a goal.[23]

One of the variables described in the literature that consistently showed a correlation with compliance is the provider-patient relationship. Most of the studies in this area were done on the physician-patient relationship and the aspects of the relationship that are important. Some of the features of this relationship that positively influence compliance include a friendly and accepting attitude of the health provider, patients' evaluations that the physician spent time with them,[15] patients' feelings that they have control in the interaction and input into the regimen,[24] the patients' feelings of satisfaction with care,[19] a regimen that is actually tailored to the individual,[25] a situation in which information is willingly shared with patients, a lack of formal disagreement with patients,[26] and continuity of the health-care provider.[22]

Although the majority of these studies have investigated the physician-patient relationship, the conclusions also may well be true for other health-care providers who work extensively with the patient. In a case-study approach, the author utilized a nurse-patient relationship that provided continuity of nursing-care provider, sharing of information with the patient, tailoring of the regimen, and acceptance of a patient's decision about the patient's own health care. This was judged to be effective by the amount the patient's behavior coincided with therapeutic prescriptions.[27]

Other variables influencing motivation to comply include patient education, a positive self-concept, and positive adaptation to illness. Although patient education alone will not necessarily result in compliance, patients cannot comply unless they know or understand the regimen they are to follow. By the same token, they will not be motivated or ready to follow advice if they are denying their health state. They may also lack motivation if their sense of self-worth and perception of ability to alter the state is low, resulting in feelings of powerlessness. Enhancing motivation should have a therapeutic effect in decreasing powerlessness.

Reports of studies that attempted to relate patient education about regimens and compliance have been conflicting, but some relationships have been identified. At times, researchers failed to define what was meant by patient teaching. Sometimes, structured versus nonstructured, or routine versus experimental teaching was the topic of study. This makes the data difficult to interpret. One such study on prenatal education found no relationship between compliance and the type of education utilized.[28]

Another study, which was well controlled, compared preoperative teaching based on a lesson plan established and approved for content, method, and visual aids with the nurse's teaching what, how, and when the nurse wanted. A significant relationship between the structured type of education and compliance was documented.[29] Two studies positively related patient education to knowledge about diabetes and skill in carrying out their treatment.[30,31] Riley found that patients need specific instructions in order to comply.[32] Two further studies on preventive health measures demonstrated that knowledge alone was insufficient, but patients' beliefs in their own susceptibility to the problem were necessary.[10]

The author successfully used a patient-education approach that included timely provision of information, resolution of problems individually identified as hampering patient learning, individualization and tailoring of the approach to the patient, and deciding with patients what the information meant in terms of their own lives. Timely provision of information and resolution of problems identified as hampering patient learning involved an individual assessment of the patient's compliance with each aspect of the patient's health deviation self-care requisites. It must be noted that reasons for not learning or changing behavior to follow health-care advice not only were different from patient to patient but also were different for various aspects of the self-care requisite. For example, the reason a person does not follow a diet may be quite different from why the person chooses not to take a medication. Problems hampering learning might also be unrelated to the specific requisite. Thus, for example, if a patient was in the denial stage of illness, nursing measures to help a patient work through the denial were taken before education about a regimen was completed. Or if a low self-concept was assessed to hinder compliance, then self-concept was addressed as a nursing diagnosis. These measures increased patient compliance in situations in which patients were previously not complying.[27]

Only a few studies have been designed specifically to evaluate the effect of self-concept on following health-care advice. Bille studied the influence of one component of self-concept, body image, on knowledge and compliance resulting from patient education in 24 men who were cardiac patients. He did not find a significant relationship between knowledge resulting from patient teaching and body image, but he did find that patients with positive body images showed increased compliance.[33] This relationship between positive self-concept and increased compliance was confirmed in one patient who was studied as part of a case-study approach to compliance.[27] This will be discussed in more detail later in the chapter.

Illness creates a change in body image. The nature of the illness as a threat, the meaning of the threat to the individual, and the ability to cope with it are important in adapting to that changed body image. The help available from care givers, family, and significant others is important.[34] Rubin says that with every bit of functional loss a person experiences, a bit of personal life space is lost. The degree of emotional response is directly related to the struggle to maintain control.[35] The purpose of patient education is to help a person manage or gain control over losses from disease or injury, thereby incorporating the illness as part of self. Compliance, then, might be seen as a way to gain control.

Combs describes the difficulty of getting patients with newly diagnosed diabetes to care for themselves. He relates this to patients' difficulty coping with or assimilating new self-concepts.[36]

Realization that something is wrong with the body causes tension and stress. Although one tension-reducing mechanism might be learning about the illness, patients will not learn effectively unless they are ready. If patients are in a stage of denial, they have not yet intellectualized what has happened or changed the self-concept to incorporate the illness. In this instance, they may reject information given to help them adjust the life-style to accommodate the condition. Coogan refers to this in describing the problems of motivating the unmotivated patient. She noted a problem when patient and nursing goals are not the same. She attributes this problem to patients being so overwhelmed by their situations that they cannot participate. She says nurses must meet patients at their level of adjustment and involve patients in decision making.[37]

It can be seen that there is a complexity and interrelationship among the variables that may influence a patient's motivation to follow therapeutic self-care demands. Sociopsychologic factors, provider-patient relationship factors, and other enabling factors likely all play roles. Although several authors have suggested various approaches to this problem, few approaches have been studied except the patient-education approaches described above. Behavior modification is another approach that has been used to help individuals gain control of behaviors; this will be discussed in more depth later in the chapter. Since a variety of potential factors influence behavior, it is clear that a thorough patient assessment and the subsequent design of an individualized approach would seem to be the best way to consider all the variables.

# NURSING STRATEGIES

## An Individualized Approach to Patient Education

A summary of the factors to consider when developing an individualized approach to patient education is found in Table 13-1. The first step should be the development of a

**TABLE 13-1.  Factors Considered in Individualized Approach**

I. Health-care Provider–Patient Relationship

Interest and friendliness
Willingness to share information with the patient
Allowing patient participation and control in the relationship
Satisfaction of the patient
Tailoring the health-care regimen to the patient
Continuity of health-care provider
Lack of formal disagreement with the patient

II. Assessment of Socio-psychologic Factors

Input from family, peers, and reference groups
Perceived susceptibility to a disease or complication
Health beliefs and motivation—acceptance of health problem
Perceived severity of the problem
Perceived benefits of following the advice
Cost of following the advice—economic, psychologic, and social
Accessibility of resources needed to follow advice
Change in life-style required to follow the advice
Duration and complexity of the health-care plan
Side effects of drugs
Family environment
Developmental needs
Career goals
Demographic factors—age, sex, marital status, culture, religion

III. Nursing Intervention—Patient Education

Focus on self-concept improvement.
  Integrate body image change into positive concept of self.
Develop patient's knowledge about the health problem, treatment.
Explore how the problem and treatment will affect the patient's life.
Provide patient-specific instruction.
Collaborate with the patient on tailoring the regimen.

relationship with the patient. Components of this relationship should include interest and friendliness, willingness to share information with the patient, allowing patient participation and control in the relationship, a desire to satisfy the patient, tailoring of the health-care information to the patient, lack of formal disagreement with the patient, and continuity of health provider.

Continuity of the relationship is hindered in some health-care settings. This is not as true in community settings as it is in large institutional settings. The advent of primary-care nursing has improved this somewhat. One method of providing continuity has been contracting. Briefly, this is an agreement with the patient with the purpose, goals, and length of the relationship clearly identified. It may be verbal or written. Some nurses have found this very effective. It provides the framework for mutual goal setting, which is essential.

Swain and Steckel[38] studied the effect of three interventions on 115 hypertensive patients' adherence to medical care, as determined by the patients' return for follow-up care. The three interventions were routine clinic care, patient education, and contingency contracting. The contingency contracting consisted of the patient establishing a goal and determining rewards for achieving the goal, with both the nurse and patient agreeing to and signing the agreement. The contingency contracting was effective in achieving patient adherence to medical care, improving knowledge, and lowering diastolic blood pressures. Patient education was not effective in lowering the patients' blood pressures. Patients receiving the education intervention had a higher dropout rate than did patients receiving routine clinic care.[38]

## ASSESSMENT

The second component of the individualized approach is assessment. It is important to assess both the self-care demands and the patient's self-care agency. Assessment results in specific identification of the therapeutic self-care requisites for the patient. If we are trying to prevent an alteration in health, then we need to assess what things affect the development of the alteration and thus the quality of life. If there is an existing health alteration, then we ask what things about the alteration will affect the quality of life of the individual. How will it affect the individual physically, emotionally, and socially? Some questions we might ask ourselves include the following:

How are the person's life processes affected?
How are the person's oxygenation, hydration, nutrition, elimination, rest, activity, comfort, solitude and social interactions, and safety altered?
What is required for this individual to integrate this illness into the life experience to prevent regression or dissociation of the event?
How will the illness change family, work, social, and sexual roles?

Next, what will aid in the control and management of the health alterations needs to be assessed. A thorough knowledge of the benefits of these control mechanisms is necessary. This approach is particularly necessary in light of the information that patient compliance is influenced by the perceived benefits of following advice and by the amount of life-style change that is incurred. We would not wish to advise a patient to change an aspect of life-style if we do not have good evidence of the benefits of that change. If the benefits are controversial, the patient has the right to know this. The more information we have to support the benefits, the better chance we should have of the patient accepting the approach.

There is much collaboration during this phase because other health-care providers, especially physicians, may have input. Even if the therapeutic demands are advised by the physician, the nurse often interprets them to the patient.

After the health alteration has been assessed and the therapeutic self-care demands have been determined, it is necessary to assess the individual's self-care agency to determine the ability to meet the demands. Assessment of the patient's present self-care actions would be the first step. This should be followed by an assessment of how the patient would need to change to meet or comply with therapeutic health-care requisites. Other sociopsychologic compliance factors should also be considered here. The patient's perception of the value of therapeutic demands and the required changes is important. Understanding the perception of family members or significant others and their influence on the patient is also helpful. The individual's own health goals are important. If they are not the same as those considered ideal in terms of health, compromise should occur. The more the nurse is able to allow patients to make their own decisions, the more freedom patients will feel to share their actual noncompliance and the reasons for it. This, in itself, offers the nurse further cues for intervention. Perhaps through compromise the patient will be able to manage more fully therapeutic self-care demands. We need to accept patient decisions even if they are not in compliance with advice given. The problem may be that our goal for the patient is different from the patient's goal. Compromise is necessary. All too often, health-care providers have judged patients as good if they follow health-care advice perfectly but have been punitive toward patients who are unable to do so.

After mutual goals have been formulated and the requisites or demands have been readjusted to meet the goals, the patient's knowledge level should be assessed. The needed knowledge level and the patient's knowledge level must then be compared. In addition, other necessary resources must be assessed. The patient's physical ability to meet the demands, the availability of others to assist and support the patient, and the availability of monetary and equipment resources are important.

The next step would be to identify existing self-care deficits—that is, those demands that exceed the capabilities of the person's self-care agency. The nurse often uses the nursing agency to act for the patient and perform interventions to meet the various therapeutic self-care demands. In an acute health alteration, the nurse may act for the patient more frequently. As the acute health situation resolves, the patient's self-care agency must be developed to enable the patient to gain more control in self-care. In a chronic health state, an individual needs long-term assistance in developing and maintaining the self-care agency.

If the patient's self-care deficit involves difficulty coping with a change in self-concept or the need to go through the grieving process, these deficits must be attended to before the patient will be able to focus attention on other therapeutic self-care requisites. For the setting-bound nurse, this can be a problem. For example, a nurse employed by a hospital usually has only the time the patient is in the hospital to develop the patient's self-care agency. Nurses may need to begin to make more referrals and collaborate with other nurses to accomplish goals. Nurses need to develop means of being directly accessible to patients for nursing care.

## Patient Education

Lack of knowledge may be one deficit. In such a case, we would give the patient necessary facts and demonstrate necessary techniques. At this point, instruction should be tailored to the patient based on the assessment data. Consider again the health deviation requisites of the patient with a newly diagnosed myocardial infarction. One of these demands is the need for rest. Rest has different meaning for different people, so specific instructions are needed. A patient who is retired and leads a sedentary life may not have to make many changes. The implications of rest would be different for an individual who plays tennis weekly, manages a busy logging firm, and is constantly under stress. Assisting this person to rest may be more difficult. Specific information about when the patient could return to work would be necessary. Relaxation training and stress-reduction strategies might be needed to help this person achieve a restful state. Both individuals might receive similar information about the need for and the importance of rest. They might also receive similar instructions in how to assess whether they are receiving adequate rest. The plan for altering their activities, however, would be different.

Continuous reassessment of all the variables affecting a patient's ability to meet therapeutic health-care demands is indicated if a patient's self-care agency is not developing in a way in which the patient can meet the demands. Compromise is important to all aspects of meeting self-care demands. Patients may choose to take risks because they do not wish to give up a given behavior. For example, an individual may choose not to give up a job that is stressful and detrimental to health because that job fulfills other needs. We can reinforce information about the risks the person is taking, but this may not help. We might take the approach of assisting the person in analyzing the role the job plays and identifying possible alternatives. This has a better chance of being successful because we are helping the person find ways to accomplish the ideal. We are assisting in not just the "what to" but the "how to." This specific information about how to meet a health-care demand can result in increased motivation. The third enabling strategy to be discussed in this chapter is one means of providing a patient with information about "how to" do something.

# Behavior Modification

The final enabling strategy to be discussed is behavior modification. This is especially helpful for patients who know what action needs to be taken but do not seem to be able to alter routine behaviors or change habits to comply with the new demands. Behavior modification uses a systematic approach to analyze the causes of a behavior and the reinforcers of a behavior, and proceeds to alter the behavior by altering either the cause or reinforcer, or both. The use of behavior modification provides the patient with a method of controlling the problem and also places the responsibility for doing so with the patient, not with health-care personnel.

Behavior therapy is a strategy that has been used by psychologists and psychiatrists to alter various problematic behavior patterns. There are basically two approaches to psychologic problems that have been dominant in American psychologic thinking. One is an introspective, or subjective, psychology in which a person's consciousness is studied to find the cause of a problem. The other, behaviorism, born in the 1900s, focuses on study of the behavior of the human being to discover causes and solutions to problems. Proponents of this latter view hold that consciousness is impossible to study objectively, whereas behavior *can* be studied and measured objectively. During behaviorism's initial use, some people reacted negatively to this approach because they felt that this consciousness is what separates man from other animals. Individuals, however, have been unable to define exactly what makes up this consciousness, and introspection is the only way to gather data about it. Behaviorists have thus attempted to throw out the old vocabulary and begin making and recording observations about behavior. This has been done by observing various stimuli and responses. A stimulus is an agent or action that elicits or accelerates a physiologic or psychologic activity. This activity is called a response. These stimulus-and-response situations may be either simple or quite complex. They can be both internal and external. Thus, for example, a stimulus or response might be chemical or hormonal, or it may enter the body through one of the sense organs such as the eyes, ears, nose, and mouth. A response might be anything from a slight change in respirations or blood pressure, to movement of a muscle, to running a 2-mile race, to experiencing feelings of joy and pleasure at winning a race. External responses are obviously far easier to measure because one can see a person write a letter, eat lunch, drive a car, and so forth. Other means of measuring internal responses need to be developed.

Responses are both learned and unlearned. Unlearned responses are often called instincts. We breathe, our heart beats, and our eyes react to light at birth. Learned responses occur with conditioning. Unlearned responses are altered by this conditioning. For example, stomach contractions from lack of food will produce crying in a newborn infant. This is different from the learned response that occurs when the sight or smell of an apple pie causes the young child's mouth to water.

Wolpe and Lazarus define a habit as a consistent way of responding to defined stimulus conditions. It is a learned response. Habits undergo extinction or cease to exist when their consequences become unadaptive, that is, they fail to serve the needs of the organism. Neurotic habits are distinguished by their resistance to extinction even in the face of unadaptiveness. Behavior therapy is the application of experimentally established principles of learning to overcoming these persistent habits. To change a habit, one must modify the responses that constitute it. Change depends on eliciting behavior that can modify these responses.[39]

Much of the research related to behaviorism has indeed been conducted on attempting to modify neuroses and various psychologic problems and phobias. Nurses assist patients to modify their behavior in order to manage health deviation self-care requisites. This often requires change in health and living habits such as overeating or smoking, which have developed over many years. Behaviorism is not the answer for all behavior, but it has been a valuable tool for modifying various types of unhealthy behavior. Thus, some of the principles of behavioral therapy might be useful in assisting the patient to change learned ways of responding.

Perhaps one of the most frequently occurring health behaviors on which these principles have been tested is the control of obesity. Stuart, in his application of behavior modification to obesity, describes four steps. *Step 1* is the analysis of the response to be controlled and its antecedent and consequent conditions. An analysis of overeating would include a precise description of the conditions under which this occurs, along with consequent events that reward and maintain the behavior. *Step 2* is the identification of behaviors that facilitate eating the proper amount of food. *Step 3* is identifying positive and negative reinforcers that control these behavior patterns. *Step 4* is the application of reinforcement to alter the probability of the preselected response. The goal is to decrease the undesired response and increase the desired response.[40]

Zifferblatt describes similar steps. He suggests that patient compliance problems are behavioral problems. These behaviors, with memorable antecedents and consequences, will have a high probability of occurrence. With effective environmental manipulations, their occurrence may be modified. Analysis of the patient's behavior will reveal cues for the behavior and assist in identifying new cues that can be integrated into the patient's environment. Establishing compliant behavior then involves identifying the target behavior, performing a functional analysis of the behavior, and rearranging the environment to facilitate the occurrence of the behavior. For example, obesity is defined behaviorally as a specific set of responses that results in eating too much. The target behaviors might be eating between meals, eating when nervous, eating in front of the television, or eating when alone. The frequency of these events may be systematically changed to solve the problem.[41] These basic steps can be used to enable patients to carry out various aspects of their health-care measures. They provide a method to show the patients "how" they can accomplish "what" they need to accomplish. The case-study example that follows will include an example of how the nurse might use this approach.

According to self-care framework, the enabling strategies discussed in the preceding paragraphs are a part of nursing agency, or the skills the nurse uses to help a person resolve therapeutic self-care deficits. In Figure 13-1, these enabling strategies would be included in the professional knowledge base. The enabling strategies of patient education, individualized approach, and behavior modification, with respective outcomes, are summarized in Figure 13-2. The ultimate outcome of developing the power resources of knowledge and motivation helps alleviate powerlessness of chronic illness.

## PATIENT ANALYSIS—APPLICATION OF ENABLING STRATEGIES

A case study demonstrates how the nurse can utilize patient education, an individualized approach to the patient, and behavior modification within the framework of self-care to empower the patient to take actions that improve a health state—alleviate powerlessness.

Mrs. A., a 51-year-old woman, was followed medically in a medical center's endocrinology clinic for diabetes and obesity. She had been overweight most of her life (she is 5 ft 1 in and weighs 290 lb). Her diabetes was diagnosed 4 years ago. She lives with her alcoholic husband, who has been on disability because of his alcoholism for 18 years. Mr. and Mrs. A. have seven children. All but two of them are married.

Mrs. A.'s physician was frustrated because Mrs. A. did not observe her diabetic diet, was gaining weight, and was experiencing high blood sugars. A nurse at the clinic said that Mrs. A. had attended diabetic instruction classes but still did not adhere to her diet. The physician said, "You tell them again and again that they should stick to their diets and threaten them with what might happen to them if they don't, but it doesn't help."

At this point, I established a nurse-patient relationship with Mrs. A. and used the self-care framework to identify her therapeutic self-care demands. The demands specific to her health deviation, diabetes, included the following: adhering to a 1200-calorie diabetic diet; injecting proper dosages of insulin in appropriate sites; paying special attention to her skin, especially on her feet; giving special attention to infections; regulating her activity level; and performing glucose tests (Clinitest) and acid tests on her urine.

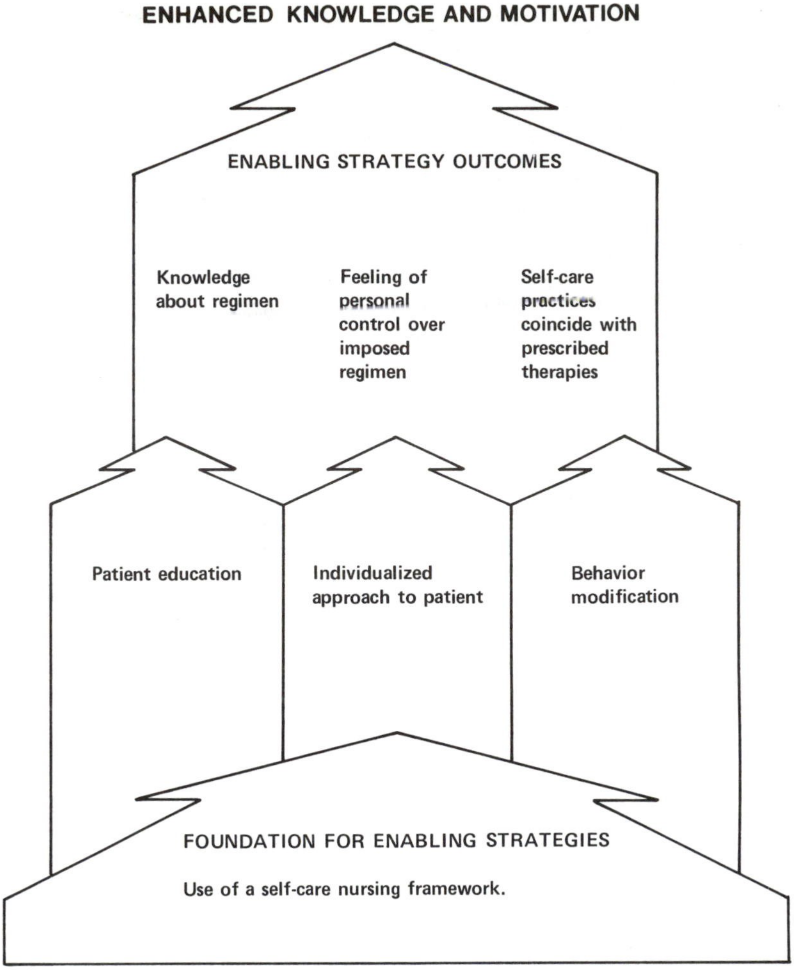

ENHANCED KNOWLEDGE AND MOTIVATION

ENABLING STRATEGY OUTCOMES

Knowledge          Feeling of          Self-care
about regimen      personal            practices
                   control over        coincide with
                   imposed             prescribed
                   regimen             therapies

Patient education     Individualized        Behavior
                      approach to patient   modification

FOUNDATION FOR ENABLING STRATEGIES

Use of a self-care nursing framework.

**FIGURE 13-2.   Enabling strategies to increase control.**

Assessment of her self-care agency revealed many limitations. In brief, she took no self-care actions to meet her demands; she did not maintain her diet, rotate insulin injection sites, or do urine glucose and acid tests. Her lack of self-care action was one manifestation of her perceived powerlessness in overwhelming social and health-deviation situations.

The next step was to appraise the knowledge base of Mrs. A. After she attended diabetic classes, was her knowledge sufficient to enable her to follow these therapeutic self-care demands? Indeed, her knowledge about what she was supposed to do was good. She understood her diet, and knew she was supposed to do the other things. Thus, some other aspect of her self-care agency was deficient, and patient education alone could not resolve the deficit.

The next step was to further individualize the assessment and the education for this patient. It was necessary to analyze what the therapeutic self-care demands entailed for

Mrs. A. It was necessary to assess her feelings about herself and her disease and her understanding of why the instructions she was given were important to her health.

During an overall assessment of how this person's therapeutic self-care demands affected her and an analysis of why, with her present self-care agency, she was unable to meet them, it was discovered that a very low self-concept seemed to hamper her ability or motivation to carry out these therapeutic measures on her own. She was very tearful during the nursing visits. Her conversation focused on how unhappy she was. She made comments about her life such as, "He (her husband) doesn't care about me or he wouldn't do this to me (referring to his drinking). Sometimes I just don't care. What difference does it make anyway? When it's God's time to take me, He will— sometimes that wouldn't be so bad."

Her appearance also reflected a lack of concern for herself, as her hair was often disheveled and her clothing untidy. When discussing her feelings about her diabetes, she said that she was upset and cried when she first found out about it, "but it was OK now." She had a diabetic niece who, she says, "even got married." It was evident that she had not worked through all her feelings about her illness. This unresolved adaptation seemed to add to her poor self-concept.

The initial attempts to discuss this patient's therapeutic needs related to her diabetes were unproductive. Her more immediate health-care deficit was her low self-concept. This deficit had to be altered before Mrs. A.'s self-care agency would be sufficient to manage other therapeutic self-care demands. It is not the purpose of this chapter to discuss improving self-concept. It is important here only because it was one aspect of an individualized approach to patient education that permitted the discovery of this self-care deficit that was hampering this patient's readiness to learn. Nursing strategies were designed to improve her self concept.[27] These included reviewing her unique assets—a good singing voice, excellent sewing ability, supportive relationship with three of her seven children, her willingness to help out by caring for grandchildren, and her continuing ability to care for her alcoholic husband. Eventually, the patient's tearfulness ceased, her appearance improved, and she began to make more positive comments about herself and to take more interest in managing her own care.

Other nursing strategies were used to meet a specific demand such as the need to rotate insulin sites. Mrs. A. gave herself insulin injections only in the abdomen because thigh injections were painful and caused bruising. She was unable to reach the sites on her arms because of her obesity. Although she knew where to rotate sites, she did not understand the importance of rotation because lack of rotation had not caused problems for her in 4 years.

Additional assessment was then done to check that Mrs. A. used the proper injection technique in her thighs. It seems her fear of sticking her leg caused her to withdraw the needle before the injection was completed, causing the insulin to be injected intradermally. This, of course, resulted in both pain and bruising. After this was corrected, Mrs. A. was able to rotate injections comfortably among the various sites on her abdomen and legs. This is a compromise from the ideals in diabetic patient-education literature; however, it was the optimum for the patient. There was no way for her to reach her arms or buttocks, and she did not wish to depend on others to assist her. She did agree to have the clinic nurse use those sites (she received her insulin there when she had clinic appointments).

Mrs. A.'s compliance with urine glucose and acid tests was also facilitated by individualizing her teaching. Initially, she did not do glucose tests at all. The use of urine glucose tests became more meaningful to her after I made a chart to show her the correlation between her blood sugars and urine sugars. At this time, Mrs. A. was proceeding with a weight-reduction program, and correlations could be seen between her weight, her urine glucose tests and blood sugars, and the amount of insulin she required. Therefore, the urine glucose tests became more meaningful to her as a reflection of changes in blood sugar levels. She never did the tests four times a day, but she did begin to do them twice a day. Mrs. A.'s progress in assuming self-care responsibility resulted in gradual alleviation of her feeling of lack of control.

One of the most important and most difficult therapeutic self-care demands of this patient was to lose weight and maintain a 1200-calorie diet. Mrs. A. understood her diet well; she said she just could not maintain it. Thus, her self-care deficit was not related to her knowledge of what to do but rather how to go about it.

The nursing strategy used to alter this deficit was behavior modification. The use of this approach was discussed with the patient, and she was amenable to it. The first step was to analyze the antecedent events—those happenings or environmental conditions that precipitated eating more than she was supposed to. Discussion with the patient revealed that she ate whenever she was nervous or lonesome. To further analyze the events related to eating, Mrs. A. was requested to keep a list of everything she ate for 1 week. Along with keeping this list of what she ate, she was to record how she was feeling when she ate, whether she was hungry, and what she was doing at the time. Analysis of her recorded data revealed that most of the time she ate her meals alone in front of the television. She never ate at the table. She ate food in large quantities, continuing to eat long after she was full. She also snacked on empty-calorie foods at frequent intervals throughout the day. She often felt lonely or restless when she was eating.

Eating was filling a big gap in this patient's life. It made her feel better when she was nervous or lonesome—at least momentarily. In the long run, the weight gain experienced was negative, but the immediate reward was more important. One of the first steps was to help manage her feelings of nervousness and lonesomeness in some other way. Some of the coping strategies identified and utilized included going for a walk to her daughter's house two blocks away, becoming more active in church groups, joining the church choir, getting out sewing projects she enjoyed, and getting a part-time job. She was encouraged to make a list of those unique talents, and in doing so, her self-concept continued to improve. She began to feel more productive and less helpless and dependent.

The next step involved identifying behavior that would facilitate the proper intake of food. It was suggested to Mrs. A. that she eat only at the table. She enjoyed watching television because it provided company for her, so she did not agree with this strategy. She did agree to eat only at mealtime, however. To help solve the problem of "shoveling" food, she was requested to set her fork down between bites of food. After doing this for a week, she was requested to swallow her food before she again picked up her fork. If she felt the urge to eat between meals, she was to stop and think about why she wanted to eat and use one of the alternative methods of coping we discovered together.

Another strategy utilized was to place everything she was supposed to eat on her plate before she began and not to go back for seconds. She was to fill her plate in the kitchen and put the additional food away.

Initially, Mrs. A. said she just could not lose weight. She continuously found excuses why suggested approaches would not work. Mrs. A. consistently used the word "can't" throughout therapeutic nurse-patient sessions. The author shared the observation of this excuse-making behavior with her. Mrs. A. was helped to realize that making excuses was counterproductive. Finally, we mutually agreed that the word "can't" would not be used. We also agreed that her excuse-making behavior would be brought to her attention when it was observed. Eventually, Mrs. A. no longer exhibited the behavior.

Positive reinforcement was provided during weekly visits for any weight lost and for any of the coping strategies Mrs. A. used to manage her loneliness that week. Eventually, after about 4 months, satisfaction from the enjoyment of the coping strategies took over as a positive reinforcer for that behavior.

The behavior modification approach was effective. Mrs. A. began to exhibit slow, progressive weight loss. She purchased a scale. By the end of 3 months, she proudly displayed clothing that was one size too large for her. Verbally, she was saying that she would go all the way with the weight-loss program. Her own satisfaction with the progress she was making and her ability to manage this need to lose weight and maintain a 1200-calorie diabetic diet served as a sustaining reinforcer to maintain the behavior.

## SUMMARY

The above examples of nursing management of the therapeutic demands illustrate the importance of an individualized approach to patients. Nurses need to do a patient-specific assessment and plan nursing care accordingly. Each patient responds differently not only to illness, but to each therapeutic demand. Patients need to know not only what to do, but how they, as unique individuals, can go about making it fit their own life-styles and needs. In an age of standardized care plans, there is a danger of overlooking individualization. Without an individualized tailored approach, patients' needs for motivation and knowledge will be missed.

The repertoire of nursing interventions must be constantly expanded so that nursing agencies grow and nurses become more efficient at increasing the self-care agencies of patients. Patients need power to manage their own health-care deviations.

Nurses need to become more involved in making and recording observations about their care and in conducting research to test new approaches to the patient in order to truly expand the professional knowledge-base component of the nursing agency. Solutions must be sought to the problems inherent in the majority of health-care settings that inhibit the development of the nurse-patient relationship. Patients need a clearer line of access to nursing in order to better develop their self-care agencies.

Enabling strategies such as patient education, individualization of that education, and behavior therapy or modification techniques utilized within the context of a nursing framework are examples of approaches that are appropriate for enhancing self-care and alleviating powerlessness. These are specific means for developing the power components of knowledge and motivation.

# REFERENCES

1. Nursing Development Conference Group: *Concept Formalization in Nursing.* Little, Brown & Co., Boston, 1973, pp. 87-89.
2. Orem, D.: *Nursing: Concepts of Practice,* ed. 2. McGraw-Hill, New York, 1980, p. 41.
3. Hokanson, J.: *The Physiological Basis of Motivation.* John Wiley & Sons, New York, 1969, pp. 1-7.
4. Darwin, C.: *The Descent of Man.* Murray, London, 1872.
5. Valle, F.: *Motivation: Theories and Issues.* Brooks/Cole Publishing, Monterey, Calif., 1975, pp. 7-10.
6. Arkes, H. and Garske, J.: *Psychological Theories of Motivation.* Brooks/Cole Publishing, Monterey, Calif., 1977.
7. Watson, J. B.: *Behaviorism.* W. W. Norton & Co., New York, 1970, pp. 1-20.
8. Maslow, A. H.: *Motivation and Personality.* Harper & Row, New York, 1954.
9. Rogers, C.: *A theory of therapy, personality and interpersonal relationships as developed in the client-centered framework.* In Koch, S. (ed.): *Psychology: A Study of a Science, Formulations of the Person in the Social Context.* McGraw-Hill, New York, 1959.
10. Marston, M. V.: *Compliance with medical regimens: A review of the literature.* Nurs. Res. 19:317, July-August 1970.
11. Davis, M. S.: *Physiological, psychological, and demographic factors in patient compliance with doctor's orders.* Med. Care 6:121, March-April 1968.
12. Kegeles, S. S.: *Why people seek dental care: A test of conceptual formulation.* J. Health Hum. Behav. 4:168, 1963.
13. Johannsen, W. J., Helmuth, G. A., and Sorauf, T.: *On accepting medical recommendations; experiences with patients in a cardiac work classification unit.* Arch. Environ. Health 12:63, 1966.
14. Rossman, J. (ed.): *Compliance: What Can Be Learned from the Patient's Point of View?* Cooper Laboratories, Wayne, N.J., 1977.
15. Stimson, G. V.: *Obeying doctor's orders: A view from the other side.* Soc. Sci. Med. 8:101, 1974.
16. Becker, M. H. and Green, L. W.: *A family approach to compliance with medical treatment.* Int. J. Health Educ. 18:178, 1975.
17. Vincent, P.: *Factors influencing patient noncompliance: A theoretical approach.* Nurs. Res. 20:511, November-December 1971.
18. Rosenstock, I. M.: *Patient compliance with health regimens.* J.A.M.A. 234:402, 1975.
19. Frances, V., Korsch, B. M., and Morris, M. J.: *Gaps in doctor-patient communication: Patient's response to medical advice.* N. Engl. J. Med. 280:535, 1969.
20. Davis, M. S. and Eichhorn, R. L.: *Compliance with medical regimens: A panel study.* J. Health Hum. Behav. 4:249, 1963.
21. Willis, F. N. and Dunsmore, N. M.: *Work orientation, health attitudes, and compliance.* Nurs. Res. 16:22, March 1967.
22. Becker, M. H. and Maiman, L. A.: *Sociobehavioral determinants of compliance with health and medical care recommendations.* Med. Care 13:20, 1975.
23. Becker, M. H.: *The Health Belief Model and Personal Health Behavior.* Charles B. Slack, Thorofare, N.J., 1974.
24. Bautista, D. E. H.: *Modifying the treatment: Patient compliance, patient control, and medical care.* Soc. Sci. Med. 10:237, 1976.
25. Fink, D.: *Tailoring the consensual regimen.* In Sackett, D. L. and Haynes, R. B. (eds.): *Compliance with Therapeutic Regimens.* Johns Hopkins University Press, Baltimore, 1976, pp. 110-118.
26. Davis, M.S.: *Variations in patients' compliance with doctors' advice: An empirical analysis of patterns of communication.* Am. J. Public Health 58:277, 1968.
27. Pfister, K.: *Factors and nursing strategies which influence a patient's inclination to follow health care advice: A case study approach.* Master's thesis, Marquette University, 1978.

28. Lowe, M. L.: *Effectiveness of teaching as measured by compliance with medical recommendations.* Nurs. Res. 19:59, January-February 1970.
29. Lindeman, C. A. and Van Aernam, B.: *Nursing intervention with the presurgical patient: The effects of structured and unstructured preoperative teaching.* Nurs. Res. 20:196, July-August 1971.
30. Bowen, R. G., Rich, R., and Schlotfeldt, R.: *Effects of organized instruction for patients with the diagnosis of diabetes mellitus.* Nurs. Res. 10:151, Summer 1961.
31. Williams, T. F., et al.: *The clinical picture of diabetes control, studied in four settings.* Am. J. Public Health 57:441, 1967.
32. Riley, C. S.: *Patients' understanding of doctors' instructions.* Med. Care 4:34, 1966.
33. Bille, D. A.: *The role of body image in patient compliance and education.* Heart Lung 6:143, 1977.
34. McClosky, J.: *How to make the most of body image theory and nursing practice.* Nursing76 6:68, May 1976.
35. Rubin, R.: *Body image and self esteem.* Nurs. Outlook 16:20, June 1968.
36. Combs, A. W., Avila, D. L., and Purkey, W.W.: *Helping Relationships: Basic Concepts for the Helping Professions.* Allyn & Bacon, Boston, 1971, p. 42.
37. Coogan, J. (ed.): *Human problems in motivating the unmotivated patient.* Nursing74 4:31, February 1974.
38. Swain, M. A. and Steckel, S.: *Influencing adherence among hypertensives.* Research in Nursing and Health 4:213, March 1981.
39. Wolpe, J. and Lazarus, A. A.: *Behavior Therapy Techniques: A Guide to the Treatment of Neuroses.* Pergamon Press, New York, 1966.
40. Stuart, R. B.: *Behavioral control of overeating.* Behav. Res. Ther. 5:357, 1967.
41. Zifferblatt, S. M.: *Increasing patient compliance through the applied analysis of behavior.* Prev. Med. 4:173, 1975.

# SELECTED READINGS

Ball, W. L.: *Improving patient compliance with therapeutic regimens: Hamilton symposium examines the problems and solutions.* Can. Med. Assoc. J. 111:268, 1974.
Benson, H.: *The Relaxation Response.* Avon Books, New York, 1975.
Benson, H., et al.: *Historical and clinical considerations of the relaxation response.* Am. Sci. 65:441, 1977.
Berkowitz, N. H., et al.: *Patient follow-through in the outpatient department.* Nurs. Res. 12:16, Winter 1963.
Berni, R. and Fordyce, W. E.: *Behavior Modification and the Nursing Process.* C. V. Mosby, St. Louis, 1973.
Bille, D.: *Practical Approaches to Patient Teaching.* Little, Brown & Co., Boston, 1981.
Caldwell, J. R., et al.: *The drop-out problem in antihypertensive treatment.* J. Chronic Dis. 22:572, 1970.
Cofer, C. N. and Appley, M. H.: *Motivation: Theory and Research.* John Wiley & Sons, New York, 1964.
Davis, M. S.: *Predicting noncompliant behavior.* J. Health Soc. Behav. 8:265, 1967.
Donabedian, A. and Rosenfeld, L. S.: *Follow-up study of chronically ill patients discharged from hospital.* J. Chronic Dis. 17:847, 1964.
Franks, C. M. and Wilson, G. T. (eds.): *Annual Review of Behavior Therapy: Theory and Practice, Vol. 4: 1976.* Brunner/Mazel, New York, 1976.
Freud, S.: *Beyond the Pleasure Principle.* Hogarth Press, London, 1948.
Green, L., et al.: *Health Education Planning: A Diagnostic Approach.* Mayfield Publishing, Palo Alto, Calif., 1980.
Gillum, R. F. and Barsky, A. J.: *Diagnosis and management of patient noncompliance.* J.A.M.A. 228:1563, 1974.
Goldfried, M. R. and Merbaum, M. (eds.): *Behavior Change through Self-Control.* Holt, Rinehart & Winston, New York, 1973.
Haber, R. N. (ed.): *Current Research in Motivation.* Holt, Rinehart & Winston, New York, 1976.

Hecht, A. B.: *Improving medication compliance by teaching outpatients.* Nurs. Forum 13:112, November 1974.

Kalisch, B. J.: *Of half gods and mortals: Aesculapian authority.* Nurs. Outlook 23:22, January 1976.

Kubler-Ross, E.: *On Death and Dying.* Macmillan, New York, 1969.

Lindzey, G.: *Assessment of Human Motives.* Rinehart & Co., New York, 1958.

Lowery, B. J. and DuCette, J. P.: *Disease-related learning and disease control as a function of locus of control.* Nurs. Res. 25:358, September-October 1976.

Meichenbaum, D.: *Cognitive-Behavior Modification: An Integrative Approach.* Plenum Press, New York, 1978.

Preston, D. F. and Miller, F. L.: *The tuberculosis outpatient's defection from therapy.* Am. J. Med. Sci. 247:21, 1974.

Sackett, D. L. and Haynes, R. B. (eds.): *Compliance with Therapeutic Regimens.* Johns Hopkins University Press, Baltimore, 1976.

Sackett, D. L., et al.: *Randomized clinical trial of strategies for improving medication compliance in primary hypertension.* Lancet 1:1205, 1975.

Stunkard, A. J.: *New therapies for eating disorders: Behavior modification of obesity and anorexia nervosa.* Arch. Gen. Psychiatry 26:391, 1972.

Weintraub, M.: *The role of industrial nurses in improving patients' adherence to therapeutic plans.* Occup. Health Nurs. 23:16, May 1975.

# 14

# DECREASING POWERLESSNESS IN THE CHRONICALLY ILL: A PROTOTYPE

## SUSAN STAPLETON

Powerlessness is a prevalent nursing diagnosis in chronically ill patients. Permitted to continue unchecked, powerlessness can have physically and mentally detrimental effects on the individual. As has been noted in previous chapters, prolonged powerlessness leads to anxiety, depression, and hopelessness. Eventually, this state may hasten physiologic deterioration and death. Therefore, alleviation of powerlessness is an important nursing goal. General categories of nursing strategies to decrease powerlessness will be discussed in this chapter, as will specific nursing measures based on the unique situation of patients with chronic renal failure (CRF). Although the strategies are related to specific factors causing powerlessness in patients with CRF, the strategy categories are general and can be used for all chronically ill patients experiencing powerlessness.

The categories of nursing strategies aimed at decreasing powerlessness include (1) modifying the environment, (2) helping the patient set realistic goals and expectations, (3) increasing the patient's knowledge; (4) increasing the sensitivity of health-team members and significant others to the imposed powerlessness, and (5) encouraging verbalization of feelings. These five general strategies provide guidance in developing specific measures to decrease powerlessness in the chronically ill individual.

# NURSING STRATEGIES

## Modifying the Environment

Chronically ill individuals can modify the environment as a means of increasing control. These measures may include simple routines taken for granted, such as having the call light and telephone within reach, arranging the environment of the hospital room for the patient's convenience, participating in decisions such as whether or not to have a roommate who smokes, and having the security of some privacy.

Other control measures relate to patients' feelings of deference and inferiority in communicating with physicians and other health-care workers. Specific measures to increase patients' security and comfort when relating to physicians decrease powerlessness. The nurse may emphasize to patients that their needs are the first priority of the health team. Reviewing with patients their medical concerns before the physician visit is helpful in assisting patients to prioritize and formulate their questions and receive needed reassurance. Nurses can interpret esoteric language for patients. Although partnership in medical-care decisions may not be accomplished, patients should not feel inferior, be unable to verbalize concerns, or be completely uninvolved in decisions made about their health.

In implementing specific measures to enhance patient control, the nurse may need to reiterate, "You do have control," and to review specific examples of that control.

Identifying situations that cause feelings of powerlessness and recognizing these feelings in oneself are examples of other control measures. If the patient realizes that long waits in an impersonal outpatient department precipitate feelings of powerlessness, substitute activities can take place during this waiting time. The patient can become resigned to the fact that the visit will take no less than $2^{1/2}$ hours and so during that time can accomplish other goals, for example, balancing the checkbook, reading a book or daily paper, writing letters, or organizing the meal plan for the week. Being sensitive to the factors causing powerlessness enables the patient to prepare for the situation. The nurse should keep the waiting patient informed as to the approximate waiting time remaining and reasons for the delay. Somehow, these courtesies are easily overlooked in institutional settings.

Mr. C. identified two aspects of his visits to the outpatient department that caused him to feel powerless. They were (1) the long wait before seeing the physician and (2) the physician's failure to supply him with all the information he wanted about his health and treatment plan. The author suggested meeting Mr. C. in the clinic waiting room before each appointment and using the time to help him write down a list of specific questions for the physician. Mr. C. was told to take the list from his pocket while talking with the physician and check off each question after it had been answered to his satisfaction. The effectiveness of this strategy in decreasing Mr. C.'s powerlessness was seen in several ways. He exhibited less anxiety during his clinic visits, as evidenced by a decrease in such motor activity as pacing, drumming his fingers, and looking at his watch. He also began to speak more positively of upcoming clinic visits, instead of dreading them. He expressed a sense of satisfaction that he had exercised some control during the visits and obtained the information he wanted. Mr. C. stated,

"Now I feel more like I have something to say about what happens to me, instead of just waiting for them to do something to me."

## Setting Realistic Goals

Individuals who can set realistic goals feel less powerless as the goals are achieved.[1] Chronically ill individuals often need assistance in setting realistic goals and in rehearsing possible outcomes. Depression and feelings of hopelessness may inhibit patients from setting goals at all. Lack of information about illness or use of denial as a coping mechanism may lead patients to set goals they are unable to achieve. Never achieving the goals reinforces powerlessness.

Patients should be given the opportunity to participate in their total plan of care by mutually identifying goals with the nurse, validating assessment of self-care skills, and confirming with the nurse that they do have unique strengths that empower them to assume responsibility to achieve desired outcomes.

Laborde and Powers[2] compared 20 patients with osteoarthritis and 20 patients undergoing hemodialysis on their ratings of past, present, and future life satisfaction using the Cantril Self-Anchoring Life Satisfaction Scale. No differences were found on past and future ratings; however, the patients on dialysis had significantly higher present life satisfaction scores (at the 0.05 level). Considering the extensive body-system involvement with multiple symptoms in chronic renal failure, this finding is surprising. The dialysis procedure provides a predictable outcome of temporary alleviation of symptoms. Patients on dialysis may have been helped to set realistic expectations of dialysis as an extension of life and a provider of temporary relief of symptoms. For some patients on dialysis, the relief of symptoms gave them a "new lease on life" compared with predialysis states. The pain experienced by patients with arthritis so interfered with present quality of life that their scores were significantly lower than those of the patients on dialysis. Nurses can use specific verbal reinforcers with the patient on dialysis to decrease powerlessness, such as "The dialysis will control symptoms by restoring fluid and electrolyte balance, eliminate wastes, and so forth." Careful explanation of the desired therapeutic effects of the medical regimen, which helps the patient have realistic expectations from the treatment, will enhance control.

The following is an example of helping the individual develop pacing behaviors to cope with the fatigue of CRF. Mrs. A. expressed feelings of powerlessness from fatigue that interfered with her ability to do her housework. She was asked to keep a list of her activities and required rest periods for a week. At the same time, Mrs. A. made a list of the things she wanted to do in order of their priority to her. Using these lists, Mrs. A. was assisted in evaluating her tolerance of specific activities and planning her activities according to her energy level. For example, she discovered that she could perform only one major task, such as grocery shopping or vacuuming, a day. She planned her weekly schedule so that these especially tiring tasks were done, one a day, on the days after dialysis, when her energy level was highest. This was a more realistic goal than trying to do several major tasks in one day, and Mrs. A.'s feeling of powerlessness decreased when she was able to reach this goal. At the same time, Mr. A. suggested that his wife plan her arrival from the grocery store to coincide with his arrival home from work so that he could carry the bags of groceries into the house. This decreased her energy expenditure so that she was still able to participate in family activities that evening. The list of activities according to priority also enabled her to determine which activities she could delegate to other family members, or eliminate completely, without damaging her self-esteem.

## Increasing Knowledge

As noted in Chapter 13, knowledge is a power resource. Control in a given situation increases with increasing knowledge about the situation. When individuals experience powerlessness, they may subsequently fail to seek information about their situations, further increasing feelings of powerlessness. Chronically ill individuals need knowledge about their illness and its management so that they can make decisions and take actions relative to the illness. This ability to make decisions and act on them gives individuals some control over what happens to them, thereby decreasing powerlessness. Being informed of physiologic changes,[3] positive responses to therapy, and expected results from therapy increases the perception of control. Nurses need to assume major responsibility for increasing patients' knowledge.

The value of providing knowledge about a situation in the reduction of powerlessness can be noted in Mr. C. When Mr. C.'s renal function deteriorated to the extent that the institution of dialysis was imminent, he began to express feelings of powerlessness about the arrangements for dialysis. He had expressed an interest in home dialysis, but the social worker, after discussing it with Mrs. C., told him, "That's not for you." Mr. C. felt that choices were being made without consulting him. A strategy for reducing this feeling of powerlessness involved providing him with information about the various dialysis alternatives: in-center, home, and in-center self-care dialysis. Mr. C. was given specific information about each type, with advantages and disadvantages of each. Mrs. C. was also involved in these discussions, as she would play an active role in the latter two types of dialysis. Mr. and Mrs. C. were helped to examine what each of the choices would mean to their lives and to discuss their individual feelings about each choice. Mr. C. came to the same decision reached by the social worker, that in-center dialysis was the best choice for him. An important distinction, however, was that now he felt the decision was his, and not one made for him by someone else. His feelings of powerlessness were decreased by providing him with information needed to make a decision about what would happen to him.

## Increasing Health Teams' and Significant Others' Sensitivity to Imposed Powerlessness

Factors within the health-care system itself are often the most significant causes of powerlessness in the chronically ill. These include unexplained delays and waiting in various hospital departments (x-ray); brisk, insensitive verbal interaction by admitting clerks or outpatient receptionists; and the sterile environment of a hospital with clearly identified boundaries (nurses' station is off limits for patients; patients cannot review their records without obtaining special permissions as established by hospital policy). Health-care professionals need to develop sensitivity to these and other causes of powerlessness. Efforts need to be made to be humanistic and to avoid depersonalizing patients.

Role playing is a valuable strategy for sensitizing health-care workers to factors in the environment that contribute to the patient's powerlessness. The more realistic the role playing the better. Placing health-care workers in a situation in which they experience an actual loss of control, and then providing the opportunity to share their feelings, can provide excellent insights into the concept of powerlessness. Role playing can be a part of planned staff conferences. A focus of the conference could be a discussion of the factors causing powerlessness (Chapter 7) and specifically how personnel can cause powerlessness. Strategies to alleviate powerlessness for specific patients could be devised in this group setting.

Health-care workers may need to review principles of therapeutic communication in addition to simply remembering to introduce themselves to the patient. Personnel need to wear name tags on which their titles and hospital departments are clearly indicated.

In order for patients to monitor physiologic progress, having access to the dialysis record on which weight, vital signs, and laboratory values are recorded is important. Some patients achieve control by keeping detailed records and graphs of blood chemistry values. By noting a controlled creatinine level and having a visual representation of the creatinine level over time on a graph, the patient realizes that no physiologic deterioration is occurring. This is a positive feedback mechanism for the patient to continue to engage in the present therapeutic plan as well as a sign of physiologic control. Teaching the patient the significance of the laboratory values must be included in this control strategy.

Those other than health-care personnel who work with the chronically ill individual can influence the amount of perceived control the ill individual has. Increasing the sensitivity of persons at home, at work, and in social settings is important to decreasing powerlessness in the patient.

Dimond[4] found a positive correlation between the hemodialysis patients' morale and the presence of social support (family environment, spouse support, and the presence of a confidant). A negative correlation was found between the family cohesion (one aspect of family environment), presence of a confidant, and the amount of change in social functioning in adjusting to the chronic illness. Social changes since beginning dialysis were less if the patient had family cohesiveness and a confidant available.[4] The nurse can work with families to help them realize how significantly they can influence adaptation and control in their ill family member. The greater the family cohesiveness and open expression, the higher the patient's morale and the fewer the medical problems that occurred.[4] Nurses can help families improve communication, increase expressions and types of support, and demonstrate caring and affection. Nurses can also devise specific mechanisms the family can use to increase the patient's perceived and/or actual control. Decisions can be referred to the patient; family can encourage the patient's resumption of family maintenance tasks, such as paying the bills. The task of planning for maximal use of leisure time and family "togetherness" activities can be assumed by the ill family member (in this case the patient on dialysis).

# Verbalization of Feelings

When the chronically ill individual is able to verbalize feelings of powerlessness, a basis for beginning problem solving to increase feelings of control is established. The patient may be able to identify factors contributing to the present state and pose alternate solutions. Through discussion, feedback is solicited from the nurse. The verbalization is a sharing of feelings and provides the nurse an opportunity to demonstrate understanding.

Open admission of feeling powerless may be too threatening to some individuals for whom control is extremely important. These patients frequently deny any feelings of powerlessness and report that they feel very much in control. Direct confrontation regarding powerlessness can increase anxiety in these patients. On the other hand, when powerlessness is due to deteriorating health that cannot be controlled, discussing these feelings enables the nurse to share them, lessening the patient's burden. When patients hear their feelings verbalized, the distortion that occurs through mental rumination about the situation is controlled. In other words, feelings and concerns may be put into perspective. Reactions from others and empathy are solicited and alternate solutions to problems are generated as a result of verbalization.

An example of a situation in which verbalizing feelings of powerlessness seemed to help decrease these feelings is that of Mr. F. His illness and the resulting financial problems forced Mrs. F. to apply for public assistance while Mr. F. was still hospitalized. She was treated rudely at the welfare office and was quite upset by her experience there. Mr. F. was extremely angry and expressed frustration regarding his powerlessness, "I'm stuck here and can't even help her! I feel like going down there and punching someone!" The strategy of encouraging him to express his feelings, not responding negatively to or denying his anger, was very effective in decreasing his feelings of powerlessness. He was visibly less agitated and stated, "It's good to get it all out." He also indicated that he felt less helpless, although the actual situation had not changed.

# Developing a Plan to Decrease Powerlessness

In using these strategies to decrease powerlessness in the chronically ill individual, the nurse must carefully develop strategies specific for each individual. The first steps are to recognize patient indicators of powerlessness and identify the factor(s) causing powerlessness (see Chapter 7). Then, specific strategies can be developed to decrease powerlessness. These strategies will fall within one or more of the five categories already discussed but must be very specific if they are to provide adequate guidance for those working with the patient. Finally, criteria for evaluation of the strategies must be identified. The criteria are specific patient behaviors that can be expected to occur if the strategies are effective.

The care plan in Table 14-1 contains examples of strategies used in working with individuals with CRF who were experiencing powerlessness. Some dealt with situations that occurred once, whereas others dealt with broader, recurring factors that caused powerlessness. The stressors or factors causing powerlessness in CRF patients discussed in Chapter 7 provide the basis for the plan. The types of factors promoting

**TABLE 14-1. Plan of Care to Alleviate Powerlessness in Patients with Chronic Renal Failure**

| Situation or factor causing powerlessness | Patient indicators of powerlessness | Strategies to decrease powerlessness | Criteria for evaluation |
|---|---|---|---|
| **PATIENT-STAFF RELATIONSHIPS** Appointments in outpatient department: a. Long waits before seeing physician. b. Difficulty in obtaining desired information from physician. | 1. Verbalizing the feeling that cannot control when patient sees physician and that patient's time is not seen as important. 2. States, "The doctor never tells me anything. I can't get him to answer my questions." | 1. Meet patient in clinic waiting room before each appointment. 2. Help patient to formulate a list of specific questions for the physician for that visit. 3. If necessary, see physician with the patient to assist patient in asking questions. 4. Suggest that patient take the list of questions out of pocket and refer to it while talking with the physician. | 1. States that patient feels the time in waiting room is spent productively. 2. Appears calm while waiting: no pacing, tapping fingers, picking at nails. 3. Makes list of questions and uses list while talking with physician. 4. Verbalizes satisfaction with the amount of information received from the physician about illness and treatment. |
| Enforced dependence during dialysis and dependence on dialysis staff and machine for life. Health-care personnel have a much greater knowledge about CRF and its management than patient. | 1. Expresses fear that some dialysis staff members are less competent than others and that patient cannot judge them. 2. Jokes that patient wants a screwdriver "so I can take the machine apart if I want to and stay in control." | 1. Provide organized, individualized teaching program that includes the following content: normal kidney function, basic CRF pathophysiology, laboratory values and their significance, purpose of dialysis, dialysis procedure, diet, medications. 2. Explain and demonstrate alarm system on machines. 3. Arrange for patient to meet some of the other patients to discuss dialysis from patients' point of view. | 1. Correctly explains dialysis to someone else in simple terms. 2. Remains calm when alarm on machine goes off. 3. Demonstrates confidence in dialysis staff. 4. Asks questions when patient does not know something about CRF and its management. |

**TABLE 14-1. Continued**

| Situation or factor causing powerlessness | Patient indicators of powerlessness | Strategies to decrease powerlessness | Criteria for evaluation |
|---|---|---|---|
| Staff expression of anger toward the patient; patient unable to show anger in return. | 3. Expresses the feeling that patient is at the "mercy" of the dialysis machine and staff. <br> 4. Refers to dialysis machine as "the monster." <br> 5. States that patient can't get angry at the staff because "I can't get along without them." | 4. Arrange for patient to observe the start and ending of dialysis on another patient (movie or in person) before beginning dialysis. <br> 5. As dialysis is started, explain each step and reinforce prior teaching. Continue to provide opportunities for questions as they occur to patient and family. <br> 6. Utilize primary nursing or assign patient to the same one or two people for the first few weeks. <br> 7. Give patient a screwdriver on the day dialysis starts. <br> 8. Keep patient informed of progress during dialysis—weight, lab values, blood pressure—and explain their significance. <br> 9. Encourage patient participation in dialysis as patient is ready—holding tubings, applying pressure to puncture sites, taking pulse. <br> 10. Give patient as much responsibility as patient is ready for—bringing any medications to be taken while on dialysis, arranging own transportation (including driving self), explaining dialysis to own family or new patients. <br> 11. Encourage patient to keep own record of blood pressure and pre- and post-dialysis weight. | 5. States present weight and range of blood pressure. <br> 6. Asks for weight, blood pressure, and lab values if this information is not volunteered by staff. <br> 7 Assists with some aspects of dialysis. <br> 8. Freely expresses anger toward staff when appropriate and in an appropriate way. |

12. Encourage verbalization of feelings about dialysis machine and staff and patient's dependence on them.
13. Allow for joking or expression of anger during dialysis as a means of maintaining some control.
14. Avoid ignoring patient's expressions of anger or responding with anger in return. Use accepting manner.
15. Avoid comments by staff, even joking ones, that emphasize the control staff has over patient during dialysis.

Physician tells patient that patient will be transferred to a different dialysis center without asking patient's approval.

1. Verbalizes feelings of not having control over where patient will go for dialysis.
2. Does not tell physician that the planned dialysis center is very inconvenient for patient.

1. Assist patient in weighing the pros and cons of each center.
2. Serve as a liaison in planning a visit to the other center to meet the staff and discuss routines.
3. Support the patient in decision to agree or disagree with the physician's decision.
4. Serve as patient advocate, if needed, in explaining patient's decision to physician.

1. States the advantages and disadvantages of each center for patient.
2. Visits the other dialysis center and asks questions there to obtain the information needed to make a decision about the two centers.
3. Questions the physician as to the rationale for switching to the other center.
4. Determines, on the basis of all the above information, which dialysis center is best for patient.
5. Discusses the decision with the physician, explaining the reasons for choice.

**TABLE 14-1.** *Continued*

| Situation or factor causing powerlessness | Patient indicators of powerlessness | Strategies to decrease powerlessness | Criteria for evaluation |
|---|---|---|---|
| Patient severely reprimanded because patient gained too much weight between dialysis runs. | Accepts reprimand and anger from staff without comment—hangs head and looks at floor.<br><br>Later remarks to me that "they're always yelling at me, but I can't afford to yell back."<br><br>When told to weigh self daily at home, did not inform staff that patient has no scale.<br><br>States, "I try to follow my diet and not drink too much, but I'm always so thirsty. I just can't help myself." | 1. State amount of weight gain in a matter-of-fact, nonscolding manner.<br>2. Explore with patient possible reasons for excess weight gain.<br>3. Ask patient to keep a list of everything eaten and drunk for 1 week—including time of day, amounts, what patient was doing at the time, and how patient felt at the time.<br>4. Explore with patient the meaning of food and drink to patient.<br>5. Assist patient to identify own eating and drinking patterns.<br>6. Teach basic pathophysiology of CRF and the physiologic effects of excess fluid retention if patient does not already know this.<br>7. Suggest that patient weigh self daily at home, keep record of weights and bring this to dialysis. Help patient get scale.<br>8. Assist patient to correlate weight changes with food and fluid intake.<br>9. Assist patient to identify how patient feels when patient has excess fluid retention.<br>10. Work with patient, dietitian, and physician to develop diet pattern that is most acceptable to patient, considering previous patterns, and meets the criteria of the medical treatment plan. | 1. Explains, in simple terms, basic CRF pathophysiology and the effects of fluid retention on the body.<br>2. Identifies various reasons for eating and drinking patterns: hunger, thirst, tension, boredom.<br>3. Verbalizes what food and drink mean to self and own feelings about food and fluid restrictions.<br>4. Keeps record of daily weights and brings to dialysis.<br>5. Correlates changes in weight with food and fluid intake.<br>6. Identifies how patient feels when has excess fluid retention.<br>7. Actively participates in development of a diet pattern.<br>8. Reports that new diet pattern is more acceptable and that patient has more success in complying with it. |

9. Practices, on a regular basis, some type of relaxation technique.

1. Looks at shunt.
2. Asks questions when patient does not know some aspect of the care of the shunt.
3. Correctly teaches shunt care to significant other.
4. Correctly describes actions to be taken if shunt comes apart and teaches this to significant other.
5. Reports that patient is able to cope with stares and questions of others about the shunt.

11. If patient eats or drinks in response to stimuli other than hunger or thirst (e.g., tension or boredom), teach other methods of coping with these feelings (e.g., relaxation techniques, self-hypnosis, physical activities).

1. Assess patient's stage in the grieving process and in adaptation to an altered body image.
2. Explore with patient the meaning of the shunt to self.
3. Observe for verbal and behavioral clues that patient is ready to learn shunt care—looking at shunt, asking questions, watching while care is done.
4. Follow this sequence to develop self-care: Explain care as done, patient assists with care, patient describes procedure verbally, patient performs care with help, patient performs care with observation by nurse, patient takes full responsibility for care.
5. Assist patient in explaining procedure to significant other—especially what to do if shunt comes apart.
6. Encourage patient to verbalize feelings and fears regarding shunt and its care.
7. Discuss ways of covering the shunt.
8. Role play with patient the explanation of the shunt to a friend.
9. Role play dealing with questions from a curious stranger.

DISEASE PROCESS
Patient expected to take care of her A-V shunt before patient felt ready.

1. Cries and states, "I don't want to do this," while shunt care is done, but does not refuse to do it if staff insists.
2. Asks no questions about shunt.

**TABLE 14-1.** *Continued*

| Situation or factor causing powerlessness | Patient indicators of powerlessness | Strategies to decrease powerlessness | Criteria for evaluation |
|---|---|---|---|
| Irritability from the central nervous system manifestations of azotemia.<br><br>Feels weak and tired constantly; must take frequent naps.<br><br>Cannot plan activities because of uncertainty of symptoms.<br><br>Cannot see printed instructions on diet, kidney disease, dialysis. | 1. States that patient cannot control moods as easily as before illness.<br>2. Expresses guilt about irritability with family.<br>3. Says, "I'm always tired, I can't get anything done."<br>4. Reports decrease in social activities, never being able to plan ahead.<br>5. States, "How can I help myself, I cannot even see the instructions?" | 1. Discuss the etiology of the irritability with patient and significant others.<br>2. Explore with patient effective ways of dealing with anger and depression without damaging relationships with family members.<br>3. Allow for verbalization of feelings of guilt about irritability.<br>4. Teach specific activities to relieve tension and help deal with stress.<br>5. Support family members in understanding and dealing with patient's mood changes.<br>6. Assist family members in identifying sources and effects of stress on each of them, and explore ways of meeting the needs of each family member.<br>7. Plan for balancing energy expenditure with energy conservation.<br>8. Set priorities; engage in activities that confirm self-worth, and have the highest value for the patient.<br>9. Provide with large print, magnifying glass, and verbal reinforcement of instructions. | 1. Correctly explains, in simple terms, the physiologic basis for the irritability.<br>2. Practices some form of relaxation technique on a regular basis.<br>3. Significant others explain physiologic basis for patient's irritability.<br>4. Significant others describe ways in which they provide for meeting their own needs.<br>5. Adheres to specific sleep-rest pattern throughout the day.<br>6. Verbalizes understanding; asks appropriate questions. |

| | | | |
|---|---|---|---|
| Inability to predict or control the outcome of renal transplantation. | 1. States, "I guess you just have to get used to the idea that you really don't have much control over how the surgery turns out." <br> 2. Does not ask questions about present health state. <br> 3. States, "It's not fair—I did everything I was told and I still rejected the kidney." | 1. Provide patient with as much data as possible about patient's level of physiologic control (lab values, weight, vital signs, results of diagnostic tests). <br> 2. Allow patient to verbalize feelings about lack of control of the outcome of the surgery. <br> 3. Explore with patient the meaning of the kidney transplant to self. <br> 4. Assist patient in recognizing and dealing with any incongruences between expectations and the actual results of surgery. | 1. Demonstrates an interest in present health state by asking for information such as test results, urine output, vital signs, weight. <br> 2. Verbalizes realistic expectations about how the transplant will affect own life. <br> 3. Indicates that patient is coping satisfactorily with the possibility of rejection and the uncertainty of prognosis. <br> 4. Expresses a sense of hope in relation to the prognosis. |
| FAMILY RELATIONSHIPS <br> Decreased ability to participate in social activities with family and friends. <br> Missed part of family activities while on vacation because of dialysis. | 1. Expresses guilt and regret that patient cannot participate in activities with family: "I used to skate with my daughters, but now I'm a real dud—all I can do is sit." | 1. Ask patient to make a list of previous activities and their importance to patient. <br> 2. Assist patient in setting priorities regarding those activities that patient would most like to continue. <br> 3. Explore with patient the meaning to self of participation in family activities. | 1. Lists activities in which patient wishes to participate according to priority. <br> 2. Identifies which activities are most important to patient and why they are important. |

**TABLE 14-1.** *Continued*

| Situation or factor causing powerlessness | Patient indicators of powerlessness | Strategies to decrease powerlessness | Criteria for evaluation |
|---|---|---|---|
| Spouse repeatedly reminds patient to rest and not to do any strenuous activities. Role reversal—spouse takes over many of the patient's roles: paying bills, shopping, yard work. | 2. "I was stuck with that machine while they were out sightseeing. Then after I'd finished, they'd already seen everything and didn't want to go back." 3. States, "Sometimes I feel like doing something, but she gets upset, so it's easier just to do nothing." | 4. Assist patient and family in realistically evaluating the patient's abilities and limitations. 5. Encourage spouse to avoid unnecessarily restricting patient's activities. 6. Explore with spouse feelings and fears that cause spouse to "shelter" the patient. 7. Assist patient in developing new interests and/or modifying previous activities according to present abilities and limitations. 8. Assist patient and family in developing new ways of interacting that are compatible with the patient's limitations. 9. Encourage family members to continue their own activities and interests as much as possible, and allow for the expression of any guilt that may be associated with these activities. 10. Provide family members with a safe outlet for the expression of any anger which might be felt toward the patient. | 3. Realistically identifies own abilities and limitations. 4. Uses the above information to decide which activities will be continued. 5. Significant others realistically identify patient's abilities and limitations and encourage patient to continue activities patient can tolerate. 6. Modifies activities as necessary to accommodate any changes in health. 7. Significant others continue with some activities that meet their own needs, even if patient is unable to participate. 8. Expresses the feeling that patient is coping satisfactorily with any changes in activities and roles required by illness. |

11. Allow for the expression of any feelings of anger or resentment the patient may have toward family members as they continue with activities in which patient cannot participate.
12. Encourage verbalization about feelings related to role reversal; determine significance of previous role expectations.

## EMPLOYMENT
Effect of dialysis on ability to retain job. Effect of CRF symptoms on job performance. Inability to work requires family to apply for public assistance.

1. Verbalizes fear that patient will be unable to continue working after starting dialysis.
2. Doesn't like job, but also fears loss of job; states, "I'm stuck here. I can never get another job with my age and kidney disease. I'm lucky to even have this one, but sometimes I feel like I'm trapped."
3. Feels that job performance has decreased. States, "I'm losing my creativity. I feel thick-headed. I forget things all the time."

1. Provide patient with specific information about dialysis: number of times a week, number of hours for each dialysis run, tentative day and time.
2. Assist patient in making plans with employer for when dialysis starts.
3. Explore meaning of job with patient and encourage verbalization of fears about being unable to continue working.
4. Ask if patient would like nurse to talk with personnel at company (supervisor or company nurse) to communicate information about dialysis schedule, symptoms of CRF, patient's health-care needs, patient's concern about retaining job.
5. Support the patient in obtaining feedback from employer about his job performance, e.g., role play how patient will approach supervisor, suggest that patient do own evaluation first.

1. Makes specific plans with employer about fitting dialysis into work schedule.
2. Indicates that patient feels a decrease in anxiety level about continuing to work after starting dialysis.
3. Identifies why job is important to self.
4. Discusses job performance with supervisor and obtains feedback as to own performance.
5. Begins to consider alternative ways of meeting needs now met by job in the event that patient is unable to continue working.

**TABLE 14-1.** *Continued*

| Situation or factor causing powerlessness | Patient indicators of powerlessness | Strategies to decrease powerlessness | Criteria for evaluation |
|---|---|---|---|
| | 4. Has made no effort to plan for dialysis with employer, even though this is a source of great anxiety for patient. | 6. Explore with patient the effects of being unemployed on self-esteem.<br>7. Allow patient to verbalize feelings regarding inability to support his family.<br>8. Allow patient and family to verbalize feelings about receiving public assistance.<br>9. Explore with patient and significant others alternate ways of enhancing patient's self-esteem (other than functioning as breadwinner in the family).<br>10. Assist patient in identifying own strengths and provide positive reinforcement to enhance self-esteem. | 6. Identifies the effects that being unemployed have had on self-esteem.<br>7. Explores alternative ways of enhancing self-esteem—what patient can do to feel better about himself. |

**TABLE 14-2. Empowerment Strategies**

Patient education
Individual approach to the patient and patient teaching
   Assessment of and emphasis on each person's uniqueness
   Emphasis on self-care assets and personal strengths
   Setting realistic goals
Behavior modification
Environment modification
   Removal of barriers to patient control
Involvement of significant others
   Sensitizing them to importance of their reactions
   Helping them devise means of permitting patient control
Facilitate verbalization of feelings

powerlessness included in the care plan are patient-staff relationships, disease process, family relationships, and employment. Although the strategies on the care plan are specific to the patient's situation or specific precipitant of powerlessness, the types of strategies used can be classified as (1) modifying the environment, (2) helping the patient set realistic goals, (3) increasing the patient's knowledge, (4) increasing the sensitivity of health-team members and significant others to the imposed powerlessness, and (5) encouraging verbalization of feelings.

The nursing strategies to decrease powerlessness provided in the care plan include strategies to modify the environment, help the patient set realistic goals, increase patient knowledge, increase significant others' sensitivity to the patient's feelings, and facilitate verbalization of patients' feelings. Sorensen and Amis[5] stress that "we must attempt to combat apathy and reawaken in the patient the feeling that he can still make decisions which affect his life inside and outside the hospital." Although the strategies discussed in this chapter were developed specifically for individuals with chronic renal failure, they provide a prototype for health professionals and significant others working with individuals with any chronic illness.

The enabling strategies discussed in Chapter 13 and the strategies to decrease powerlessness in patients with CRF described in this chapter are collectively labelled *empowerment strategies* and are summarized in Table 14-2.

The empowerment strategies listed in Table 14-2 are specific for strengthening the power resources of psychologic stamina and social support network, motivation, and knowledge. Specific strategies related to the remaining components of the power resource model (self-esteem and hope) are included in chapters 15 and 16. (Refer to the power resource model, Chapter 1.)

# REFERENCES

1. Roy, Sister Callista: *Introduction to Nursing: An Adaptation Model.* Prentice-Hall, Englewood Cliffs, N.J., 1976, p. 229.
2. Laborde, J. and Powers, M.: *Satisfaction with life for patients undergoing hemodialysis and patients suffering from osteoarthritis.* Research in Nursing and Health 3:19, 1980.

3. Roberts, S.: *Behavioral concepts and nursing throughout the life span.* Prentice-Hall, Englewood Cliffs, N.J., 1978, p. 140.
4. Dimond, M.: *Social support and adaptation to chronic illness: The case of maintenance hemodialysis.* Research in Nursing and Health 2:101, 1979.
5. Sorenson, K. and Amis, D.: *Understanding the world of the chronically ill.* Am. J. Nurs. 67:816, April 1967.

## SELECTED READINGS

Dimond, M.: *Patient strategies for managing maintenance hemodialysis.* Western Journal of Nursing Research 2:555, Summer 1980.
Finkelstein, F. and Kitsen, J.: *Quality assurance and the care of patients with end-stage renal disease.* J. Chronic Dis. 32:605, 1979.
Greenberg, I., et al.: *Factors of adjustment in chronic hemodialysis patients.* Psychosomatics 15:178, 1975.
Luke, B.: *Nutrition in renal disease: The adult on dialysis.* Am. J. Nurs. 79:2155, December 1979.
MacElveen, P., Hoover, P., and Alexander, R.: *Patient outcome success related to cooperation among patient, partner and physician.* Journal of Nephrology Nurses and Technicians 2:148, 1975.
Oberly, T. and Oberly, E.: *Learning to live with dialysis: A personal perspective.* In Lancaster, L. (ed.): *The Patient with End-stage Renal Disease.* John Wiley & Sons, New York, 1979, pp. 83-93.
Perlmuter, L. and Monty, R.: *Choice and Perceived Control.* Lawrence Erlbaum Associates, Hillsdale, N.J., 1979.
Rhodes, V.: *Promoting patient independence: Self-care dialysis.* Nephrology Nurse 1:37, January-February 1979.
Rusk, G.: *Psychological aspects of self-care and home dialysis.* Journal of Dialysis 2:165, 1978.

# 15

# ENHANCING SELF-ESTEEM

## JUDITH FITZGERALD MILLER

Self-esteem is the evaluative component of self-concept; it is the individual's judgment about one's own worth. Rosenberg[1] states that self-esteem is an attitude of approval or disapproval of self. Individuals with high self-esteem perceive themselves as worthwhile and significant; they feel confident in influencing desired outcomes. However, persons with low self-esteem feel worthless, of little importance, and unable to affect outcomes. Wells and Marwell[2] reviewed the theoretical bases of self-esteem and present other labels for self-esteem such as self-love, self-confidence, self-respect, self-acceptance, self-satisfaction, self-regard, self-evaluation, self-appraisal, self-worth, sense of adequacy or personal efficacy, sense of competence, self-ideal congruence, and ego or ego strength.

While self-acceptance is fundamental to high self-esteem, illness challenges self-acceptance. Chronic illness presents lifelong demands for coping with a health alteration and imposed health regimen. The diagnosis of a chronic illness may be accompanied by a change in the individual's view of self (self-perception). If the individual's view of self is one of physical strength, endurance, and wholeness, there is a greater likelihood for the individual to have a higher self-esteem than if the self-perception is one of physical weakness, lack of energy, and altered body function. A change in self-perception occurs in chronically ill persons when previous aspirations need to be modified, roles changed, and other adjustments made because of altered physical reserve. When physical ability deteriorates, individuals may conclude they are worthless, undeserving of self-respect, and generally inadequate. This lowered self-esteem is present in all patients during some phase of the health problem.

How self-esteem serves as a power resource for chronically ill individuals will be discussed in this chapter. Nursing assessment of the patient's level of self-esteem and nursing strategies to enhance self-esteem are presented.

# POWER RESOURCE

Self-esteem is a power resource. High self-esteem empowers the chronically ill individual in the following ways:

—It enables the person to be an active participant in care.
—It helps the person develop confidence in interpersonal communication.
—It provides the person with accurate feedback as opposed to the inaccurate, derogatory feedback that occurs in persons with low self-esteem.
—It enhances the potential for successful role performance.

Being an active participant in care decisions and assuming responsibility for care to hasten independence in self-management depend on many factors, one of which is self-esteem. Self-esteem enables the patient to assume an active role in controlling care. Being a self-care agent requires the patient to have motivation, knowledge, and self-worth.[3] Patients with high self-esteem feel that they are worth the time and effort needed to maintain and improve health and eagerly take responsibility to meet self-care needs. Conversely, individuals with low self-esteem may be unable to make self-care decisions and assume responsibility for care outcomes. For example, an obese individual with low self-esteem may feel undeserving of better health, and unworthy of close dietary monitoring, health-care personnel's time, and the patient's own effort.

The confidence and competence individuals have in their interpersonal relationships are positively influenced by high self-esteem. Interactions with significant others (those from whom acceptance is sought) and with strangers provide feedback about self. If the individual feels worthwhile and demonstrates self-approval during interactions, others will respond with similar feelings of respect and approval. Patients with high self-esteem feel worthy of using nurses' and physicians' time. These patients feel confident that their own concerns are not petty or foolish but are deserving of professional consultation.

High self-esteem enables individuals to more accurately interpret feedback about self, whereas low self-esteem causes individuals to distort feedback. Persons with low self-esteem may consistently engage in an internal dialogue that results in a negative interpretation about self. Guilt and self-pity may be induced. For example, consider Mr. C., who has a colostomy. When his dressing is changed on a particular day, his nurse is less talkative than usual. Mr. C. interprets this as being due to her repugnance of him. The patient may carry on a silent dialogue to reaffirm his false interpretation. It seems as though the patient seeks reinforcement for his own negative feeling of low self-worth. Instead of being open in interactions and validating the meaning of the feedback, the patient may interpret the message in a way that is destructive to self.

High self-esteem breeds success in performing life roles. Self-esteem provides confidence in undertaking new roles (such as assuming the role of self-care agent) and a recognition of personal potential for accomplishing goals associated with familiar roles.

The belief in one's own ability to be successful operates as a self-fulfilling prophecy. The patient with high self-esteem confidently anticipates success, which in fact does materialize.

Coopersmith[4] describes three conditions that foster high self-esteem in children. These conditions include (1) acceptance of the children by parents, (2) enforcement of clearly defined limits set by parents, and (3) respect for the individual child's initiative and latitude within the set limits.

Coping mechanisms of persons with high and low self-esteem may be distinctly different. Cohen[5] stated that preferred defenses (mental coping mechanisms) of persons with high self-esteem include denial and repression or ignoring conflicting impulses. Persons with low self-esteem used projective and expressive defenses. Persons who had low self-esteem before the onset of chronic illness may experience greater threats to self-esteem as a result of the illness than do persons with high premorbid self-esteem. This may be especially true if development of the illness is viewed as a personal shortcoming or a negative component of self.

Because self-esteem is a power resource, nursing efforts to enhance self-esteem help to increase the patient's perceived power (alleviating powerlessness). Ascertaining the patient's level of self-esteem is an important first step.

# ASSESSMENT OF SELF-ESTEEM

To determine the nature of the patient's self-esteem, information is gathered through observation, an interview, analysis of the patient's role performance, and identification of changes in social interaction.

# Observation

Nursing observations of patient behavior include noting the pattern of verbal comments by the patient over time. Self-derogatory verbal comments indicate low self-esteem. Examples are the following statements:

I feel I am no longer a good person.
I can't do anything anymore. Now I am good for nothing, useless.
I feel guilt and embarrassment when I have to ask for help.
I've lost my independence, that is mighty rough.
I've lost faith in myself.
Sometimes I feel my body has turned against me.
I don't like myself this way.

These comments indicate feelings of insignificance, uselessness, and worthlessness.

Other observations of patient interaction may indicate low self-esteem. The patient may be hesitant to bother the nurse or ask for help. The person with low self-esteem may avoid direct eye contact when communicating with others, especially when interacting with authority figures. The patient's reluctance to participate in the medical plan may also indicate low self-esteem.

# Interview

After a trusting nurse-patient relationship has been established, specific questions can be raised to gather information about the patient's self-esteem. Besides gathering data for self-esteem assessment, interview questions enable the patient to review existing abilities and develop self-insight, thereby providing an opportunity to enhance self-esteem. The following questions are helpful in gathering self-esteem information:

How has having arthritis (or whatever the health problem is) changed the way you feel about yourself?
In evaluating your abilities, how would you describe yourself?
Would you say you had a positive or negative attitude toward yourself?
What do you like best about yourself?
What are your weak points?
What do you do to feel good about yourself?

Information gathered by using patient self-report (responses to the above or similar questions) can be validated with the patient by asking the questions again or by confirming responses later. The self-report is compared with observations, social interaction, and role performance.

# Role Performance

Role changes may be imposed by illness. Sometimes, previous work roles are no longer possible. The more important the role is in determining the person's self-concept, the more devastating the role loss is to the person's self-esteem. For example, if a symphony pianist suffered a traumatic amputation of three fingers, the concept of self as a pianist is threatened. The patient's breadwinning capacity may be threatened temporarily until the patient can accept a substitute role, for example, teaching piano or developing a related talent such as vocal music performance. Questions to be considered in assessing role performance include the following:

How threatening is the health problem to the individual's definition of self or self-concept?
Will the health problem interfere with established career goals or the present employment role?
Does the health problem cause the patient to feel less sexually attractive? (Joint deformities and decreased mobility of arthritis may limit activities the individual views as important for developing and maintaining sexual relationships.)
Does the patient perceive self to be less adequate in social relationships because of the health problem? (Patients with chronic diarrhea from Crohn's disease may hesitate to become involved in group activities to avoid embarrassment of frequent trips to the rest room.)

# Changes in Social Interaction

Although information about self-esteem and social interaction relates closely to role performance, specific changes in social interaction can be noted. Have social activities been eliminated, leisure activities changed, or relationships with family and significant others altered?

Patient's family and friends may relate that the patient's interaction themes focus on negative self-talk. That is, self-derogatory, self-condescending comments by the patient may dominate communication with others. Friends may eventually withdraw. The resulting social isolation may contribute to further lowering of self-esteem.

Valued social activities may be eliminated. For example, the patient with severe emphysema may avoid the weekly card party at the senior citizens' center to avoid exposure to crowds and respiratory infections. Although the decision may be a good one in terms of health maintenance, unless acceptable substitutes are found, positive feelings about self may diminish. The nurse can help the patient find an alternative activity; for example, the patient could select three friends to meet weekly at the patient's home to play cards.

Low self-esteem indicators (verbalizations and behaviors) can be summarized in three categories: changes in role performance, changes in interpersonal relationships, and presence of negative self-talk. See Table 15-1.

Assessment of self-esteem is important for designing appropriate individual strategies to enhance self-esteem. Individuals evaluate themselves highly in situations in which they achieve a sense of mastery. A sense of mastery is based on the person's behavior

## TABLE 15-1. Indicators of Low Self-Esteem

| Interpersonal Relationships | Negative Self-talk | Role Performance |
| --- | --- | --- |
| Feels unworthy of nurses' time, care, attention. Hesitant to ask for help. Pessimistic. Feels undeserving of praise. Resentful of others who are well. Lacks assertiveness. Lacks self-confidence in one-to-one and/or group interactions. Self-conscious. Expresses a sense of worthlessness. | Verbalizations convey: —Self-blame. —Guilt over disease. —Self-derogatory comments. —Negative attitude toward self (physical self, personal self, and spiritual self). —Feeling of uselessness. —Lack of self-respect. | Expresses having few accomplishments. Expresses doubts about ability to fulfill roles. Feels inferior; compares self to others. Feels own actions will have little effect on an outcome (feels ineffective). Feels insignificant. Unable to take pride in accomplishing goals. Unable to set goals. Feels has failed in life's mission. Lacks a sense of competence. |

being consistent with self-expectations and the expectations of others.[6] Nursing strategies that develop patient insight into feelings about self and self-expectations need to be used. Nursing strategies should also focus on developing the patient's self-care abilities (agency). This results in patients achieving mastery of care needs and a perceived sense of control; consequently, self-esteem is enhanced. Developing self-care skills in order to manage the care regimen is the foundation for designing other strategies to enhance self-esteem.

# NURSING STRATEGIES

Patients with chronic illnesses may feel that their bodies or they themselves have somehow failed. The nursing goal of helping patients overcome this feeling of failure is important in allowing the patient to achieve a sense of control and, thereby, heightened self-esteem. What the nurse can do to enhance patients' self-esteem will be discussed in terms of interpersonal relationships, negative self-talk, and role disturbance.

## Interpersonal Relationships

### NURSE-PATIENT RELATIONSHIP

The nature of the helping relationship established by the nurse will influence the patient's self-esteem. The helping relationship should be characterized by caring, concern, empathy, unconditional acceptance, and respect. Respect is communicated by letting patients know they have much to contribute to others, including the nurse. The nurse is responsive to patients' unique abilities. Ways in which the nurse benefits from the relationship should be shared with patients. Nurse benefits may include greater understanding about the central topic discussed. The goal for the interaction may have been to discuss a topic about which the patient has some expertise, such as world events, governmental policies, and historical events. Recognition is given for the patient's knowledge. The nurse expresses appreciation to the patient for new insights gained. Nurse responsiveness to the patient's unique abilities enhances the patient's feelings of worth. It communicates to the patient the nurse's sincerity in that the nurse is interested in the patient as a whole person, not just the present health problem. The patient's awareness that the concept of self extends beyond the health problem is renewed. Other nurse benefits that can be shared with the patient include a sense of joy over being able to share time and self with the patient, appreciation for learning what it is like to have a chronic health problem, and increased understanding about the lives of patients with similar problems.

### FAMILY

Family members need to realize the importance of their reactions to the patient. The patient may be vigilantly watching for their reactions, thinking "If they reject me, what will the people who care less about me do?" The patient may falsely interpret the family members' response as repugnance. It has been well documented that persons with low self-esteem are more sensitive to negative information about self and persons with high self-esteem are more sensitive to positive information about self.[7-11] The ill person's self-esteem is lowered by the illness and its impositions. Patients may misinterpret nonverbal cues, resulting in further lowering of self-esteem; for example, a facial expression may be misinterpreted as a reaction of disgust. The nurse can help family members become sensitive to their interactive styles. Family members can be helped to interact in ways that make the patient feel lovable, respected, and enjoyable to be with. Letting the patient know how much the patient is needed by the family renews the patient's self-worth.

## SOCIAL ACTIVITIES

If the patient is feeling socially isolated, the nurse may need to review with the patient what has happened with family and friend relationships. The following questions can be considered:

Has the health problem influenced the nature of the patient's social relationships?
Does the patient spend so much time on symptom control that no time is provided for friends and social activities?
Does the patient repeatedly review physical ailments when interacting with family?

Affirmative answers to these questions may cause family and friends to withdraw. Besides being helped to develop insight into the interactive situation, the patient can be helped by being asked to select one or more significant others in whom to confide, disclosing information about symptoms without repetitious review of the troublesome symptoms with each loved one.

The patient may withdraw from social activities because the patient feels unworthy of involvement. The nurse can help the patient become aware of the benefits of successful social interaction to self-esteem. The nurse can review appropriate social activities that are available to the patient. These may range from joining a church group, volunteering at a school, taking an art appreciation class, working with the elderly in a nursing home, or becoming involved in a political campaign, to sharing a daily cup of coffee with a neighbor. Positive social experiences reinforce the individual's sense of worth. Making the effort to engage in appropriate social activities will enhance self-esteem.

Patients with chronic illnesses may have more leisure time and less physical ability than they did in the past. Helping the patient develop new activities may be necessary. These activities contribute to self-satisfaction and a sense of fulfillment. A feeling of accomplishment can be gained from activities such as reading a book, designing a greeting card, writing a poem, or compiling favorite recipes.

# Negative Self-talk

Helping patients eliminate negative self-talk will eliminate this self-initiated message of low self-esteem. The self-derogatory statements are a consistent reinforcement to patients that they *are* really worthless. For example, the patient may state, "I'm not able to play ball with my grandson now that I have only one good leg. I can no longer be the strong man I want to be. My grandson will not accept me." Negative self-talk may cause a feeling of guilt when the patient begins to make plans for an improved psychologic state. Negative self-statements precipitate self-pity.

At the onset, the nurse needs to help the patient become aware of the harmful effects of negative self-talk on self-esteem. A direct reflective communication technique is useful in helping patients hear what they are saying. After the nurse repeats patients' self-derogatory statements, patients can reappraise what has been said. A substitute positive verbalization can then be made. Meichenbaum[12] refers to this as changing the client's internal dialogue. A three-phase process is used to eliminate negative self-talk:

Phase 1 The patient listens to the self-derogatory statements that are reflected by the nurse.

Phase 2 The patient cognitively reappraises the negative statements by asking, "Do I really believe that? Does that accurately describe me?" The patient is helped to think, "What could be the most positive statement I could make about myself?"

Phase 3 The patient substitutes the newly accepted positive statement about self. The substitute statement is rehearsed with the nurse.

If need be, the patient can set aside time each day to review the substitute positive self-talk. Some patients benefit from listening to a tape or a self-recorded message of the positive self-talk statement. The nurse may have to help the patient formulate some positive statements such as the following:

Today, I am the best me possible.
Because I am human, I am worthwhile.
I was created in the image of God; therefore, I am lovable.
People like me for what I am.
I am special; there is no one like me in the entire world.

Giving the patient feedback about negative self-talk not only develops patient insight but also stimulates reappraisal. Keeping track of the number of negative self-statements the patient makes during one interaction is helpful. At the completion of the interaction, the nurse should give the patient feedback about these statements, including the number of negative statements used, nature of the statements, and how these statements contribute to low self-esteem.

It is recognized that eliminating the negative self-talk may not completely alleviate the patient's internal feelings of low self-worth. The patient's unique strengths should also be reviewed. Often, the intact roles the patient plays are an appropriate starting point to renew continuing valued abilities.

## Role Performance

Helping patients recognize the existing roles they will continue to play successfully in life helps renew a feeling of worth. If some roles are eliminated, substitutes can be

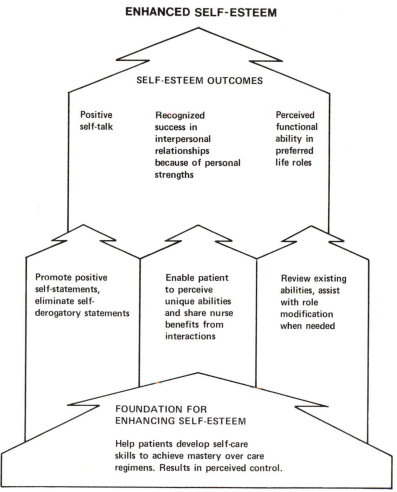

FIGURE 15-1.  Nursing strategies for enhancing self-esteem.

found. For example, if a woman with ankylosing spondylitis of the spine had been an avid horsewoman, instead of riding horses, she may now have to be involved in show-ing horses, stable work, grooming, horse-care supervision, speaking at functions spon-sored by horseman groups, writing for horse journals, and so forth. If the patient who enjoyed jogging suffers a traumatic injury to the hip, use of a stationary bicycle may be an appropriate substitute physical outlet. Other roles that individuals will continue to fill despite the illness are reviewed, for example, husband, father, accountant, church board member, neighbor, organizer of the summer block parties, and household handy-man.

In addition to the review of existing abilities and strengths, the patient's potential may need to be discussed. Individuals should be encouraged to develop unique interests and untapped latent talents.

In this book, the health problem is considered the precipitating factor in lowering the patient's self-esteem. The nurse's challenge is to help the patient achieve mastery over the health problem. A self-care nursing framework has as its central purpose the development and maintenance of the patient's (family's) ability to care for self so as to sustain life and health, recover from disease or injury, cope with their effects,[13] and/or achieve a better state of wellness. Self-care is needed to face demands of an altered health state and prescribed regimen, as well as to face the patient's own desire for better health when illness is not present. The patient's self-care abilities need to be developed through teaching (role modeling, role playing, supporting, and evaluating). It is through developing the patient's self-care abilities that the patient's sense of control is enhanced, self-esteem is heightened, and powerlessness is alleviated. Through nursing efforts, negative self-talk can be eliminated, interpersonal strengths can be identified, and ability to resume functions in life roles can be reviewed, as shown in Figure 15-1. These roles can be accomplished after the patient has confidence and ability to manage the health problem.

Self-esteem preserves psychologic integrity. It serves as a power resource in that individuals have a need to feel good about themselves and value their worth before they invest in improving their situations, such as enhancing their state of health. Illness threatens a patient's self-concept and lowers self-esteem, which leads to feelings of powerlessness. Enhancing self-esteem is a high priority for nursing care and research.

# REFERENCES

1. Rosenberg, M.: *Society and the Adolescent Self-Image.* Princeton University Press, Princeton, N.J., 1965.
2. Wells, L. E. and Marwell, G.: *Self-Esteem: Its Conceptualization and Measurement.* Sage Publications, Beverly Hills, Calif., 1976.
3. Kearney, B. and Fleisher, B.: *Development of an instrument to measure exercise of self-care agency.* Research in Nursing and Health 2:25, 1979.
4. Coopersmith, S.: *The Antecedents of Self-Esteem.* W. H. Freeman, San Francisco, 1967.
5. Cohen, A.: *Some implications of self-esteem for social influence.* In Hovland, C. and Janis, I. (eds.): *Personality and Persuasibility.* Yale University Press, New Haven, Conn., 1959, pp. 102–120.
6. Brissett, D.: *Toward a clarification of self-esteem.* Psychiatry 35:255, 1972.
7. Stotland, E., et al.: *Group expectations, self-esteem and self-evaluations.* J. Abnorm. Soc. Psychol. 54:55, 1957.
8. Stotland, E. and Zander, A.: *Effects of public and private failure on self-evaluation.* J. Abnorm. Soc. Psychol. 56:223, 1958.
9. Silverman, I.: *Self-esteem and differential responsiveness to success and failure.* J. Abnorm. Soc. Psychol. 69:115, 1964.
10. Fitch, G.: *Effects on self-esteem, perceived performance and choice on causal attributions.* J. Pers. Soc. Psychol. 16:311, 1970.
11. Shrauger, J. and Rosenberg, S.: *Self-esteem and the effects of success and failure feedback on performance.* J. Pers. 33:404, 1970.
12. Meichenbaum, D.: *Toward a cognitive theory of self-control.* In Schwartz, G. and Shapiro, D. (eds.): *Consciousness and Self-Regulation: Advances in Research,* Vol. 1. Plenum Press, New York, 1976.
13. Orem, D.: *Nursing: Concepts of Practice,* ed. 2. McGraw-Hill, New York, 1980.

# SELECTED READINGS

Barksdale, L. S.: *Building Self-Esteem.* Barksdale Foundation, Idyllwild, Calif., 1976.

Bowden, M.L., et al.: *Self-esteem of severely burned patients.* Arch. Phys. Med. Rehabil. 61:449, 1980.

Brandon, N.: *The Psychology of Self-Esteem.* Nash Publishing, Los Angeles, 1979.

Breytspraak, L.: *Measurement of self-concept and self-esteem in older people: State of the art.* Exp. Aging Res. 5:137, 1979.

Buscaglia, L.: *Personhood: The Art of Being Fully Human.* Charles B. Slack, Thorofare, N.J., 1978.

Christian, K.: *Aspects of the self-concept related to level of self-esteem.* J. Consult. Clin. Psychol. 46:1151, 1978.

Elkins, D. P.: *Glad to Be Me: Building Self-Esteem in Yourself and Others.* Prentice-Hall, Englewood Cliffs, N.J., 1976.

Fitts, W.: *The Self-Concept and Behavior: Overview and Supplement.* William H. Fitts, Nashville, Tenn., 1972.

Germain, R.: *Self-concept and self-esteem reexamined.* Psychology in the Schools 15:386, 1978.

Kellerman, J., et al.: *Psychological effects of illness in adolescence. I. Anxiety, self-esteem and perception of control.* J. Pediatr. 97:126, 1980.

Maltz, M.: *Psycho-cybernetics and self-fulfillment: A guide to confidence and self-respect.* Grosset & Dunlap, New York, 1970.

Rosenberg, M.: *Conceiving the Self.* Basic Books, New York, 1979.

Rynerson, B.: *Need for self-esteem in the aged: A literature review.* J. Psychiatr. Nurs. 10:22, 1972.

Sullivan, B.-J.: *Adjustment in diabetic adolescent girls II. Adjustment, self-esteem, and depression in diabetic adolescent girls.* Psychosom. Med. 41:127, 1979.

Wylie, R.: *The Self-Concept,* Vol. 1. University of Nebraska Press, Lincoln, Neb., 1974.

# 16

# INSPIRING HOPE

## JUDITH FITZGERALD MILLER

## POWER RESOURCE

One of a human being's most valued, private, and powerful resources is hope. Hope is an intrinsic component of life. Hope provides dynamism for the spirit,[1] saving individuals from apathetic inaction. Hope is the affect that accompanies faith (belief system). Although faith could not be sustained without hope, the basis of hope is faith. Hope means anticipating success but having a feeling of uncertainty. Hope is the negation of the worst possible outcome.[2] Stotland[3] defines hope as an expectation greater than zero of achieving a goal. Beyond these views, hope is considered to be a state of being. "Hope is an inner readiness, that of an intense but not yet spent activeness."[4] Everything human beings do in life is based on some level of hope.

Three levels or intensities of hope can be described, as shown in Figure 16-1. The first level is the most elementary type of hope, in which superficial wishes, as for basic material goods or a nice day, are included. Shallow optimism characterizes this level. When this level of hope is not actualized, little despair occurs and little psychic energy is spent.

The second level of hope includes hoping for relationships, self-improvement, and self-accomplishments. When hope at this level is thwarted, the resultant level of despair is characterized by anxiety. The anxiety is relieved with new goal establishment. Psychic energy investment is greater than at the first level but less than at the next stage. Thoughts about goal achievement occupy considerable time and energy.

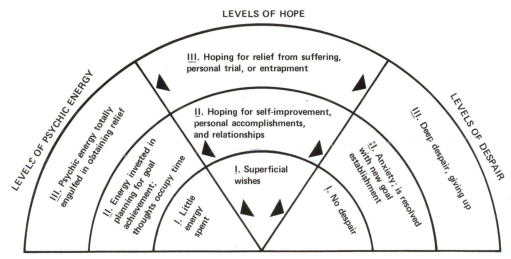

FIGURE 16-1.  Levels of hope, despair, and psychic energy.

The third level of hope arises out of suffering, personal trial, or state of captivity. Marcel[5] states that it is in a situation tempted by despair that hope has its true meaning. Deep despair, or giving up, occurs when, according to the individual's evaluation, relief is not imminent. Total engulfment of psychic energy occurs at this point.

This chapter deals with the third level of hope—hope at its most intense and powerful level. Maintaining hope despite a downward physical course is a challenge (coping task) of the chronically ill. Included in this chapter is a discussion of assessment of hope-hopelessness and nursing strategies to inspire hope. Nursing strategies that inspire hope also decrease powerlessness.

Chronic illness, by virtue of its unpredictable nature and concomitant losses, precipitates powerlessness. When powerlessness is not contained, hopelessness can result. As shown in Figure 16-2, the cycle of powerlessness leads to depression and low self-esteem, causing hopelessness that in turn immobilizes the individual. The cycle continues until the giving up of prolonged hopelessness leads to death. See Chapter 6 for a clinical description of hopelessness leading to death. Power is restored to a degree when the patient's hope is restored. Hope can be viewed as a potent power resource.

The losses suffered by chronically ill patients can lead to hopelessness. Not only does the chronically ill individual suffer from loss of health status and body-function control—for example, coordination—but also the person may suffer loss of body parts, loss of roles, loss of self-esteem, loss of certainty, loss of sexual attractiveness, loss of social relationships, loss of independence, and loss of finances. Categories of losses recorded in 81 chronically ill adults are included in Table 16-1.[6] Grieving over these losses is a crucial process for the chronically ill person. Grief resolution may be needed to prevent the accumulated losses from becoming overwhelming, thereby causing hopelessness.

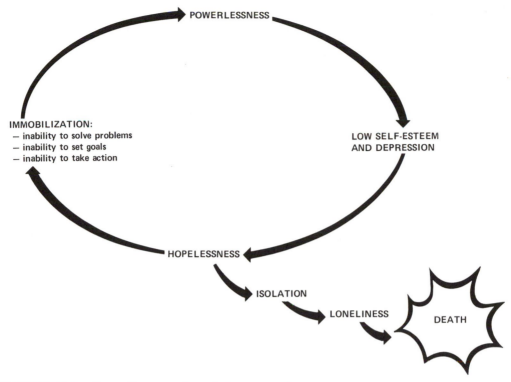

FIGURE 16-2. Powerlessness-hopelessness cycle.

## ASSESSMENT OF HOPE-HOPELESSNESS

The patient's degree of hopelessness can be understood by determining the patient's perceived sense of powerlessness, duration of powerlessness, and the severity of losses suffered. A concrete analysis of hope-hopelessness behavior according to Isani's[7] nine-stage progression of hopelessness is helpful in a specific hope-hopelessness assessment. In Table 16-2, patient behaviors indicative of moving toward hope or moving toward despair are identified for each stage of hopelessness.

Alleviating hopelessness is a crucial nursing concern not only because it contributes to the patient's sense of power but also because it prevents other harmful consequences of illness and therapy. Hopelessness affects the patient's response to therapy, can hasten death, and has been identified as a factor in the development of cancer.[8,9]

Schmale and Iker[8] studied 40 women who had abnormal Pap smears but were asymptomatic for cancer, to determine the relationship between feelings of hopelessness and the disposition to develop cancer. The subjects were interviewed on the day of their cervical cone biopsy to determine their general attitudes, concerns, and ambitions. Patients receiving high hopelessness scores (based on the interview) were predicted to have cancer, whereas patients receiving low hopelessness scores were predicted to have

**TABLE 16-1. Losses of Chronic Illness**

| *Categories of losses of the chronically ill* |
|---|

Health status losses—functions
  Energy
  Strength-vitality
  Ability to communicate verbally
  Muscle coordination
  Bowel and bladder control

Loss of body parts
  Organs
  Hair
  Weight

Loss of roles
  Loss of breadwinner role
  Loss of secure future

Loss of self-esteem, dignity

Loss of certainty, predictability from day to day

Loss of sexual performance abilities
  Loss of intimacy

Loss of relationships with others

Loss of independence—ability to care for self

Loss of finances

---

no cancer. The predictions of cancer or no cancer were correct in 31 cases and incorrect in 9 (significant at the 0.007 level). Three subscales (ego strength, depression, and masculinity-feminity) of the Minnesota Multiphasic Personality Inventory (MMPI) were also administered. Only depression correlated with cancer. In 1971, Schmale repeated this study with 68 women and made correct predictions in 50 of the 68 patients. In his discussion of carcinogenesis, cell dysplasia is labeled the initiator of cancer, and the psychologic experience of hopelessness acts as the promoter of cancer.

Responses of 69 women treated for early breast cancer were studied 3 months and 5 years after their initial surgical treatment.[10] Those women who had reacted to cancer with denial or who had a "fighting spirit" were significantly free from recurrence of the disease as compared with those women who responded with stoic acceptance or feelings of helplessness and hopelessness.

The MMPI was administered to three groups of 47 male renal dialysis patients to determine psychologic correlates of survival on dialysis.[11] Subjects in group A died within 1 year of initiating dialysis; group B subjects lived 3 to 7 years; subjects in group C lived 7 to 10 years. Subjects in group A were characterized by feelings of helplessness, high levels of depression, anxiety, and preoccupation with somatic difficulties. Subjects in groups B and C tended to be dependent, have mild levels of depression, and have a sense of hopefulness about the future. Similar findings were noted in a study on survival of burned children. Positive factors of survival were coping mechanisms of denial, withdrawal, splitting of the ego, somatic responses, and *hope* in parents and/or staff.[12]

**TABLE 16-2. Analysis of Patient Behavior According to Nine-Stage Progression of Hopelessness**

| Patient Behavior Indicates Moving Toward Hope | Definition of Hopelessness[7] | Patient Behavior Indicates Moving Toward Despair |
|---|---|---|
| Readily establishes personal goals and anticipated positive outcomes | 1. The person has anticipations of an improved state of affairs relating to achievement of goals | Unable to set goals |
| Continually modifies goals to allow perceived success | 2. Repeatedly fails to achieve goals | Perceives unachieved outcomes as personal failure |
| Focuses on past successes as a sustaining force | 3. Makes unfavorable comparisons of present situation of failure with past anticipations of success | Emphasizes failure in light of accomplishments while well |
| Modifies goals without self-punishment | 4. Fails to modify goals or selected routes to goal achievement | Rigidly adheres to achieving goals possible only during healthy state |
| Plans for alternative action if one plan does not produce expected results | 5. Reduces anticipations of finding clear cut solutions | No effort is made to consider alternatives |
| Promotes peace of mind through activity and motivation toward goal | 6. Increasingly limits efforts to achieve goals | Becomes increasingly agitated over accomplishing nothing |
| Rationalizes why solution not found | 7. Despairs of finding solutions | Verbalizes doubt in self, therapy, and life |
| Consensually validates with friends their belief in patient | 8. Loses faith in self and others | Verbalizes giving up as the only solution |
| Persists in motivating self, clings to positive signs and encouragement from respected others | 9. Gives up trying, becomes hopeless | Gives up |

Hopelessness has also been correlated with external locus of control and depression.[13] Rotter's Internal-External Locus of Control Scale and Beck's Depression Scale were used in studies of 67 and 44 undergraduate subjects to arrive at these correlations.

Engel[14] has labeled the failure of coping mechanisms as the ''giving-up–given-up complex.'' This complex includes (1) feelings of being at the end of the rope, at an impasse, helpless, and hopeless; (2) having a poor self-image, and feeling incompetent and out of control; (3) having a loss of gratification from roles and relationships; (4) feeling a sense of disrupted continuity among past, present, and future; and (5) recalling memories of previous helpless states. Engel proposes that this psychologic state creates a psychobiologic condition that contributes to the emergence of disease. Engel[15] also attributes deaths of subjects after experiencing sudden losses (e.g., death of a spouse) to the giving-up–given-up complex.

The serious consequences of hopelessness have been documented. Although it is easier to prevent hopelessness than to reverse it,[16] nurses are able to inspire hope.

# NURSING STRATEGIES

Nursing strategies to inspire hope are characterized by sensitivity and understanding of the patient's plight. Sweeping into the patient's world with good wishes and optimism is not helpful. Nurses can be realistic without losing the capability to dream and without becoming bitter or cynical because of reality. An existential frame of reference will be used to describe nursing strategies to inspire hope. Three categories of nursing strategies are helping the patient engage in reality surveillance, devising and revising goals, and hoping in God.

## Existential Frame of Reference

Inspiring hope does not mean hope for cure or hope for return to previous ways of living and working. Rather, the nurse inspires patients with hope "to be."[17] In an existential framework, human beings have a never-ending possibility of improving their own being.[5] Vaillot[17] states that nurses can help patients reach for a fullness of being, in spite of physical limitations. Dwelling on physical limitations only precipitates helplessness. An individual's hope can be fostered by utilizing the internal resources and strengths of another. Nurses can radiate hope. Nurses can demonstrate faith and confidence in patients, letting patients realize their unique adaptive resources are perceived by others. The expectations for the patient to live life fully, rallying forth untapped strengths, is conveyed to the patient. The patient may not have felt this expectation before the relationship with the nurse. The cliche "no one can give to others what he himself does not have" applies here. Patients are quick to sense the nurse's feelings of hopelessness. Nurses must make a conscious effort to work with patients to display hope for living or an improved state. The expectation for living life fully is conveyed in the open, loving, helping nurse-patient relationship.

### MAXIMIZING THE EXPERIENCE

It is clear, then, that inspiring hope is not confined to hope for renewed physical being but rather focuses on hope to live life fully. This includes fully appreciating even the smallest experiences. These esthetic experiences may prevent the patient from being smothered by despair. Maximizing experiences includes countless examples, such as helping the patient:

—savor the richness of black coffee at breakfast.
—feel the tartness of grapefruit wake up the taste buds.
—note the crystal-clear blue of the sky.
—feel the warmth of a sunbeam.
—watch activities of animals in a tree outside the window.
—benefit from each encounter with another human being.
—share experiences children are having.
—note loving characteristics of spouse.
—appreciate expressions of caring concern.
—work out intricate plans, such as for rebuilding the summer cottage.
—plan to rearrange the living room furniture.
—build highlights into each day, such as meals, visits, Bible reading.
—write messages to grandchildren, nieces, or nephews.
—plan for volunteer work to help others.
—study a favorite painting.
—listen to a symphony as an escape to another world.

It is recognized that not all patients will benefit from isolated reconstructed experiences such as the melting of snowflakes on their cheeks. However, all patients will benefit from renewed appreciation of making the most of the moment, not letting the moment pass by without appreciating its beauty. Using these experiences helps to achieve a sense of personal fulfillment.

Jourard[18] describes inspiriting and dispiriting persons to live. "To inspirit a person is to augment and confirm his values and purposes, to increase his experience of meaning in his existence ... to render him more resistant to both 'physical' and 'mental' diseases."[19] Individuals need to realize the freedom to create a new self when the old self has caused despair.

The patient may be searching for meaning in the experience, defining something to live for, and looking for clues that encourage hope. The nurse can help the patient in this search.

# Reality Surveillance

Reality surveillance is a cognitive task in which the individual searches for clues that confirm that maintaining hope is feasible. Wright and Shontz[20] described reality surveillance (also called reality or phenomenal grounding) as an important element in the hoping process in adults. The phenomenal grounding of reality refers to what the person in the situation believes provides grounds for hopes. It is the phenomenal grounding of reality, not whether the person is actually being realistic, that provides reassurance to the individual. The components of reality surveillance have relevance for identifying nursing strategies to inspire hope. Table 16-3 presents an analysis of categories of reality surveillance, patient behaviors related to each component, and examples of nursing's role. It must be recognized that some patients need to delay reality surveillance while maintaining a future orientation, having uncertain hopes, and not using any of the hope-grounding strategies indicated in Table 16-3.

**TABLE 16-3. Analysis of Reality Surveillance**

| Select Categories of Reality Surveillance Adopted from Wright and Shontz[20] | Examples of Patient Behavior Indicative of the Category | Nursing Role |
|---|---|---|
| Reviewing changing environmental conditions. | "I must be improving; the nurses are not monitoring me as closely; they come less often." | If patient's interpretations are accurate, confirm them; that is, the V.N.A. will visit less frequently because of these signs of improvement. Review indicators of improvement. |
| Reviewing assets. | "I have a good health history; I have never been hospitalized before." "I still have one good leg." "I have always exercised to keep physically fit." "Now that I have an ileostomy, at least I won't get cancer of the bowel." | Help patient review assets, which include physical, interpersonal, and role-function abilities. |
| Comparing self with other individuals or groups. | "It took my neighbor longer to recover from his heart attack." "I didn't realize I would be able to wear my same clothes after my colostomy surgery." "The patient representative from the ostomy association was so helpful." | Information on self-help groups can be provided. Listen to patient's need to compare own better progress to other patients with slower progress. |
| Planning for assuming self-care responsibilities. | "I realize now, the diabetes will not be going away. I'd better start learning to take care of myself." | Provide assistance through teaching and support so patient gradually assumes responsibility for care and realizes that self-care is not an impossible overwhelming task. |
| Avoiding confrontation with negative outcomes. | "The chemotherapy has got to be effective after all this suffering with side effects. It's got to be killing something." | Listen with empathy; help patient with internal dialogue to increase patient's insight. |
| Plans are contingent upon if-then events. | "If I remain in remission until Christmas, I will plan the trip." | Foster positive expectations for remaining physically stable. Teach importance of optimistic mind set, influencing body response. Inform patient of mind-body pathways and holistic response to health. |

**TABLE 16-3.** *Continued*

| Select Categories of Reality Surveillance Adopted from Wright and Shontz[20] | Examples of Patient Behavior Indicative of the Category | Nursing Role |
|---|---|---|
| Holding out for future discoveries. | "Who knows, maybe they will find a cure for multiple sclerosis." | Share knowledge of advances in caring for patients with debilitating diseases. Acknowledge discoveries in medicine that were unheard of years ago. |
| Using statements of uncontestable truisms. | "God will help me through this." "All that is needed is for me to do my best and to follow the medical orders." | Recognize that this verbalization is comforting to the patient and the patient is watching the nurse's response. |
| Making testimonials. | "I've read of miraculous cures of arthritis." | Demonstrate interest without scientific interrogation or "putting the patient down," repudiating the patient for the claims. |

Affective mechanisms accompany the cognitive task of reality surveillance. The affective mechanisms include encouragement, worry, and mourning.[20] When the individual finds basis for hope through reality surveillance, encouragement is felt. The encouragement in turn sustains hoping. Uncertainty about realizing hopes provokes worry. Worry causes the individual to reexamine reality, which may result in sustaining hope or dissolving it. Mourning occurs when hopes are abandoned and deep loss is felt.[20] Mourning accompanies hopelessness or despair.

# Devising and Revising Goals

Hope means having something to look forward to, anticipating an outcome. Hope is energized by the belief in accomplishing goals.[3,21] Patients may need help in devising goals. Types of goals that are helpful in inspiring hope include goals that reflect (1) physical strides for the patient, (2) work to be accomplished, (3) responsibility to discharge, and (4) love relationships to renew and/or sustain.

The significance of unsophisticated goals, as indicators of patient progress, may be overlooked; yet these goals provide hope for the patient. Nurses can help patients formulate goals such as being able to tolerate sitting up in the chair for an additional 15 minutes, being able to take a walk outside, using one less dose of analgesic during a 24-hour period, and reading one additional chapter of a new book. When the goal is accomplished, nurses can discuss this with the patient as a sign of progress—a positive, hope-mobilizing force.

Work to be accomplished refers to determining with the patient any work (job or other role-related) pressures the patient may be feeling and setting up goals to alleviate these pressures. Determining the work that is feasible for the patient to complete in spite of hospitalization or an altered health state can be done. For example, an executive vice-president of a business, hospitalized in traction owing to low back pain, uses the telephone for participation in ongoing business decisions and has a messenger deliver mail and return completed projects to the office. A housewife facilitates ongoing household management by use of the telephone to support her husband and children in completion of household tasks. She is also able to fulfill her role as mother by having daily after-school telephone conferences with each of her children.

Responsibility to discharge means helping the patient make use of human resources available to take care of work pressures. Being reassured that responsibilities are not neglected helps the patient avoid the feeling of despair from, "This is too much for me. I will never be able to catch up with the demands when I am able to function again."

Renewing and making efforts to sustain love relationships maintain hope. Having someone and something to live for is a strong inspiration. Lynch[21] states that hope cannot be achieved alone; it results from an act of community (two or more people working together). The future is tolerable if the patient feels there is unconditional love from someone and someone with whom the future can be shared. With hopelessness, the future is intolerable. This does not mean that the nurse is the significant other; however, the nurse can determine, with the patient, the network of support present in the patient's family, review the nature of the relationships, and emphasize their significance in terms of inspiring hope. The nurse's role is to help the patient realize that hope depends on a firm "I-Thou" relationship that includes sharing and feeling with another.[5]

The first three categories of goals discussed (simple goals as marks of physical strides, work to be accomplished, and responsibility to discharge) will need constant revision to act as continuous hope-mobilizing forces. New goals need to be established as old goals are successfully met. For some individuals, establishing action plans to accomplish goals is founded in belief in God.

# Hoping in God

Individuals who have used religious beliefs and practices as coping mechanisms throughout their lives easily turn to God for hope when the uncontrollable nature of long-term illness precipitates hopelessness. Heagle[22] states the goal of hope is not the things we hope for but the persons we trust in, the person of God and human persons who represent Him. Hope is reified when suffering is thrust upon individuals. Heagle[22] says that when hope is transformed into a personal bond, it becomes trust. Trust is hope in a relationship. The greatest of bonds, the one that provides the most hope, is the bond with God.

When individuals think poorly of themselves, they may feel unworthy of renewing their love, faith, and hope relationship with God. Strategies to enhance self-esteem (discussed in Chapter 15) may need to be employed.

Patients may need to be encouraged to use religious practices that provide hope. At times, patients are hesitant to openly read scripture, display religious articles, or request chaplain visits. This hesitancy stems from a fear of being ridiculed by professionals whose decisions are founded on scientific rather than theologic principles. The patient can be encouraged to share passages from the Bible with the nurse, clarifying meanings of the passage in doing so. An environment must be created in which the patient feels comfortable expressing hope in God and renewing this hope.

Nurses can support the patient's hope by emphasizing that nothing is impossible with God. A reminder is needed about the boundless, infinite love God has for each human being. The strength of God's love is beyond our human ability to describe.

Arriving at inner peace with the human experience is the ultimate result of turning over the despair to God. Marcel[5] states, "Hope is the radical refusal to set limits." When all in life looks grim—that is, what is happening is beyond the individual's influence—hopelessness is prevented by turning to God.

Figure 16-3 summarizes the nursing strategies used to inspire hope. These include reality surveillance, devising and revising goals, and hoping in God, using an existential frame of reference.

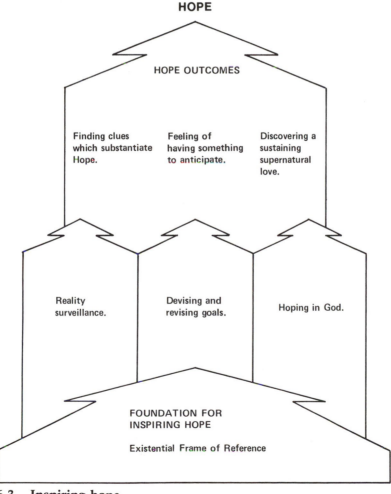

**FIGURE 16-3.  Inspiring hope.**

Throughout this chapter, a deliberate effort was made to avoid referring to hoping during the final stage of life. Our focus is on inspiring hope in people who are chronically ill. Chronic illness is not synonymous with dying; on the contrary, it means individuals will be *living* with a health problem that will not be cured. These patients must be helped to envision some quality in their lives with hope to become more fully developed human beings. Hope is not directed at complete restoration of physical stamina and return of lost body parts or function. These are aspects of life that are beyond control, hopelessly irreversible. Lynch[21] stresses that patients and helpers need to differentiate aspects of life that are hopeless from those in which hope can be a sustaining force.

Marcel[5] emphasized that "to hope" is different from "to hope that." To hope transcends all possible disappointments because of a security in BEING. To "hope that" subjects individuals to vulnerable insecurity of not having the expectation met according to a defined timetable. For example, the 21-year-old man who suffered a spinal cord injury at the T-3 level announces he will be able to void without self-catheterization by the end of the week. Despair occurs when bladder function does not return. When the patient is assisted to grieve over the loss, he is actually liberated from the anguish and can use his freedom from this anxiety to work toward other aspects of life. Hope transcends imagination. Inspiring hope is a means of empowering chronically ill individuals.

# REFERENCES

1. Fromm, E.: *The Revolution of Hope.* Harper & Row, New York, 1968.
2. Dembo, T.: *Sensitivity of one person to another.* Rehabil. Lit. 25:231, 1964.
3. Stotland, E.: *The Psychology of Hope.* Jossey-Bass, San Francisco, 1969.
4. Fromm, op. cit. pp. 11–12.
5. Marcel, G.: *Homo Viator* (translated by Craufurd, E.). Harper & Row, New York, 1962.
6. Miller, J. F.: *Losses of chronic illness.* Unpublished material.
7. Isani, R.: *From hopelessness to hope.* Perspect. Psychiatr. Care 1:15, 1963.
8. Schmale, A. and Iker, H.: *The affect of hopelessness and the development of cancer.* Psychosom. Med. 28:714, 1966.
9. Schmale, A.: *Hopelessness as a predictor of cervical cancer.* Soc. Sci. Med. 5:95, 1971.
10. Greer, S., Morris, T., and Pettingale, K. W.: *Psychological response to breast cancer: Effect on outcome.* Lancet 2:785, 1979.
11. Ziarnik, J., et al.: *Psychological correlates of survival on renal dialysis.* J. Nerv. Ment. Dis. 164:210, 1977.
12. Seligman, R., MacMillan, B., and Carroll, S.: *The burned child: A neglected area of psychiatry.* Am. J. Psychiatry 128:84, 1971.
13. Prociuk, T., Breen, L., and Lussier, R.: *Hopelessness, internal-external locus of control and depression.* J. Clin. Psychol. 32:299, 1976.
14. Engel, G.: *A life setting conducive to illness: The giving-up–given-up complex.* Ann. Intern. Med. 69:293, 1968.
15. Engel, G.: *Sudden and rapid death during psychological stress: Folklore or folk wisdom?* Ann. Intern. Med. 74:771, 1971.
16. Schneider, J. S.: *Hopelessness and helplessness.* J. Psychiatr. Nurs. 18:12, March 1980.
17. Vaillot, Sister Madeleine Clemence: *Living and dying: Hope the restoration of being.* Am. J. Nurs. 70:268, February 1970.
18. Jourard, S.: *Living and dying: Suicide an invitation to die.* Am. J. Nurs. 70:269, February 1970.

19. Ibid. p. 273.
20. Wright, B. and Shontz, F.: *Process and tasks in hoping.* Rehabil. Lit. 20:322, 1968.
21. Lynch, W.: *Images of Hope.* University of Notre Dame Press, Notre Dame, Ind., 1974.
22. Heagle, J.: *Contemporary Meditation on Hope.* Thomas More Press, Chicago, 1975.

# SELECTED READINGS

Adams, C. and Proulx, J.: *The role of the nurse in the maintenance and restoration of hope.* In Schoen-
berg, B., et al. (eds.): *Bereavement: Its Psychosocial Aspects.* Columbia University Press, New York,
1975, pp. 256–263.

Beck, A. T.: *The development of depression: A cognitive model.* In Friedman, R. and Katz, M. (eds.):
*Psychology of Depression: Contemporary Theory and Research.* Winston-Wiley, Washington, D.C.,
1975.

Beck, A. T., et al.: *The measurement of pessimism: The hopelessness scale.* J. Consult. Clin. Psychol.
42:861, 1974.

Buehler, J.: *What contributes to hope in the cancer patient?* Am. J. Nurs. 75:1353, August 1975.

Davies, R., et al.: *Organic factors and psychological adjustment in advanced cancer patients.* Psychosom.
Med. 35:464, 1973.

Day, J. P.: *Hope.* American Philosophical Quarterly 6:89, April 1969.

Erickson, R., Post, R., and Paige, A.: *Hope as a psychiatric variable.* J. Clin. Psychol. 31:324, 1975.

Frank, J.: *The role of hope in psychotherapy.* Unpublished material.

Gottschalk, L.: *A hope scale applicable to verbal samples.* Arch. Gen. Psychiatry 30:779, 1974.

Lange, S. P.: *Hope.* In Carlson, C. and Blackwell, B. (eds.): *Behavioral Concepts and Nursing Intervention.* J. B. Lippincott, Philadelphia, 1978, pp. 171–190.

LeShan, L. L.: *Some observations of the problem of mobilizing the patient's will to live.* In Kissen, D. M.
and LeShan, L. L. (eds.): *Psychosomatic Aspects of Neoplastic Disease.* J. B. Lippincott, Philadelphia, 1969, pp. 109–119.

Melges, F. and Bowlby, J.: *Types of hopelessness in psychopathological processes.* Arch. Gen. Psychiatry
20:690, 1969.

Menninger, K.: *The Vital Balance.* Viking Press, New York, 1963.

Pruyser, P.: *Phenomenology and dynamics of hoping.* Journal of Scientific Study of Religion 3:86, 1963.

Richter, C.: *On the phenomenon of sudden death in animals and man.* Psychosom. Med. 19:191, 1957.

Shea, F. and Hurley, E.: *Hopelessness and helplessness.* Perspect. Psychiatr. Care 2:32, 1964.

Werner-Beland, J.: *Nursing and the concept of hope.* In Werner-Beland, J. (ed.): *Grief Responses to Long-
Term Illness and Disability.* Reston Publishing, Reston, Va., 1980, pp. 169–188.

# EPILOGUE

While medical science research has brought about dramatic advances in treatment technologies for diseases, the concomitant research on the behavioral impact of the diseases and technologies has been lagging. Nurses are charged with providing psychologic comfort to chronically ill patients who are undergoing sophisticated treatments. With continuing study and development, nursing science will provide this research base on psychosocial needs and interventions for the chronically ill. Little data have been amassed to develop understanding about the coping tasks and coping strategies of the chronically ill.

Although certain aspects of chronic illness are beyond the ill person's control, much can be done to prevent powerlessness from becoming a pervasive emotional response that induces hopelessness. Developing those aspects of patient control that the patient retains is uniquely within the realm of nursing practice.

Nurses are the professionals who display sensitivity to the dilemmas of illness and therapy. The effect of the intrusiveness of illness on self-concept (especially body image and self-esteem) is buffered by nursing. Efforts to help the patient recognize existing strengths and capabilities and avoid defining self with emphasis on the disease entity are appropriate nursing actions. General positive self-concept is related to motivation for rehabilitation and successful vocational rehabilitation.[1] Nurses help chronically ill patients obtain security through ongoing caring, trusting relationships that promote patient self-regard and permit patient self-disclosure. Helping patients with role supplementation by referring them to reference groups (e.g., ostomy group) also promotes security with new role enactment. Reference groups help patients realize others have similar health problems and have adjusted well to their plight. Patients will gain confidence from seeing others enjoy quality of life despite the illness.

Nurses are challenged to humanize a somewhat dehumanizing event—the occurrence of illness and continuous surveillance of the patient within a health-care system. Experiences of depersonalization and dehumanization may result in chronic anxiety and hopelessness.[2] Efforts to avoid dehumanization may help to minimize powerlessness. Failure of coping mechanisms also leads to hopelessness.[3,4]

Nurses provide comfort to the patient and family by helping them with their anxiety over the uncertainty of illness. Certainty is provided when possible, for example, by keeping them informed about treatments and desired outcomes. The capacity to be one's self-care agent is developed by nurses' working with family members as well as the patient. Developing self-care agency enables the patient and family to have a sense of control.

After a family member receives a diagnosis of a chronic disease, the family is never quite the same again.[5] Specific needs of the ill member will demand family attention, disrupt plans for travel, and cause uncertainty in the family's use of leisure time. The stress of the illness may promote a new closeness in relationships[6] or so severely tax relationships that other family members' needs are not met and the family unit dissolves. Family members play a key role in enabling the ill member to have quality of life. The family is the focus of nursing care of the chronically ill because the family is the source of hope, self-esteem, social support, and in some instances, motivation. Nurses can help alleviate family tension, fears, overprotection, resentment of altering routines, or jealousy of ill member's attention. The impact of chronic illness on the family is a fertile area for nursing research. The family influences whether or not the patient can achieve quality of life.

Attaining and maintaining quality of life in chronic illness mean being able to:

—engage in roles that are important to the individual.
—perceive oneself as worthwhile.
—achieve a sense of independence.
—feel satisfaction with self, accomplishments, and relationships.
—have a sense of well-being despite illness limitations.

Perceived powerlessness interferes with achieving these goals. The focus of this book has been to develop understanding about the concept powerlessness by presenting a theoretical base in Chapter 3 and by providing measures to alleviate powerlessness throughout the book. Alleviating powerlessness potentiates quality of life.

This book has emphasized viewing the chronically ill person as one who has resources and coping skills that first are to be recognized by nurses, then supported, and in some cases developed. In a plan to alleviate powerlessness, intact power resources are supported or developed. See Figure 1-1, Chapter 1. It is important for nurses to understand that nursing approaches to patients are to be tailored not only to the patient's biologic, psychosocial, and cultural variables, but also to the unique power resources and coping style of the individual. While the unique strengths present in human beings are diverse and situations vary dramatically, generalized patient power resources are developed in this book. The select power resources include physical strength and reserve; psychologic stamina and social support network; positive self-concept, especially self-esteem; energy; knowledge; motivation; and belief system—hope.

Nurses collaborate with other health disciplines to provide various physical aspects of care of the chronically ill. Promoting positive adaptation to the chronic illness, developing self-care abilities of the patient and family, and promoting quality of life are unique to nursing practice. Quality of life can be developed despite widespread incapacitation caused by illness. Enthusiastic, yet sensitive and compassionate, nursing care could make a difference between patients' self-imposed invalidism and their return to productive roles.

The American dream is having *freedom* to become all that one can, to realize one's potential.[7] Perceived powerlessness is incongruent with feelings of freedom. The individual's premorbid potential and levels of aspiration are changed by illness. This realization alone may lead to despair.

Finding purpose and meaning in life is at best difficult when one is faced with a lifetime of illness. The limitations imposed by illness are to be transcended to reach meaning and purpose in life.[8] Nurses assist patients with this transcendence by enabling them to realize that the human capacity to love, feel, and share is without boundaries, and that this capacity is present in all human beings.

# REFERENCES

1. Litman, T. J.: *Self-conception and physical rehabilitation.* In Rose, A. M. (ed.): *Human Behavior and Social Processes.* Houghton Mifflin, Boston, 1962, pp. 550-574.
2. Leventhal, H.: *The consequences of depersonalization during illness and treatment.* In Howard, J. and Strauss, A. (eds.): *Humanizing Health Care.* John Wiley & Sons, New York, 1975, pp. 119-161.
3. Gaylin, W.: *Caring.* Alfred A. Knopf, New York, 1976.
4. Engel, G.: *A life setting conducive to illness: The giving-up–given-up complex.* Ann. Intern. Med. 69:293, 1968.
5. Wishner, W. and O'Brien, M.: *Diabetes and the family.* Med. Clin. North Am. 62:849, 1978.
6. Levy, N.: *The chronically ill patient.* Psychiatric Quarterly 51:189, Fall 1979.
7. Hall, B.: *The change paradigm in nursing. Growth versus persistence.* Advances in Nursing Science 3:1, July 1981.
8. Feldman, D.: *Chronic disabling illness: A holistic view.* J. Chronic Dis. 27:287, 1974.

# SELECTED READINGS

Braham, S., et al.: *Evaluation of the social needs of nonhospitalized chronically ill persons.* J. Chronic Dis. 28:401, 1975.
Davis, A.: *Disability, home care and the care-taking role in family life.* J. Adv. Nurs. 5:475, 1980.
Hyman, M.: *Social psychological factors affecting disability among ambulatory patients.* J. Chronic Dis. 28:199, 1975.
Krulik, T.: *Successful "normalizing" tactics of parents of chronically ill children.* J. Adv. Nurs. 5:573, 1980.
Mercer, S. and Kane, R.: *Helplessness and hopelessness among the institutionalized aged: An experiment.* Health Soc. Work 4:90, February 1979.

Stephenson, C.: *Powerless and chronic illness: Implications for nursing.* Baylor Nursing Educator 1:17, 1979.

Strain, J.: *Psychological Interventions in Medical Practice.* Appleton-Century-Crofts, New York, 1978.

Strauss, A.: *Editorial comment.* Soc. Sci. Med. 14:351, 1980.

Valentine, A.: *Caring for the young adult with cancer.* Cancer Nursing 1:385, October 1978.

# INDEX

6541 19 89